DENTAL ASSISTING PROGRAM
SOUTH PUGET SOUND COMM COLLEGE
754-7711

PHOTOGRAPHY BY CLIFFORD L. FREEHE

ILLUSTRATIONS BY VIRGINIA E. BROOKS

AN
ATLAS
OF
PEDODONTICS

DAVID B. LAW, B.S.D., D.D.S., M.S.
*Professor and Chairman,
Department of Pedodontics,
University of Washington School of Dentistry,
Seattle, Washington*

THOMPSON M. LEWIS, D.D.S., M.S.D.
*Assistant Dean and Associate Professor of Pedodontics,
University of Washington School of Dentistry;
Co-Director, Dental Department, Children's Orthopedic
Hospital and Medical Center, Seattle, Washington*

JOHN M. DAVIS, D.D.S., M.S.D.
*Assistant Professor of Pedodontics,
University of Washington School of Dentistry*

W. B. SAUNDERS COMPANY / PHILADELPHIA
LONDON / TORONTO

W. B. Saunders Company: West Washington Square
Philadelphia, Pa. 19105

12 Dyott Street
London WC1A 1DB

833 Oxford Street
Toronto, Ontario M8Z 5T9, Canada

Listed here is the latest translated edition of this book together with the language of the translation and the publisher.

Japanese (1st Edition) — Igaku Shoin, Ltd.,
Tokyo, Japan
French (1st Edition) — Julian Prelat,
Paris, France

An Atlas of Pedodontics   ISBN 0-7216-5655-2

©1969 by W. B. Saunders Company. Copyright under the International Copyright Union. All rights reserved. This book is protected by copyright. No part of it may be duplicated or reproduced in any manner without written permission from the publisher. Made in the United States of America. Press of W. B. Saunders Company. Library of Congress catalog card number 69-17820.

Print No.:   9   8   7

To

Dean Maurice J. Hickey

ACKNOWLEDGMENTS

The authors wish to express their appreciation to Mr. Clifford Freehe, R.B.P., Director, Health Sciences Television and Dental Photography at the University of Washington. It was his high standard of dental photography that originally inspired this text. To his assistant, Mr. David Andrews, go thanks for many hours of preparation. Our thanks also for photographic contributions go to Mrs. Ada M. Pepin, R.B.P., Director of Photography at Children's Orthopedic Hospital and Medical Center.

Miss Virginia Brooks, scientific illustrator for the Health Sciences at the University of Washington, is to be highly commended for her excellent illustrations.

We are indebted to the clinicians and educators from whom we have borrowed special material. They have been acknowledged individually in the appropriate legends. Of vital importance to this text have been the contributions of the Pedodontic Faculty and Graduate Pedodontic students at the University of Washington. Also to Dr. Edward Funk for his special assistance with the chapter on Exodontia, appreciation is extended.

To Mrs. Norma Norton go our heartfelt thanks for the excellent and tedious task of typing this entire text in all of its many drafts.

Saving the best till last we thank our wives for their patience, understanding and support.

PREFACE

The purpose of this book is to give the practicing dentist a photographic presentation of clinical pedodontics characterized by clarity and brevity. There are several fine textbooks on pedodontics but there is need for the pictorial type of reference which can supply immediate and practical assistance to the clinician, who in turn can pass this knowledge on to both his patients and their parents.

The field of pedodontics is so all inclusive that it is impossible for any one book to portray everything that might be considered pertinent and worthwhile. Improvements in intra-oral photography, however, make it possible to show clinical material in a far more easily understood fashion than by the printed word alone. A good example of this is the recognition and diagnosis of dental anomalies. The subject of patient management, on the other hand, does not lend itself to the photographic format of an Atlas and therefore has been presented in abbreviated form.

There are many different ways of accomplishing most clinical procedures in pedodontics; the authors, however, have presented their method of choice, fully cognizant that other techniques may be equally acceptable.

Time is the most precious factor in the life of the precise, conscientious and understanding dentist. It is hoped that this Atlas will provide a readily accessible source of information that will be frequently used.

DAVID B. LAW

THOMPSON M. LEWIS

JOHN M. DAVIS

CONTENTS

Chapter 1
GROWTH AND DEVELOPMENT 1

Chapter 2
ORAL DIAGNOSIS 25

Chapter 3
ANOMALIES OF THE DENTITION 51

Chapter 4
RADIOGRAPHY 113

Chapter 5
CARIES PREVENTION 131

Chapter 6
ANESTHESIA 143

Chapter 7
RUBBER DAM 153

Chapter 8
OPERATIVE DENTISTRY 163

Chapter 9
PULP THERAPY 187

Chapter 10
EXODONTIA IN THE PRIMARY DENTITION 209

Chapter 11
SPACE MAINTENANCE AND INTERCEPTIVE ORTHODONTICS 221

Chapter 12
PROSTHODONTICS 249

Chapter 13
TRAUMA TO THE PRIMARY DENTITION 269

Chapter 14
TRAUMA TO THE PERMANENT DENTITION 281

Chapter 15
THE HANDICAPPED CHILD 307

Chapter 16
MANAGEMENT OF THE CHILD PATIENT 319

INDEX 325

GROWTH AND DEVELOPMENT

Chapter 1

    A thorough understanding of the fundamental principles of growth and development of the facial complex is essential in the practice of pedodontics. Without knowledge of the manner in which teeth calcify and erupt, it would be difficult to differentiate between a hypoplastic condition induced by local factors and an inherited syndrome. Normal stages in the development of the dentition can be mistaken for malocclusion by the untrained observer. It is not within the scope of this book to treat the subject of growth and development in all of its ramifications. Rather, the purpose is to focus attention on some of the key areas in which the clinician who treats children should be knowledgeable. It is the responsibility of the practitioner to give accurate answers to the questions frequently asked by parents concerning tooth position, spacing, labial frenum, and effect of traumatic injuries, to mention only a few. More exhaustive information, if needed, can readily be obtained from textbooks of orthodontics and pedodontics.

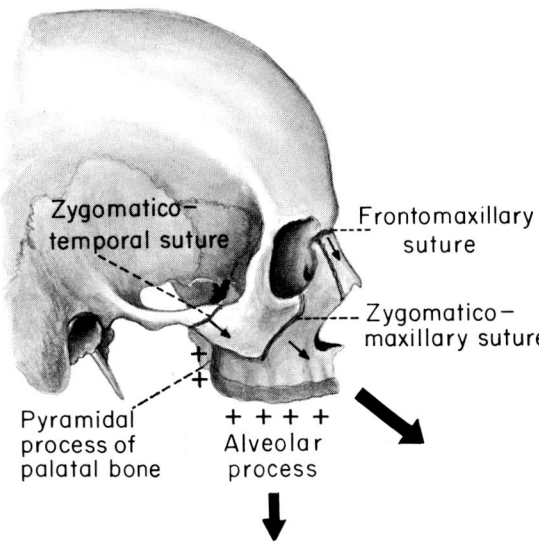

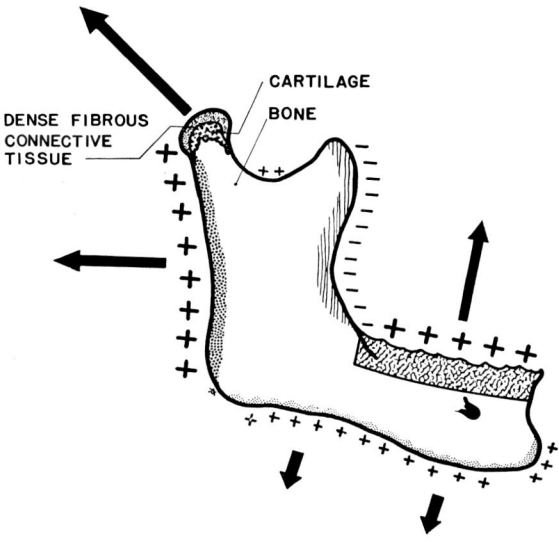

Figure 1-1 Maxillary growth sites. The primary centers of growth contributing to the downward and forward direction of the maxilla are:
  A. Growth at the spheno-occipital and sphenoethmoidal junctions.
  B. Growth of the nasal cartilaginous septum.
The following sutures are considered secondary or accommodating growth sites for the primary centers of growth:
  A. Frontomaxillary suture.
  B. Zygomaticomaxillary suture.
  C. Zygomaticotemporal suture.
  D. Pryramidal process of palatal bone.
  E. Alveolar process.

Figure 1-2 Mandibular growth sites. Growth in the condyle increases the anterior-posterior (downward and forward pattern of growth) dimension of the mandible. Anterior-posterior dimension of the mandible is also increased by resorption of bone on the anterior border of the ramus and apposition of bone on the posterior border of the ramus. Appositional growth of alveolar bone increases the superior-inferior dimension of the mandible. (From Graber, T. M.: *Orthodontics*, 2nd ed., 1966, p. 60.)

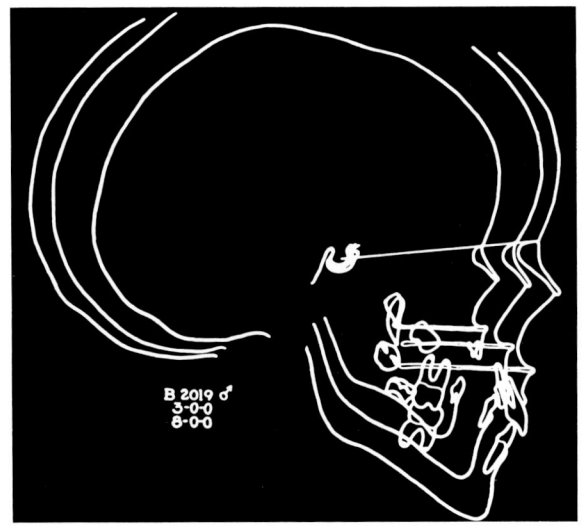

Figure 1-3 Tracing of superimposed films of head showing the normal downward and forward facial growth pattern. Ages 6 months, 3 years, and 8 years.

GROWTH AND DEVELOPMENT 3

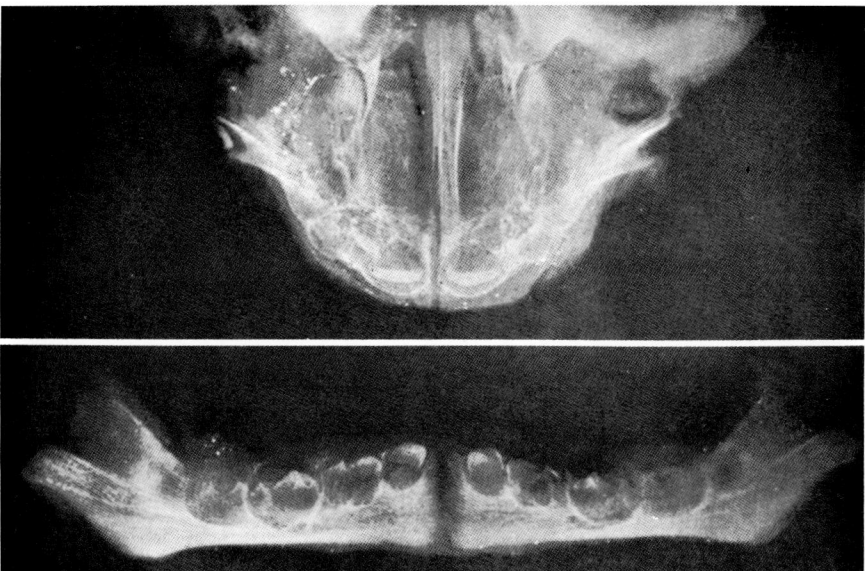

Figure 1-4 Eight-month fetus (wet specimen). Note areas of dental calcification in the mandibular incisors, cuspids, and first primary molars as well as the maxillary centrals, laterals, and first primary molars. There is only slight calcification in the maxillary cuspids and cusp tips of the second primary molars. (From McCall, J. O., and Wald, S. S.: *Clinical Dental Roentgenology*, 4th ed., 1957, p. 153.)

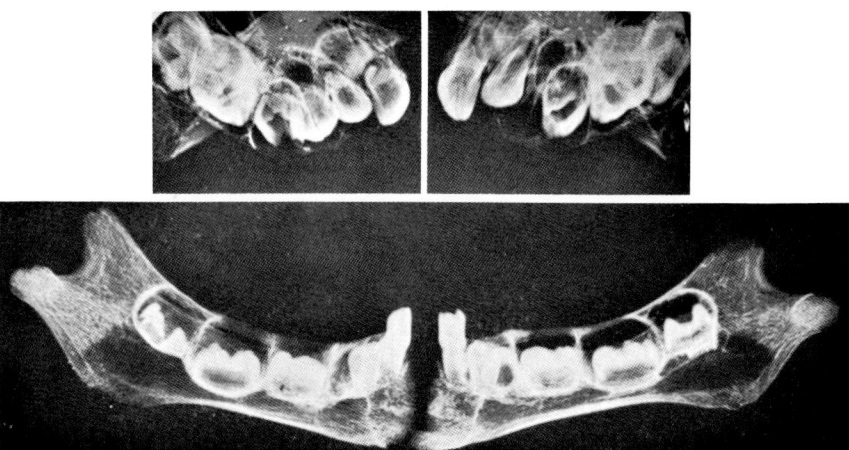

Figure 1-5 Infant at birth (wet specimen). Note areas of dental calcification similar to those shown in Figure 1-4. Maxillary calcification is slightly less advanced. (From McCall, J. O., and Wald, S. S.: *Clinical Dental Roentgenology*, 4th ed., 1957, p. 154.)

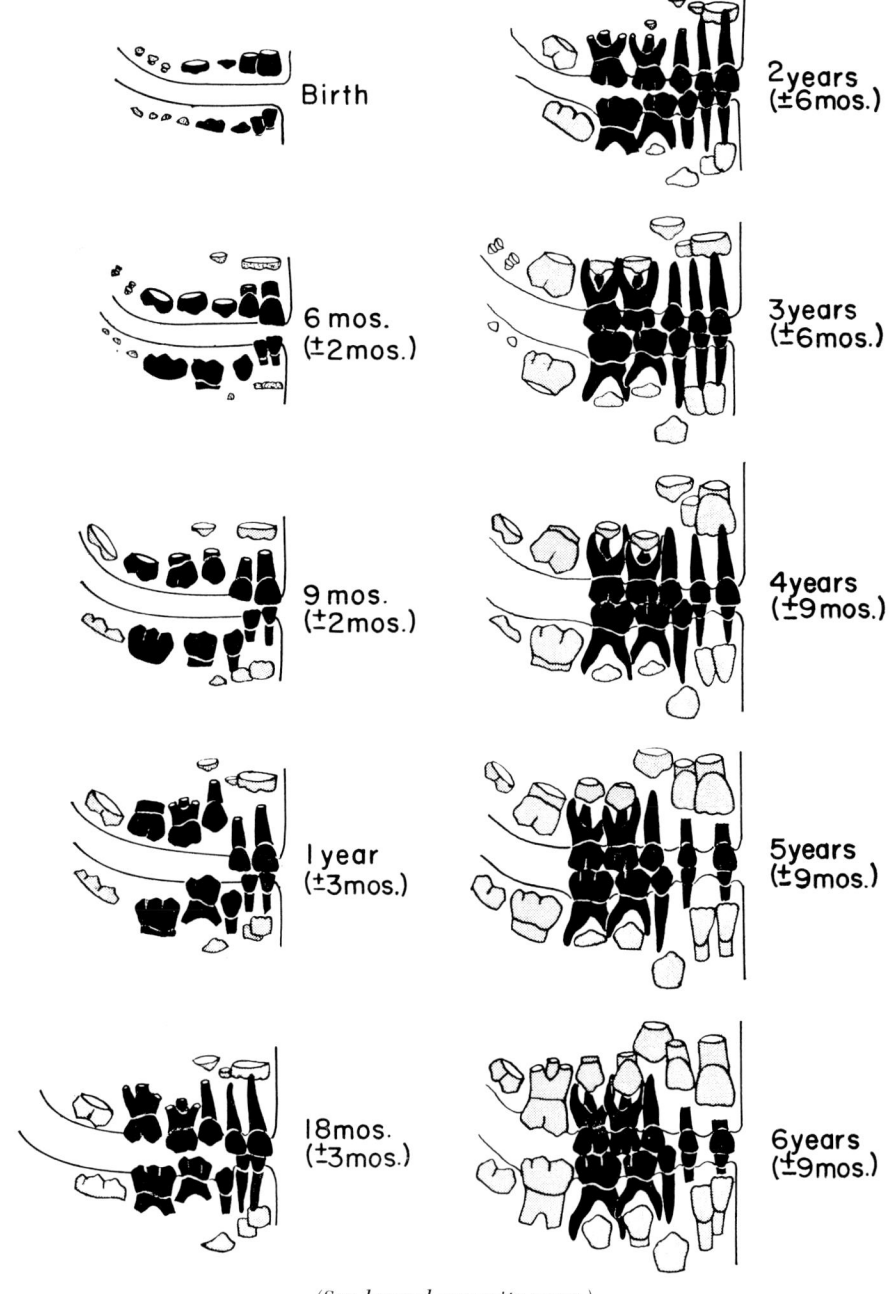

(See legend opposite page.)

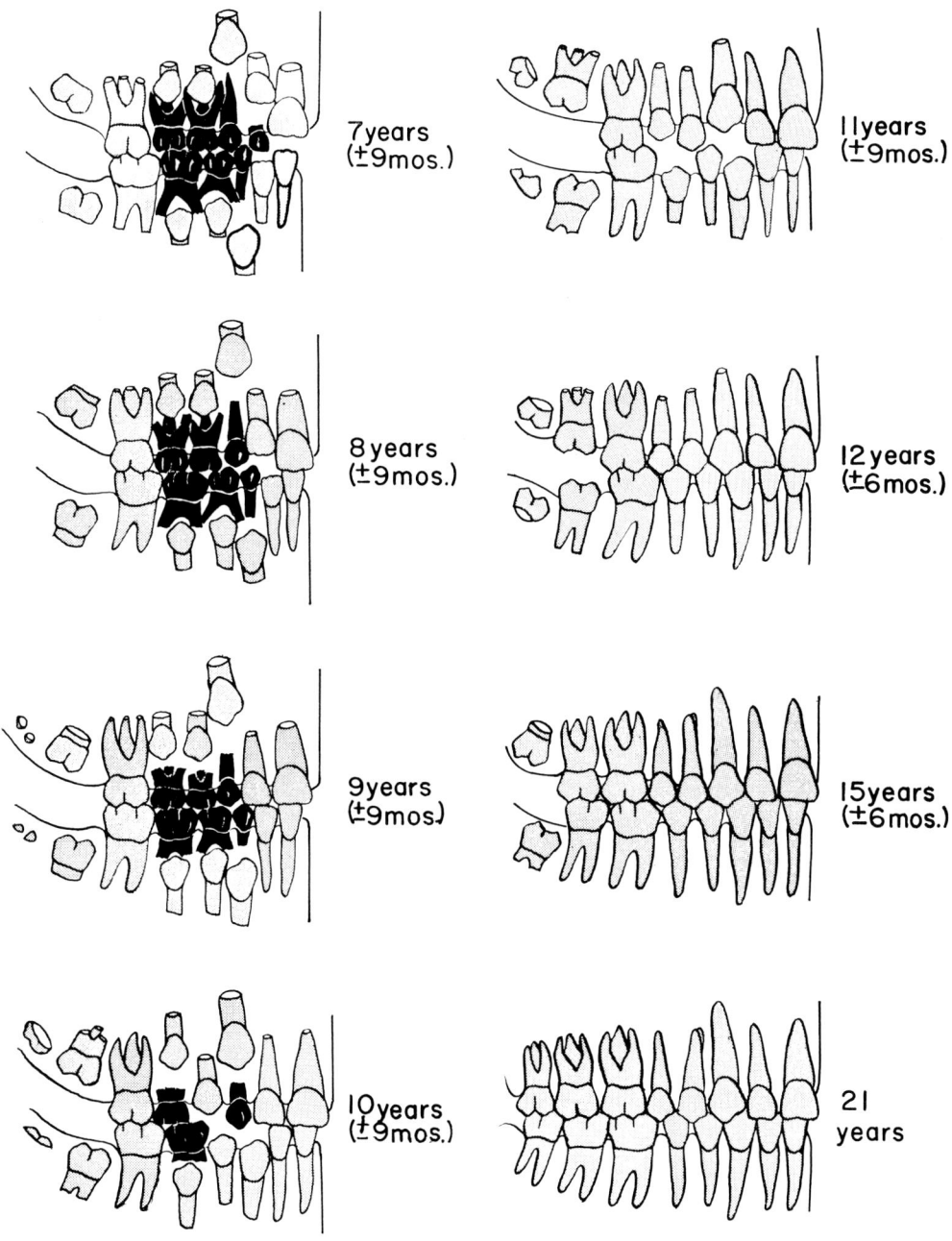

Figure 1-6 Development of human dentition. (Modified from Schour and Massler, from Graber, T. M.: *Orthodontics*, 2nd ed., 1966, pp. 44 and 45).

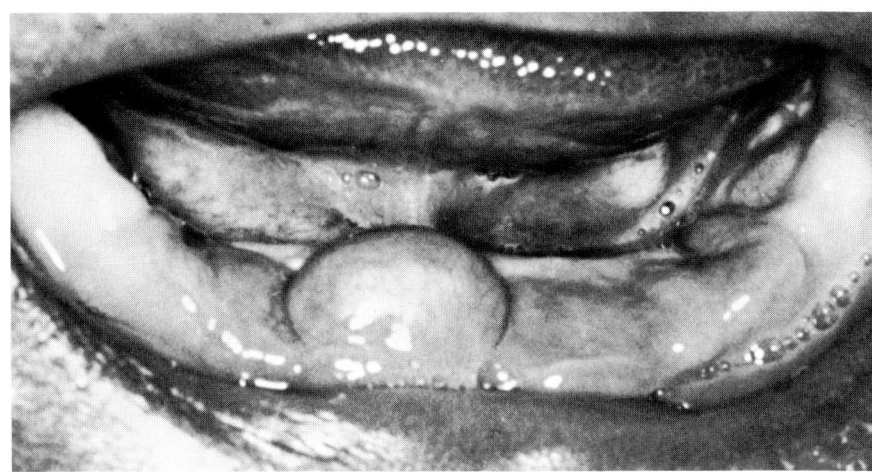

Figure 1-7 Eruption cyst in newborn infant. Note primary incisor visible through cyst. (Courtesy Dr. James R. Hooley.)

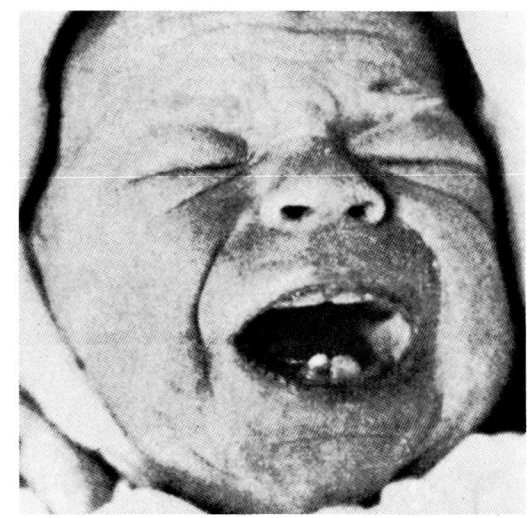

Figure 1-8 Male child, 1 day old. Mandibular right primary central incisor erupted at birth (natal tooth). Natal teeth are present in oral cavity at birth. Mandibular left primary central incisor did erupt on tenth day of life (neonatal). Neonatal teeth erupt within first 30 days after birth. Most natal and neonatal teeth are normal primary central incisors and should be left in the mouth. (From Bodenhoff, J.: Dentition connatalis et neonatolis. Odont. Tids. 67:645-695, Dec., 1959.)

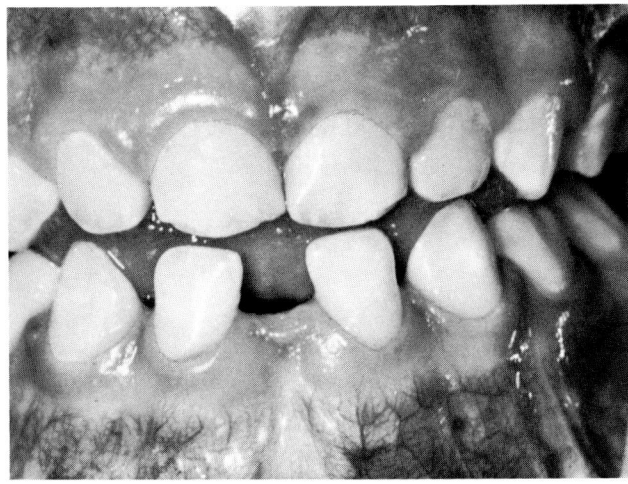

Figure 1-9 Natal mandibular primary central incisors in this 4-year-old girl were extracted the first week after birth. Note the position of the mandibular primary lateral incisors and cuspids in relation to the maxillary primary lateral incisors and cuspids. A possible loss in mandibular arch length may occur.

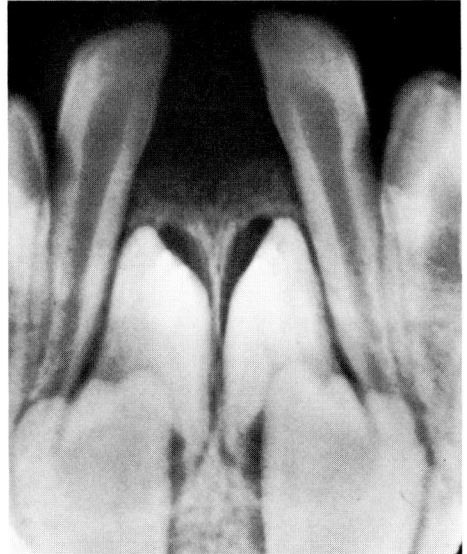
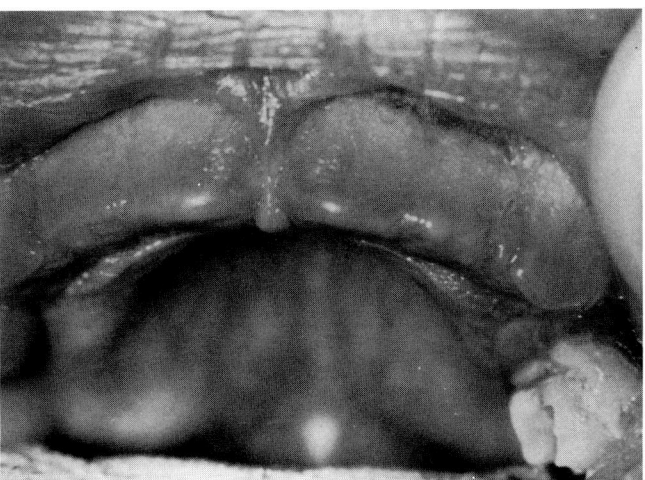

Figure 1-10 Radiograph of patient seen in Figure 1-9, showing space closure. Extraction of natal or neonatal teeth should be avoided if possible.

Figure 1-11 An 8-day-old male with a natal maxillary left primary molar and an epithelial cyst in the area of the maxillary right primary molars.

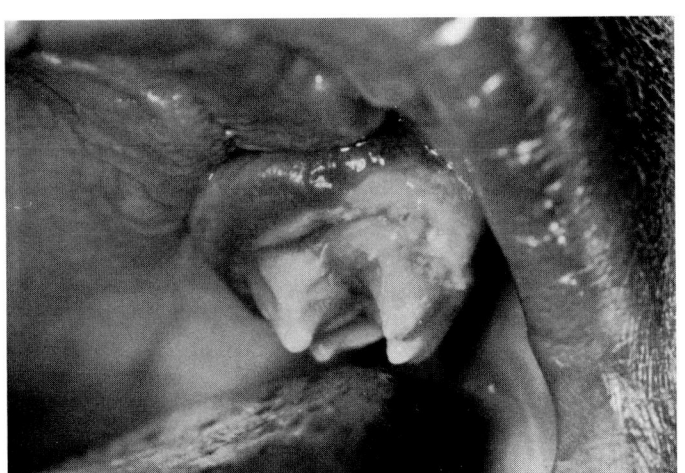

Figure 1-12 Close-up view of the natal maxillary left primary molar illustrated in Figure 1-11.

Figure 1-13 Close-up view of the epithelial cyst in the maxillary right primary molar area seen in Figure 1-11. According to Hooley, pea-sized cysts may form over one or more of the first primary molars. These cysts are shed during the first 2 months of life.

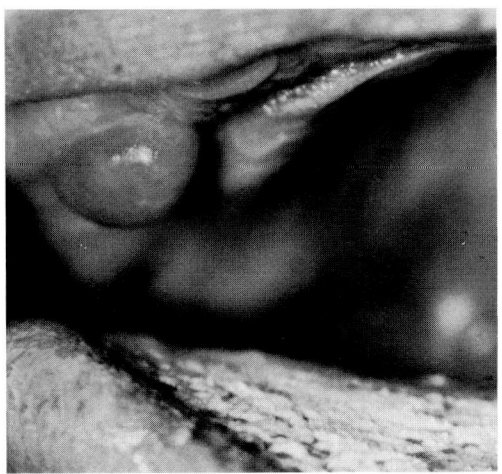

8   GROWTH AND DEVELOPMENT

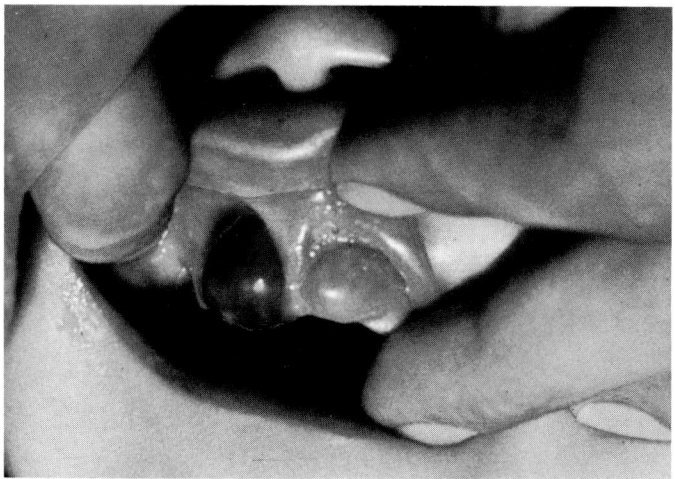

Figure 1-14 Eruption hematoma in the area of the maxillary right primary central incisor on a 7-month-old infant. This is nonpathologic and may occur prior to the eruption of some teeth. No treatment is indicated unless child is extremely irritable. Lancing of tissue should be avoided. Gentle rubbing with a teething ring may be helpful.

Figure 1-15 Slight eruption hematoma prior to the eruption of the maxillary left primary first molar on a 14-month-old child.

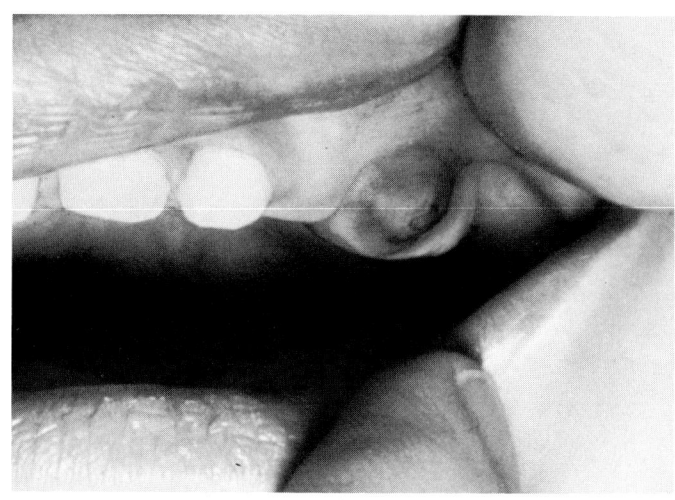

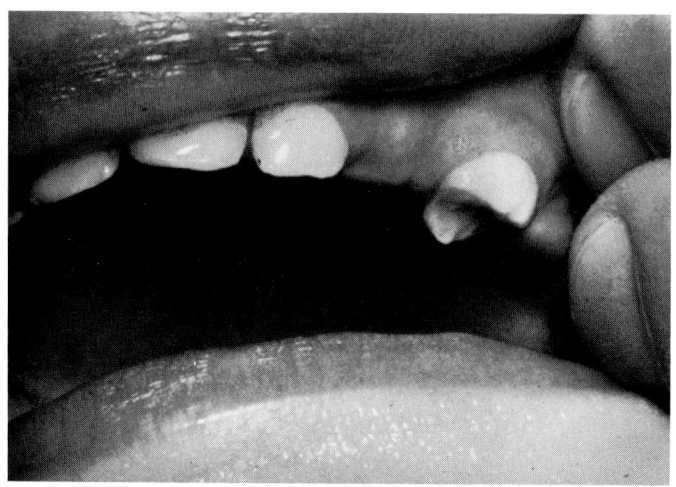

Figure 1-16 Same patient as seen in Figure 1-15 after eruption of the maxillary left primary first molar. Note the normal sequence of eruption of the first primary molar ahead of the primary cuspid.

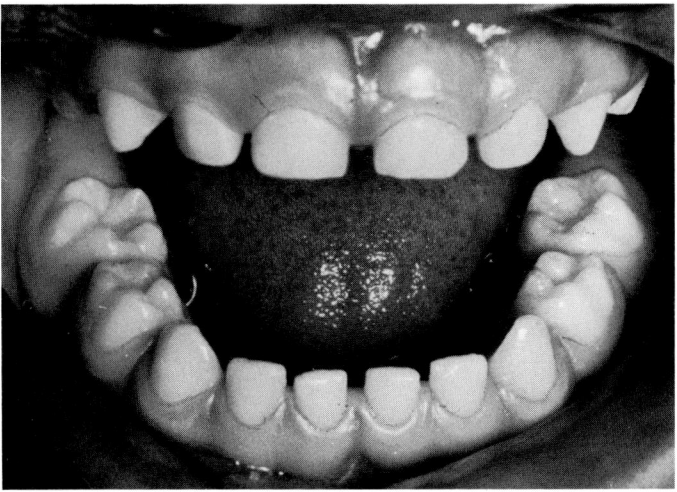

Figure 1-17 A 4-year-old child with normal healthy teeth and supporting tissues. Note the desirable spacing of the anterior teeth in the primary dentition.

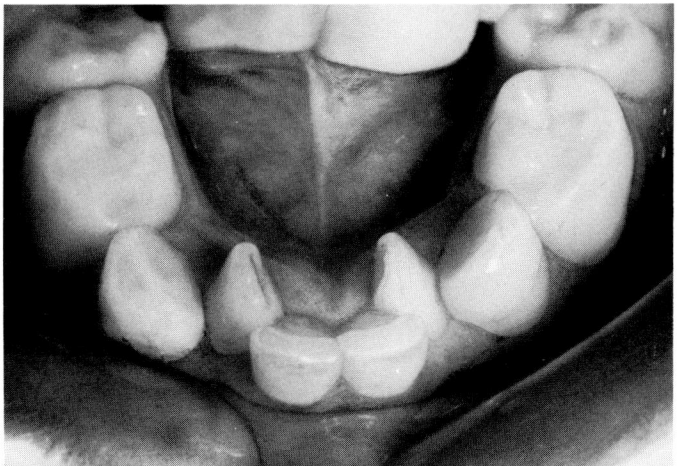

Figure 1-18 A 4-year-old child with abnormal crowding of the primary dentition. Most children with primary anterior teeth in contact or crowded will eventually require orthodontic care.

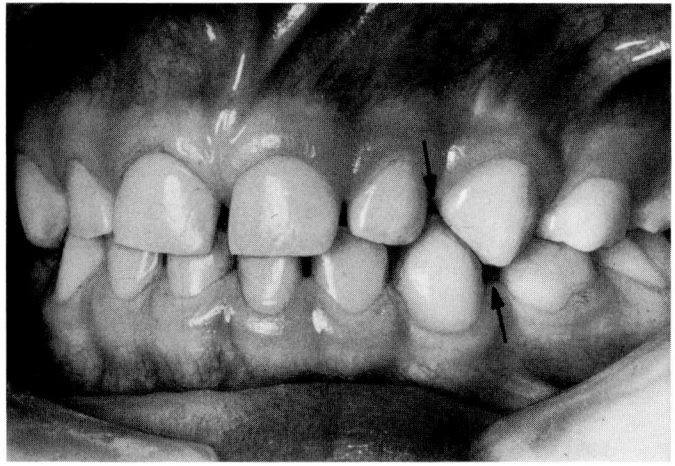

Figure 1-19 Normal dentition of preschool child showing maxillary primate space between lateral and cuspid, and mandibular primate space between cuspid and first primary molar.

Figure 1-20 Step relationship of distal surfaces of maxillary and mandibular primary second molars and its effect on the occlusion of the first permanent molars. Note the permanent molars erupting into normal occlusion. (Hitchcock, P. H., from Finn, S. B.: *Clinical Pedodontics*, 3rd ed., 1967, p. 256.)

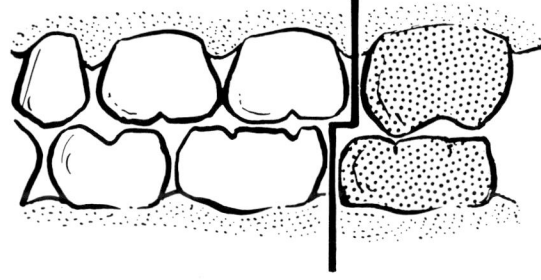

Figure 1-21 Flat plane relationship of distal surfaces of maxillary and mandibular primary second molar and its effect on the occlusion of the first permanent molar. Note the end-to-end occlusion of the permanent molars. (Hitchcock, P. H., from Finn, S. B.: *Clinical Pedodontics*, 3rd ed., 1967, p. 256.)

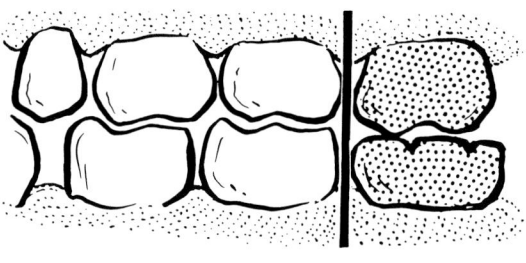

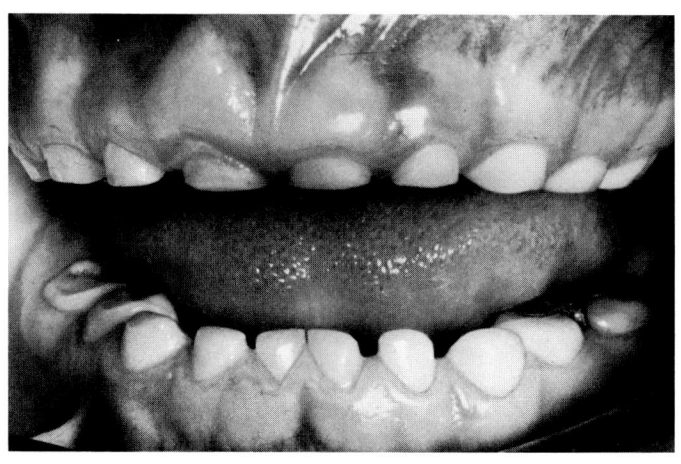

Figure 1-22 Five-year-old child with occlusal wear due to bruxism. Bruxism is common in the primary dentition, resulting in varying degrees of occlusal wear.

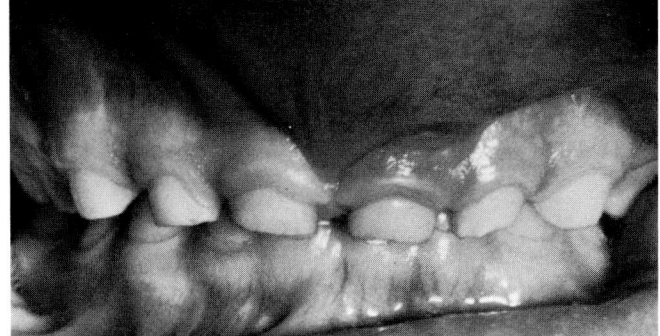

Figure 1-23 Five-year-old child with a deep overbite in the primary dentition.

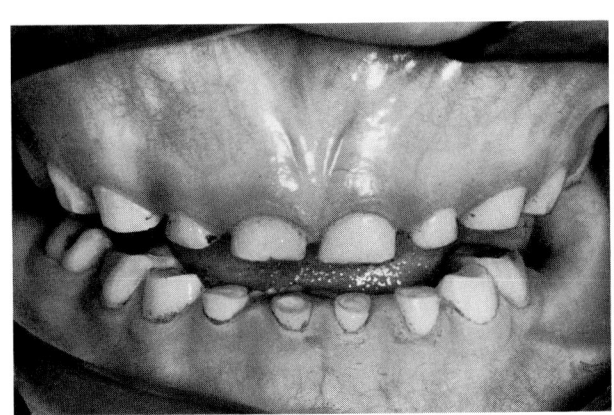

Figure 1-24 Six-year-old child with extreme incisal wear of the mandibular primary incisors. Note the erupting mandibular right permanent central incisor. Bilateral extraction of primary central incisors is indicated.

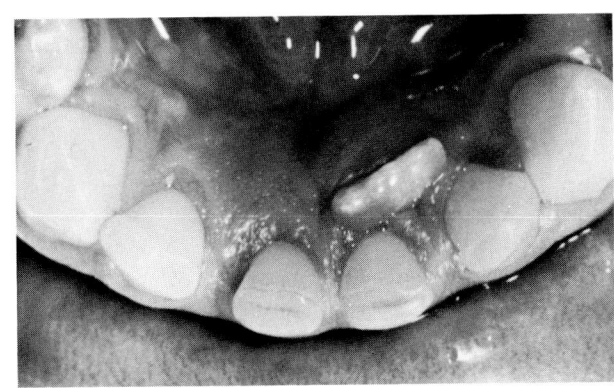

Figure 1-25 Six-year-old child with mandibular left permanent central incisor erupting lingually. Since neither of the mandibular *primary* central incisors was loose and ready to be naturally exfoliated, the dentist extracted them, allowing the permanent incisor to erupt into normal position. After the primary incisor or incisors are exfoliated or extracted, the action of the tongue usually moves the permanent incisor labially into a normal labiolingual position.

12   GROWTH AND DEVELOPMENT

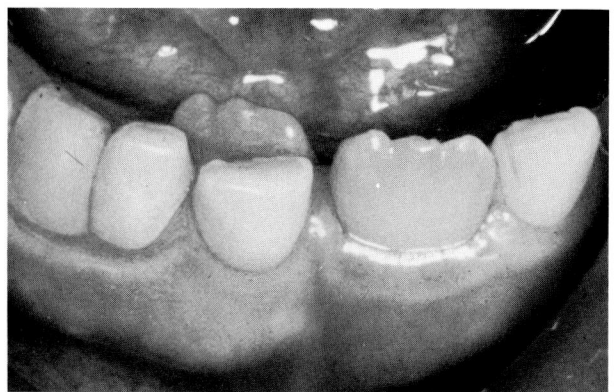

Figure 1-26 A 6½-year-old child with a lingual erupting mandibular right permanent central incisor. Immediate treatment is extraction of the mandibular right primary central incisor.

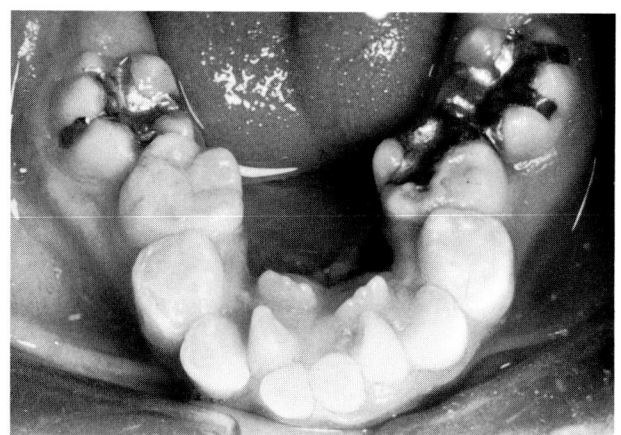

Figure 1-27 Seven-year-old child with extreme crowding of primary and permanent teeth in the mandibular arch (same child as shown in Figure 1-18). A complete orthodontic evaluation should be done at this time prior to any treatment.

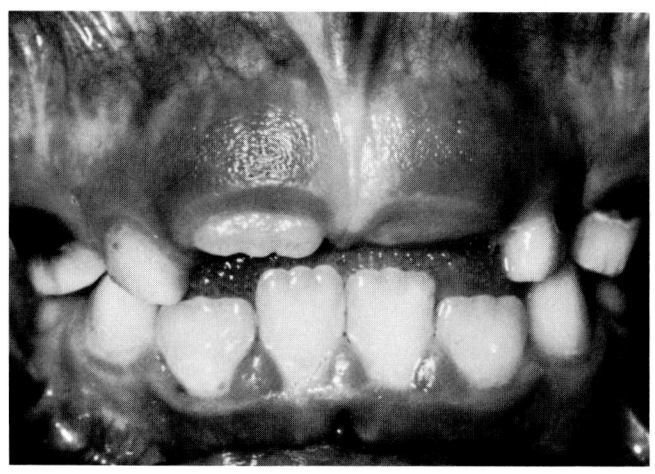

Figure 1-28 A 7½-year-old child with normal beginning of mixed dentition. Note swollen gingivae around erupted mandibular teeth and bulging tissues over erupting maxillary permanent central incisors.

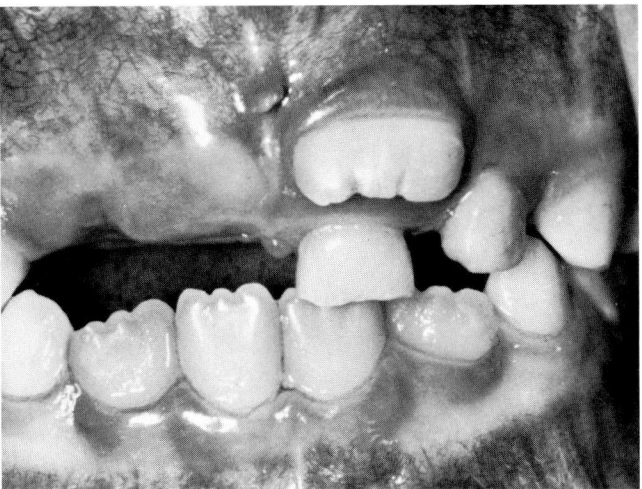

Figure 1-29 A 7½-year-old child with a maxillary left permanent central incisor erupting labially. Maxillary permanent central incisors often erupt labial to the *primary* central incisor. The maxillary primary central should be extracted to provide room for the permanent incisor. Pressure from the lip will usually move the permanent incisor lingually into better alignment.

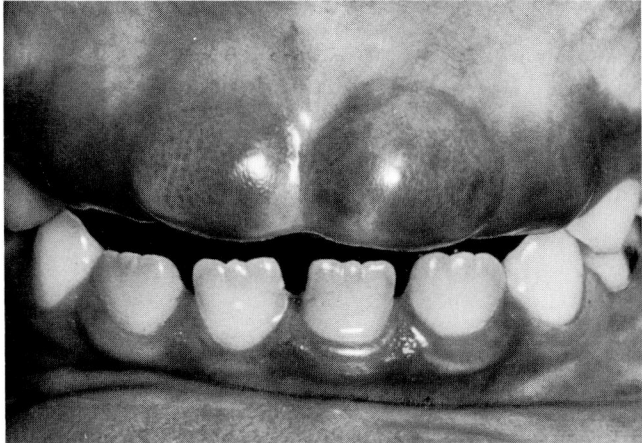

Figure 1-30 An 8-year-old child with delayed eruption of maxillary permanent central incisors. Treatment consists of removing tissue from incisal one-third of crown on labial and lingual.

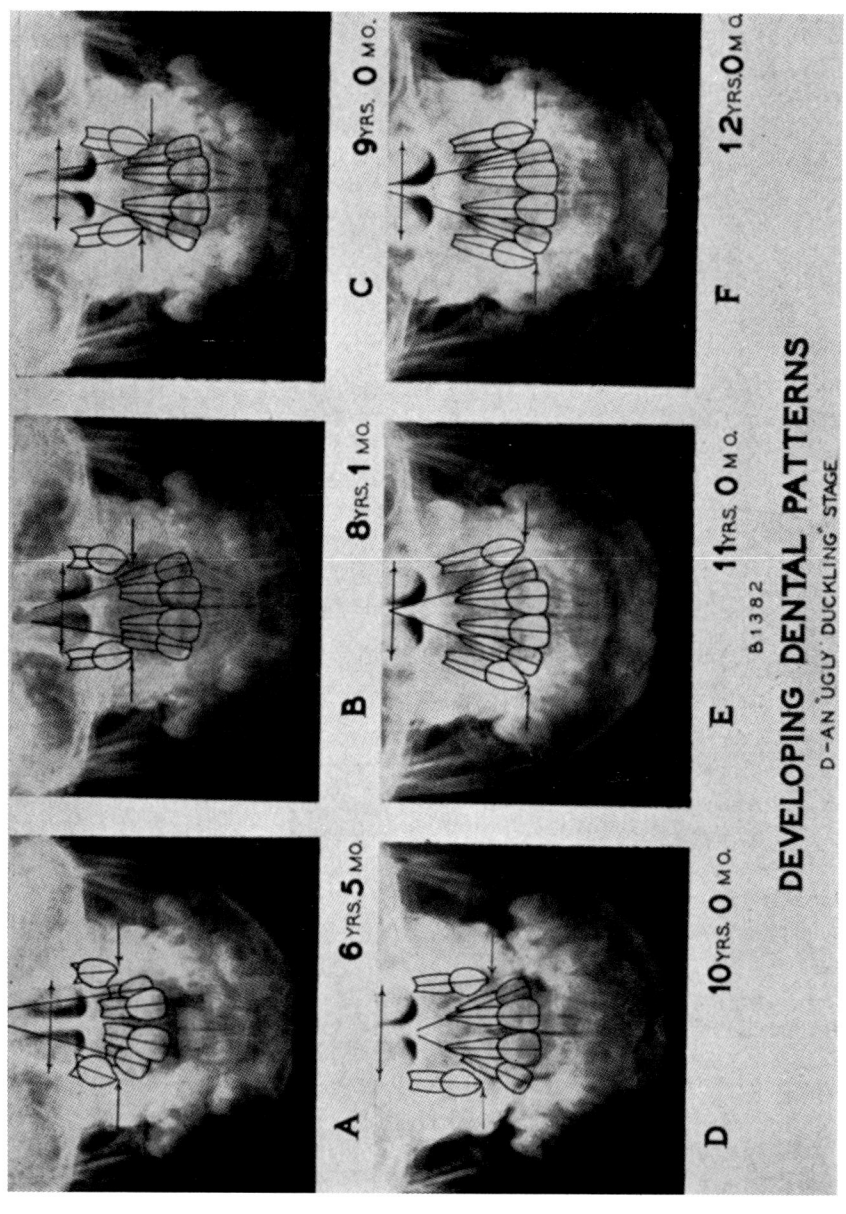

Figure 1-31 Normal developmental pattern of maxillary permanent teeth in children between 6 and 12 years of age. The central diastema and distally flaring laterals are usually self-correcting with the eruption of maxillary permanent cuspids. (From Broadbent, H. B.: The face of the normal child. Angle Orthodontist 7:183-208, Oct., 1937.)

GROWTH AND DEVELOPMENT 15

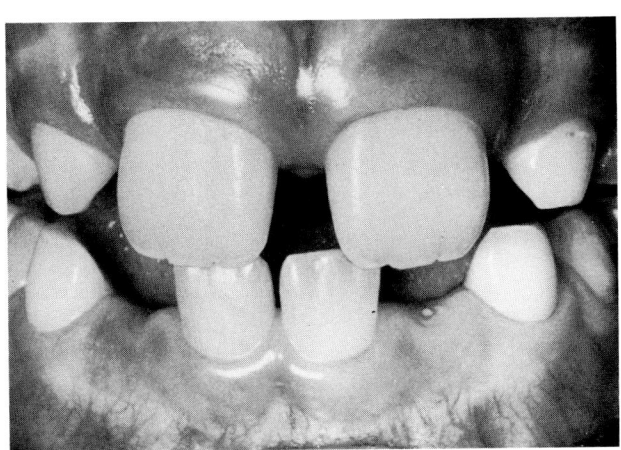

Figure 1-32 A 7½-year-old child. Note diastema between the maxillary permanent central incisors. Radiographs are indicated to determine presence or absence of maxillary permanent laterals.

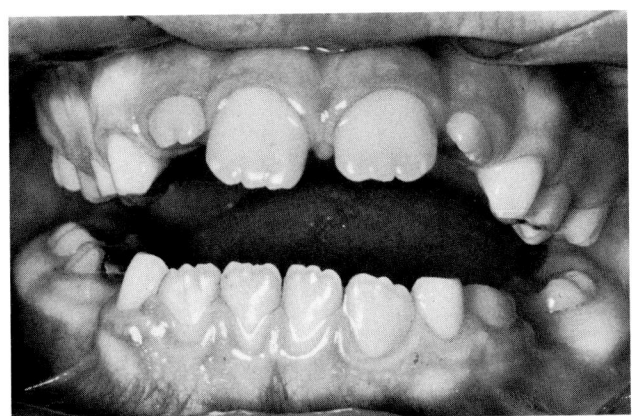

Figure 1-33 An 8-year-old child. Note eruption of maxillary permanent lateral incisors. Frenectomy is usually not considered until permanent cuspids have erupted. Mamelons on incisal edges of teeth are very prominent but will become less noticeable as wear occurs.

Figure 1-34 A 9-year-old patient. Maxillary and mandibular centrals and laterals are well erupted but primary cuspids are still present. Interdental spaces usually close with eruption of permanent cuspids.

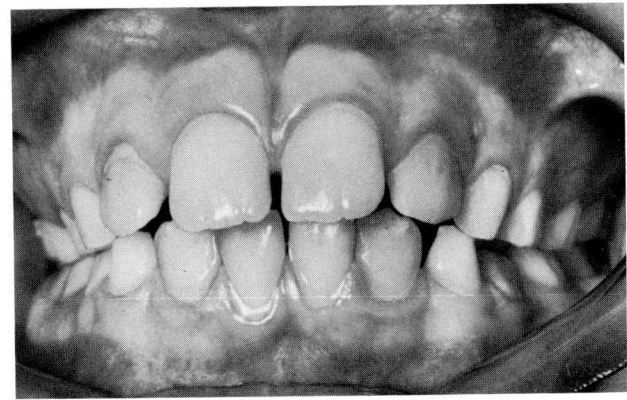

16 GROWTH AND DEVELOPMENT

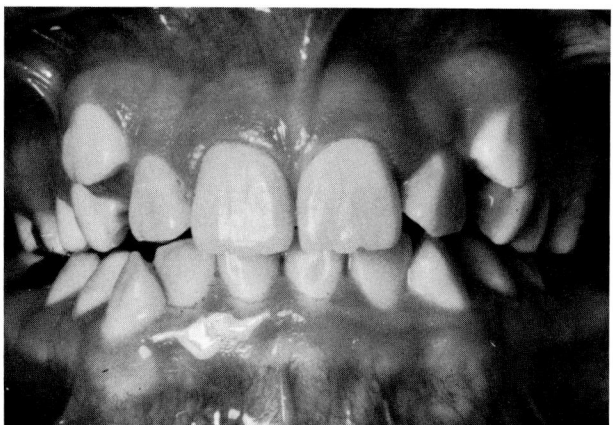

Figure 1-35 A 14-year-old patient. Note the lack of room for the maxillary permanent cuspids as the result of disharmony between tooth size and available arch length.

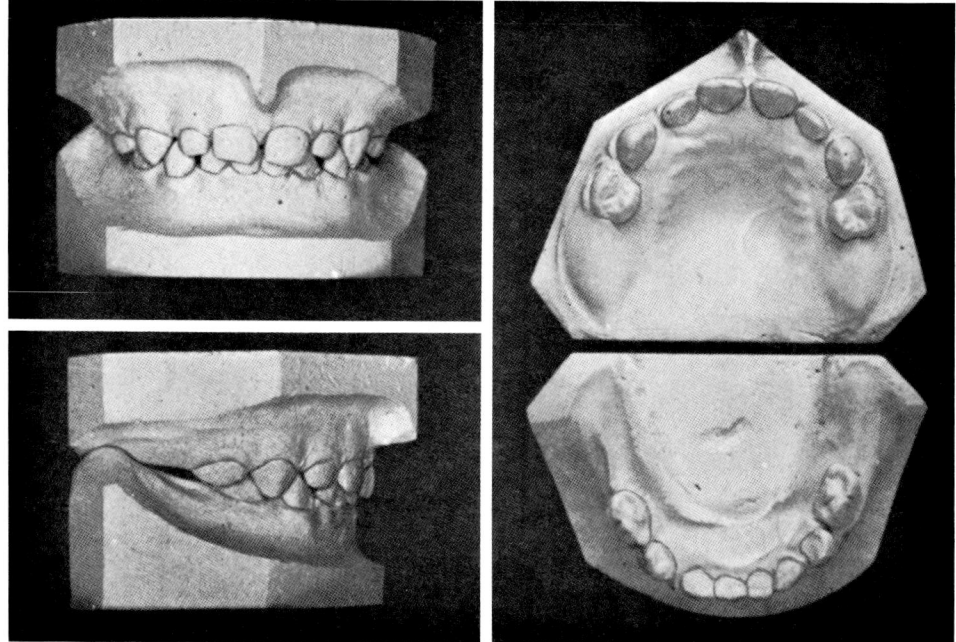

Figure 1-36 Patient D. M.; 2 years old. Second primary molars not yet erupted. Overbite appears excessive, but is normal for this age. (Sillman, J. H., from Graber, T. M.: *Orthodontics*, 2nd ed., 1966, p. 58.)

GROWTH AND DEVELOPMENT 17

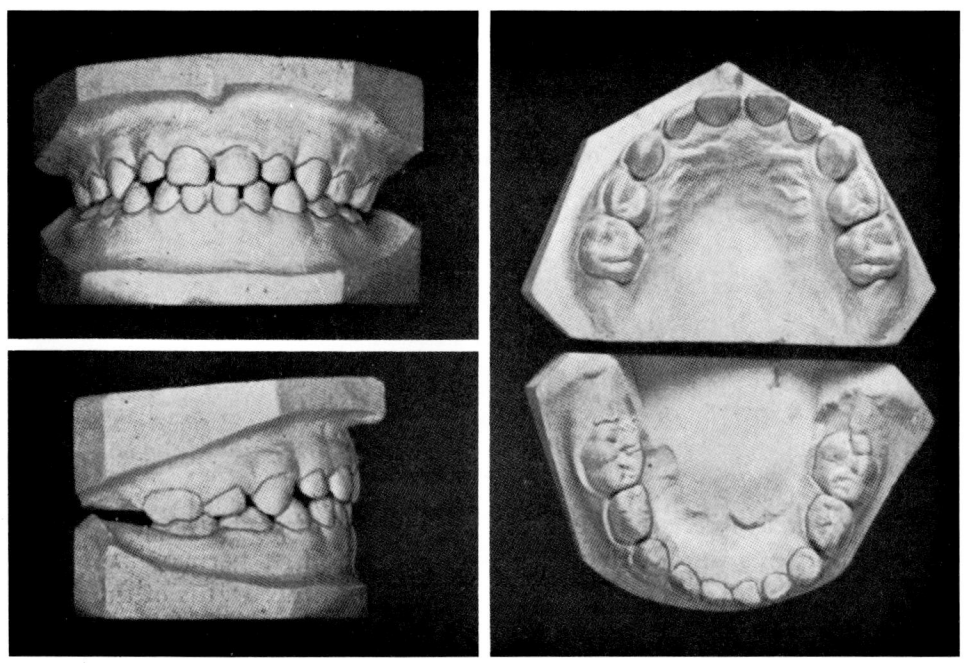

Figure 1-37 Patient D. M.; 4 years, 1 month, 20 days. There has been some reduction in overbite. (Sillman, J. H., from Graber, T. M.: *Orthodontics*, 2nd ed., 1966, p. 60.)

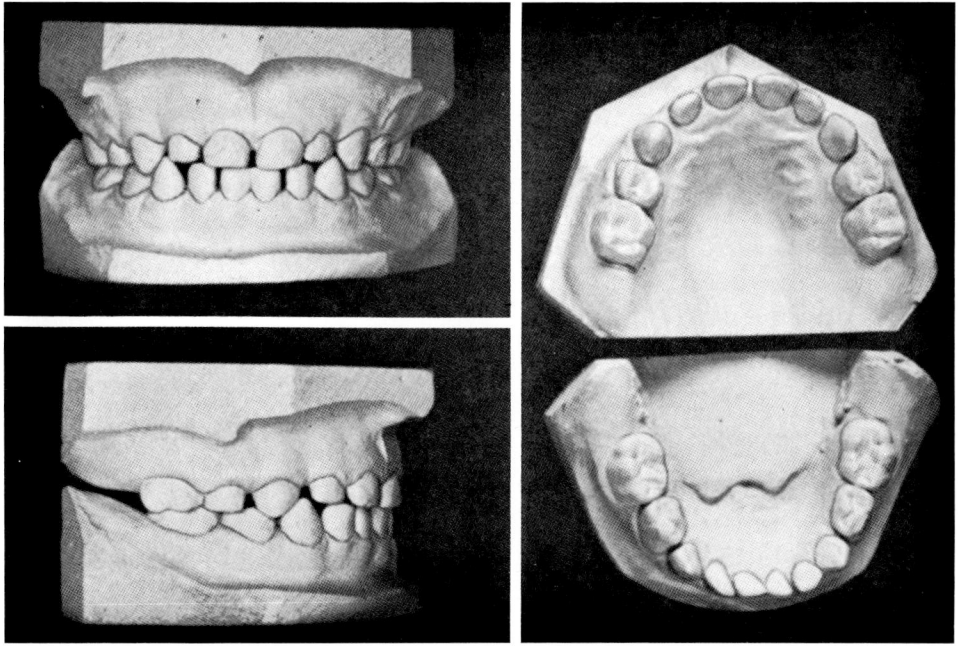

Figure 1-38 Patient D. M.; 5 years, 6 months. (Sillman, J. H., from Graber, T. M.: *Orthodontics*, 2nd ed., 1966, p. 63.)

18   GROWTH AND DEVELOPMENT

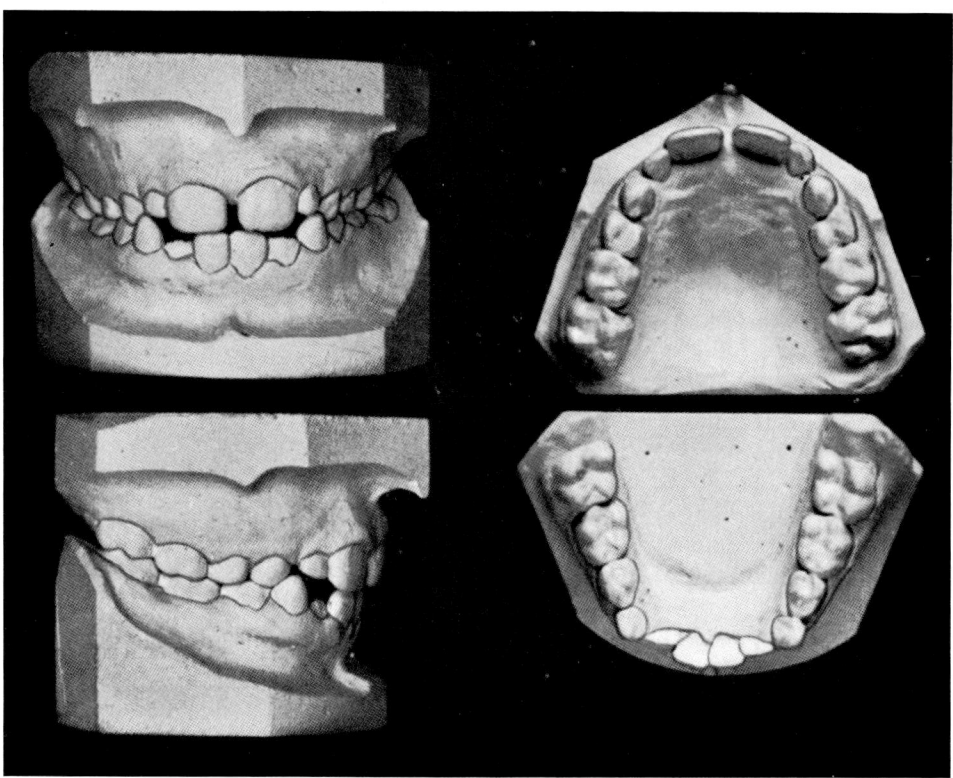

Figure 1-39 Patient D. M.; 7 years, 4 months, 8 days. Observe the irregularity of the erupting mandibular incisors. (Sillman, J. H., from Graber, T. M.: *Orthodontics*, 2nd ed., 1966, p. 68.)

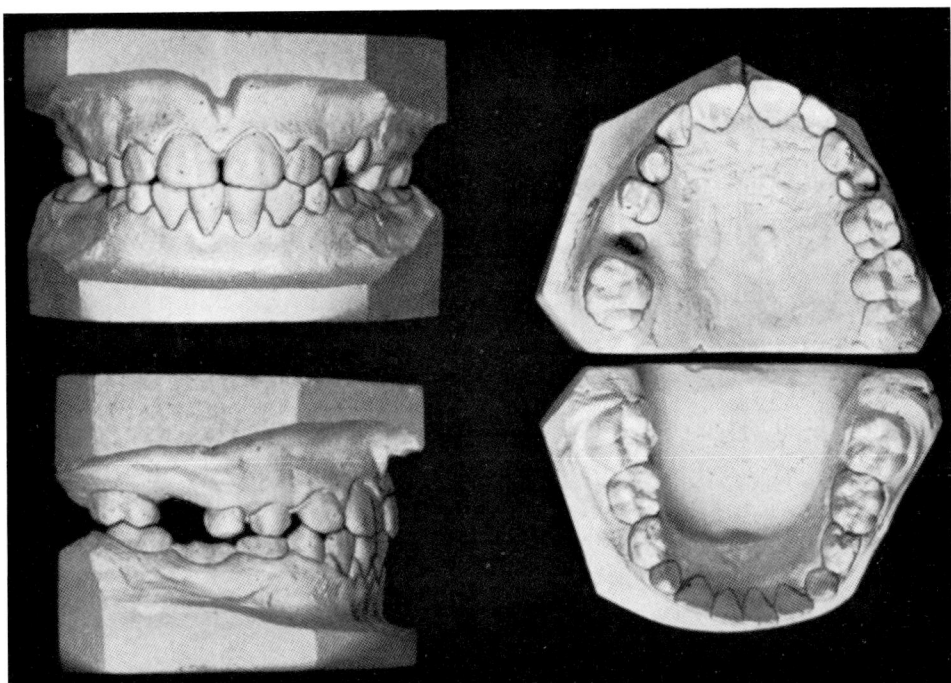

Figure 1-40 Patient D. M.; 8 years, 8 months, 9 days. The irregularity in the mandibular incisor segment has lessened. Eruption of the maxillary first premolars at this time indicates a precocious developmental pattern. The maxillary right second deciduous molar has been lost prematurely due to caries. (Sillman, J. H., from Graber, T. M.: *Orthodontics*, 2nd ed., 1966, p. 69.)

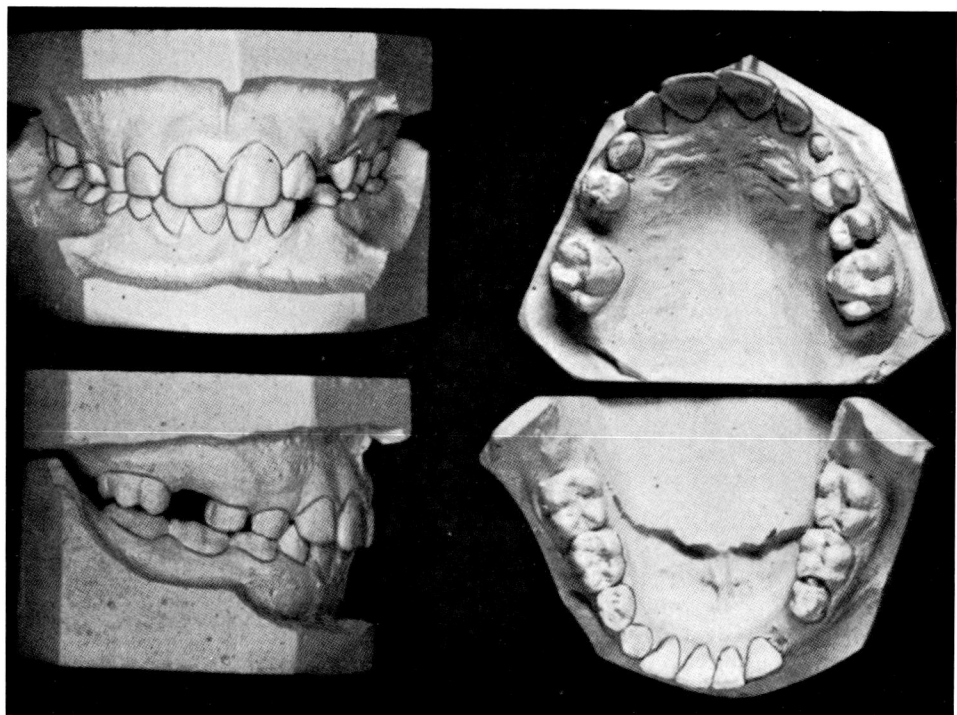

Figure 1-41 Patient D. M.; 10 years, 1 month, 17 days. Despite the premature loss of the maxillary right second deciduous molar, the second premolar has not erupted (though it has come into place on the opposite side). The maxillary right first permanent molar has drifted mesially and rotated slightly, but space is still adequate for the second premolar to erupt. (Sillman, J. H., from Graber, T. M.: *Orthodontics*, 2nd ed., 1966, p. 71.)

GROWTH AND DEVELOPMENT 21

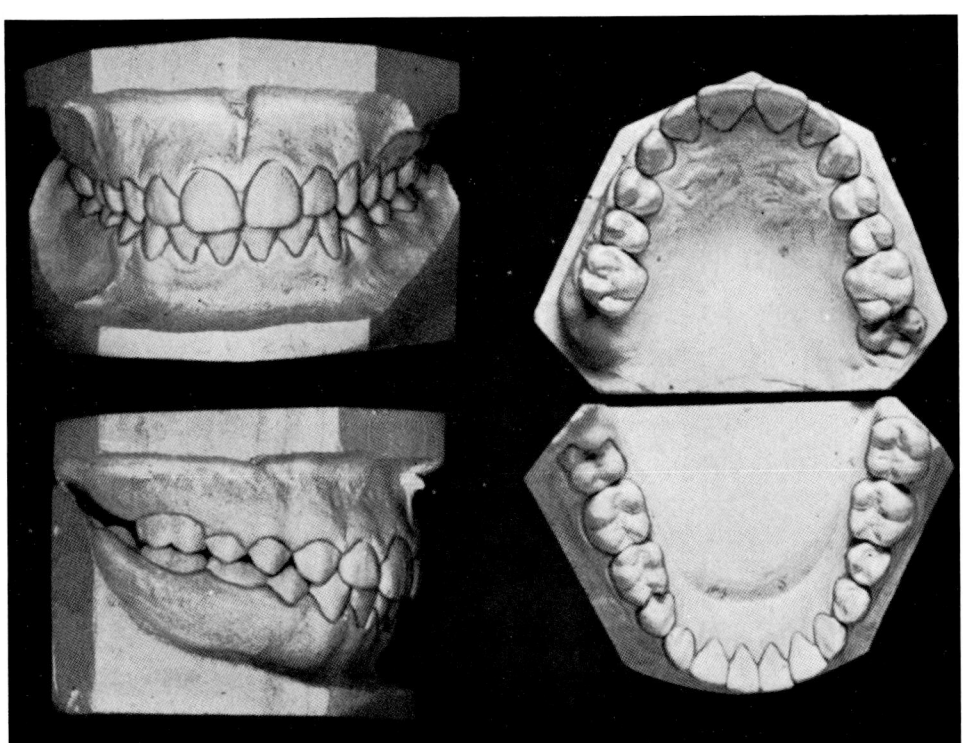

Figure 1-42 Patient D. M.; 12 years, 1 month, 24 days. The maxillary right second premolar has finally erupted and the second molars are making their appearance. Mandibular irregularity has disappeared. (Sillman, J. H., from Graber, T. M.: *Orthodontics*, 2nd ed., 1966, p. 73.)

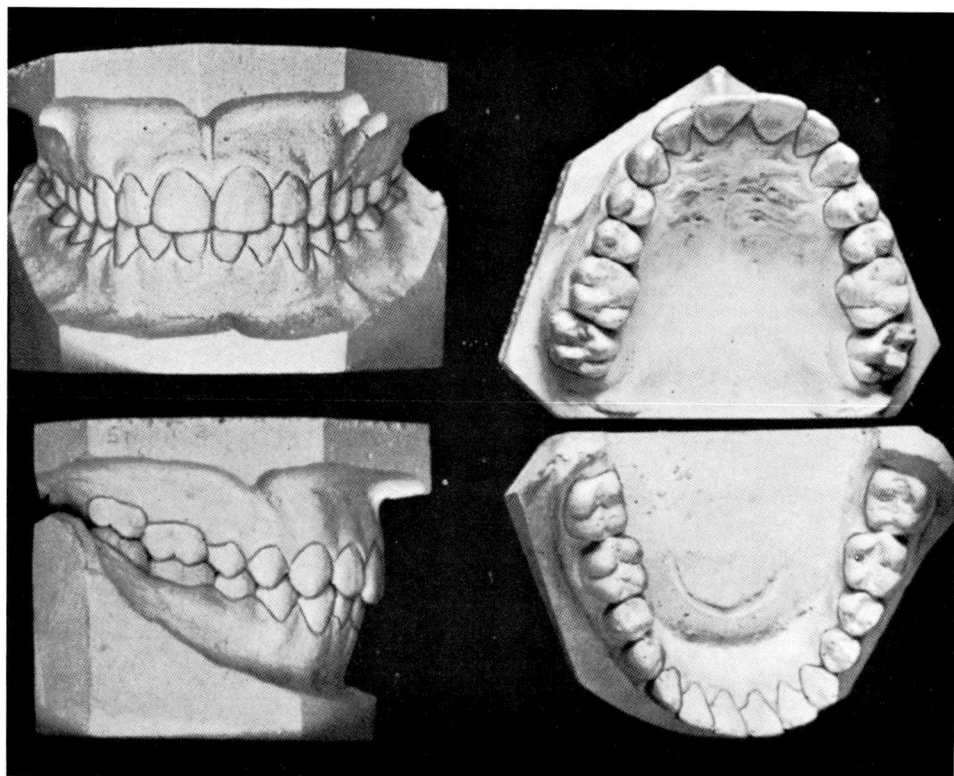

Figure 1-43 Patient D. M.; 14 years, 0 months, 17 days. Second molars are fully erupted at this time. (Sillman, J. H., from Graber, T. M.: *Orthodontics*, 2nd ed., 1966, p. 73.)

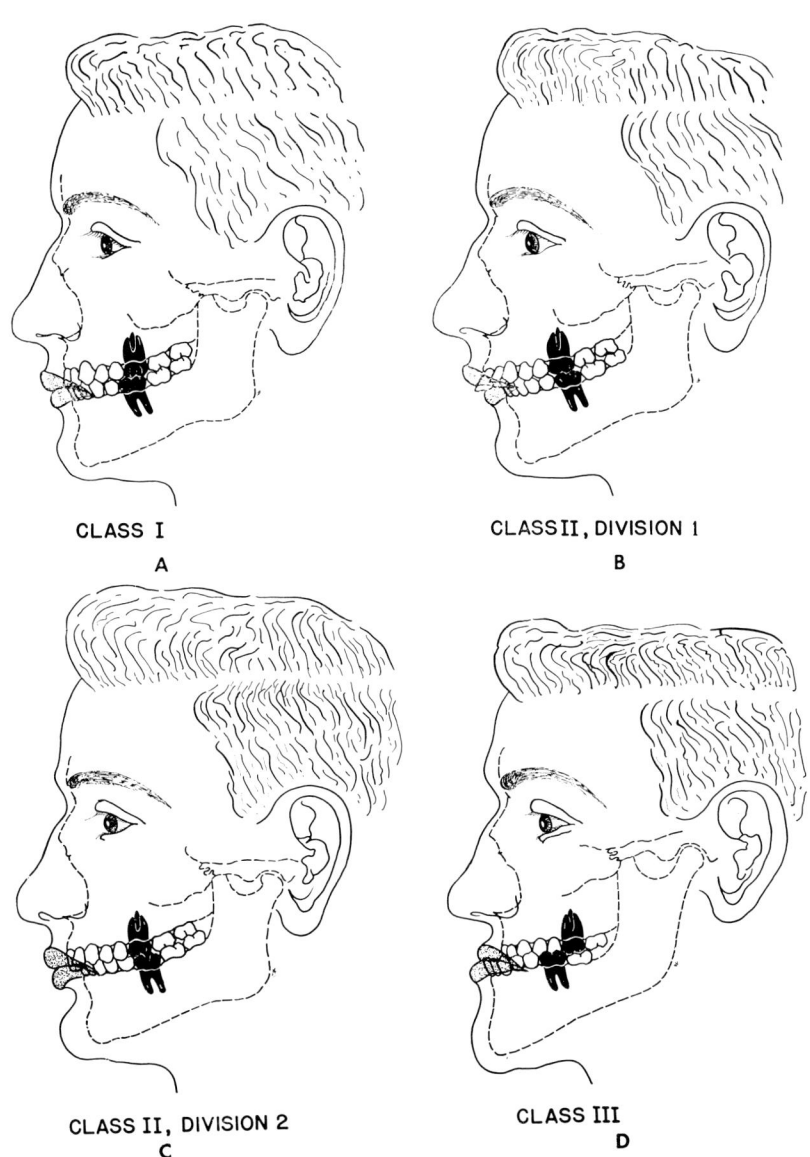

Figure 1-44 Angle's classification of malocclusion:
A, Class I. Mesiodistal first molar relationship normal; tooth irregularities elsewhere.
B, Class II, Division 1. Lower first molar distal to upper first molar. Mandibular retrusion usually reflected in patient profile.
C, Class II, Division 2. Lower first molar distal to upper first molar. Deep overbite often reflected in patient profile.
D, Class III. Malocclusion. Lower first molar mesial to upper first molar. Mandibular prognathism usually reflected in patient profile.
(From Graber, T. M.: *Orthodontics*, 2nd ed., 1966, p. 226.)

ORAL DIAGNOSIS

Chapter 2

A good diagnostician evaluates all aspects of a child's appearance and behavior before arriving at any conclusions concerning his oral condition. From the moment a youngster walks into the office for the first time, until the termination of his appointment, a great deal of pertinent information can be elicited by the alert clinician. The gait and stance of the child may be an indication of medical problems, as may be his complexion, hair, and other physical features. It is important to get into the habit of always noting these obvious physical characteristics before narrowing down to the area of particular interest to the dentist, which is the oral cavity. Such evaluation is not necessarily time-consuming if the observer is perceptive.

Some kind of health questionnaire or past medical and dental history should be completed in writing by the parent prior to the child's introduction to the dentist. The nature of the questions on this form will reflect the individual dentist's ideas and concepts of diagnosis. Good examples of adequate health questionnaires are the Cornell Medical Index and the Minnesota Multiphasic Personality Inventory. The health questionnaire should provide basic information such as the child's name, nickname, age, weight, and place of birth, in addition to the chief complaint and past medical and dental history. Using this type of form as a guide, the dentist can then complete his own case history in conference with the parent, securing additional facts as indicated by the answers previously supplied.

The oral examination of the child patient should consist of a detailed inspection of the soft and hard tissues of the mouth and a radiological survey. When this is completed the need will be established for special tests, diet surveys, medical reports, or consultation with specialists. A systematic approach to examination of soft and hard tissues is essential. A good order of sequence is to inspect the lips, externally and internally, the buccal mucosa and mucobuccal fold, the hard palate, the pharyngeal area, the sublingual area, the tongue, and the gingivae. An evaluation of the occlusion should be performed next, noting both the position of teeth in contact and the path of closure. The individual condition of each tooth may then be verified with respect to color, mobility, caries, and other abnormalities. All information should be accurately recorded on the patient's chart and later augmented by careful examination of the radiographs. Regardless of the dentist's individual preference for a particular type of radiographic survey, there should be sufficient exposures to include periapical areas as well as the customary interproximals. It is particularly important in treating children to make an early determination of missing teeth, supernumeraries, and similar abnormalities, which will be missed if only bitewing radiographs are obtained.

The dentist who sees children should have as his goal the ability to make an accurate diagnosis of every case that he treats. To meet this challenge he will have to keep abreast of the professional literature, utilize all known methods of examination, and above all maintain close relationships with allied specialists who can cooperate with him on his referrals.

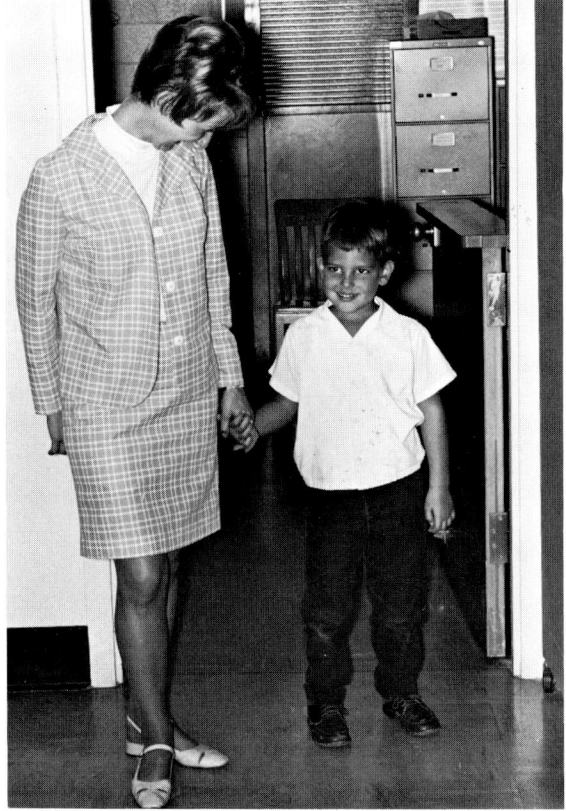

Figure 2-1 Child and mother walking into office. Note the child's gait, stature, dress, and speech.

ORAL DIAGNOSIS 27

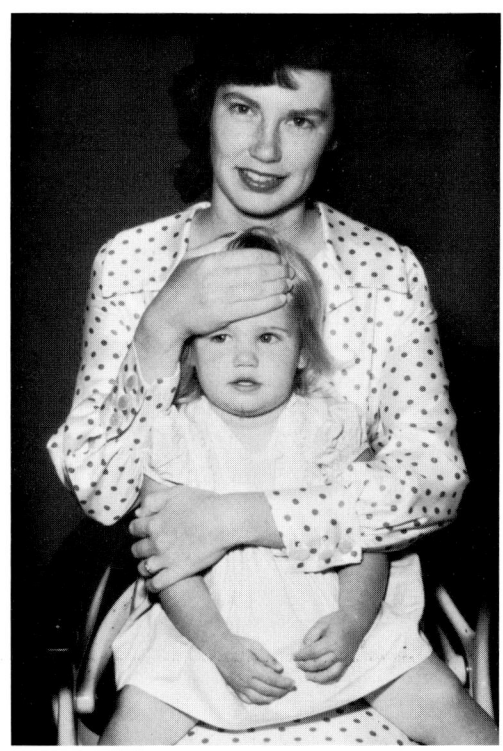

Figure 2-2 Young child seated on mother's lap for dental examination. Note position of mother's arms and hands to stabilize the child during the examination. This approach may be used on the very young child who feels more secure when seated in the mother's lap.

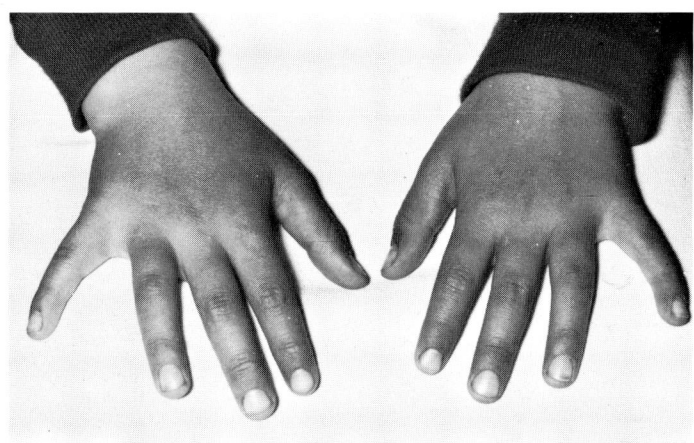

Figure 2-3 Fingers being examined. Look for abnormalities of shape that may be an indication of an oral habit, a systemic disease, or other condition.

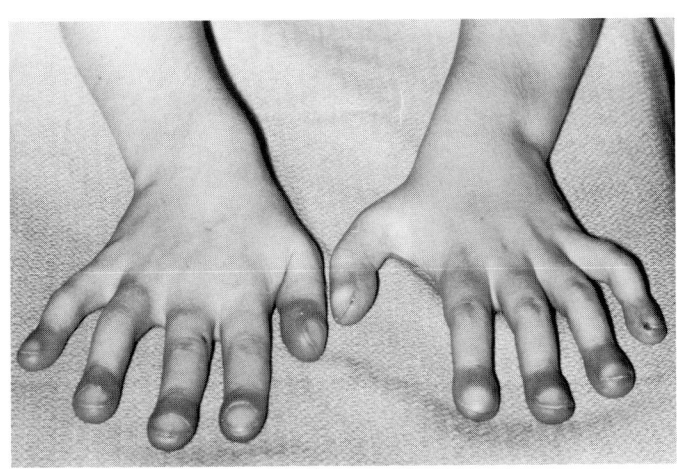

Figure 2-4 Fingers of a child with a congenital heart defect. Note clubbing of the ends of the fingers.

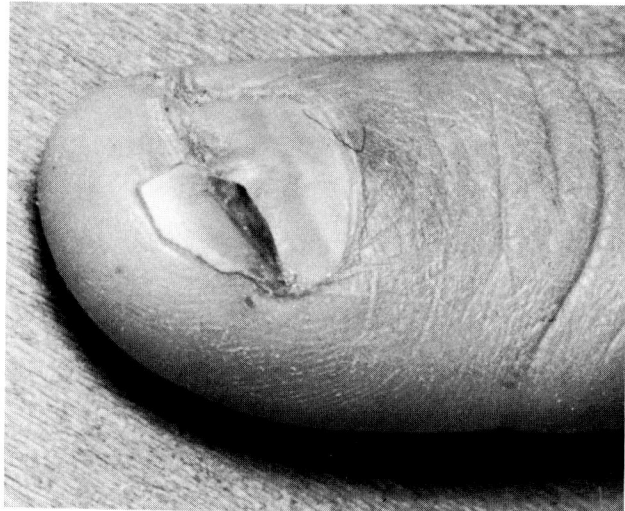

Figure 2-5 Thumb of a child with sucking habit.

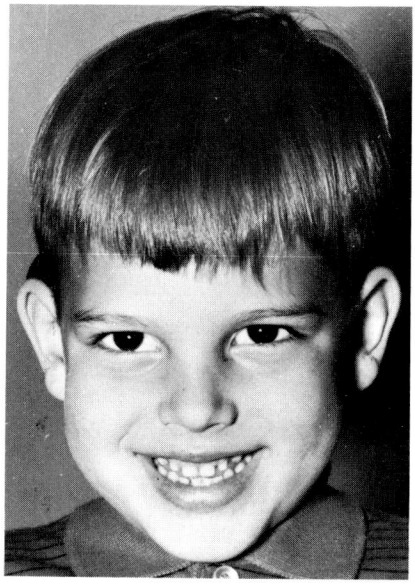

Figure 2-6 Anterior view of the head. Examine the skin, eyes, nose, and lips, and check for facial asymmetry.

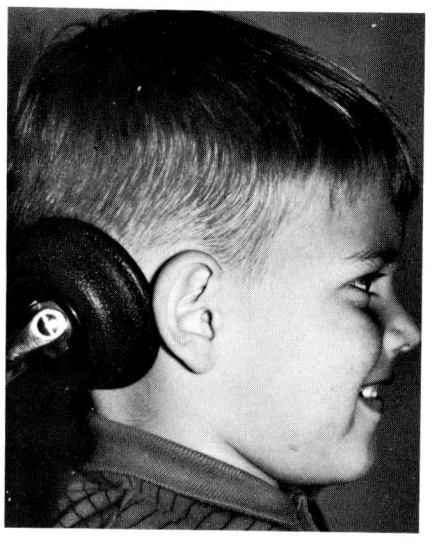

Figure 2-7 Lateral view of the head. Observe the shape of the head and nose. Note the quality and distribution of hair.

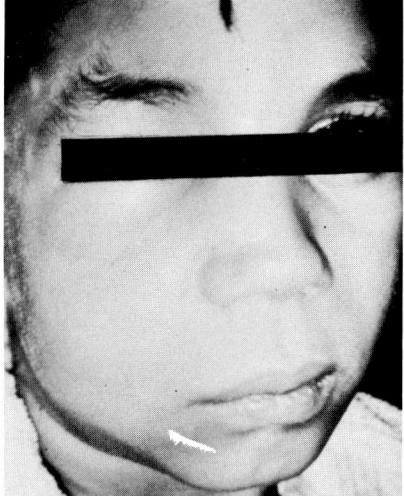

Figure 2-8 Severe swelling of the right side of the face extending from lower border of mandible to the orbital region as a result of a periapical abscess of the maxillary right primary second molar.

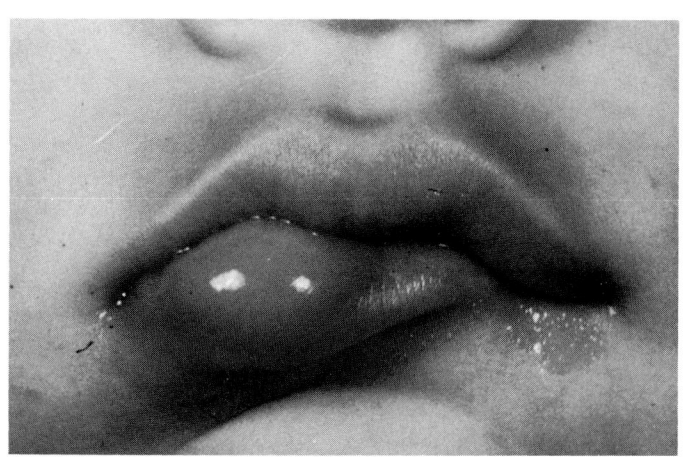

Figure 2-9 Bulbous area on the lower right side of the lip associated with a lip-sucking habit.

Figure 2-10 Child sucking on lip (same child as shown in Figure 2-9).

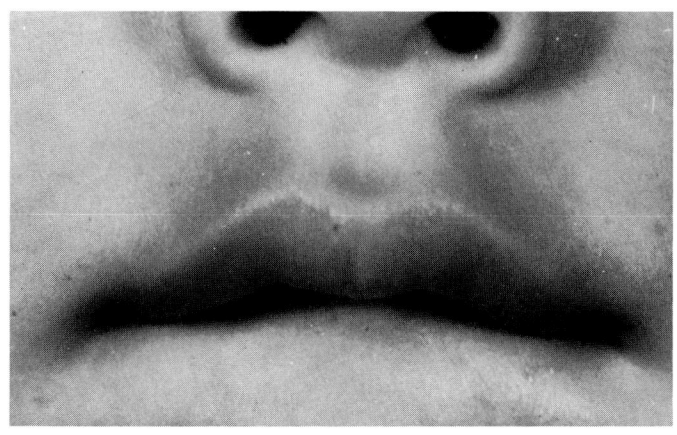

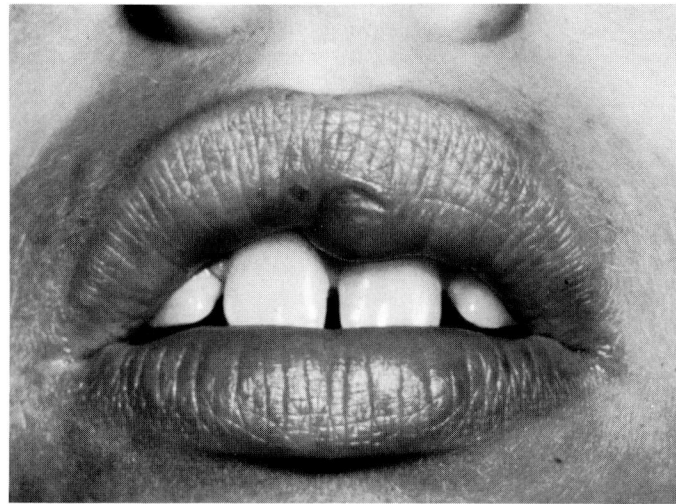

Figure 2-11 An 8½-year-old child with a history of falling and biting the upper lip.

Figure 2-12 Typical appearance of mouth in a child with lip-biting and lip-sucking habit.

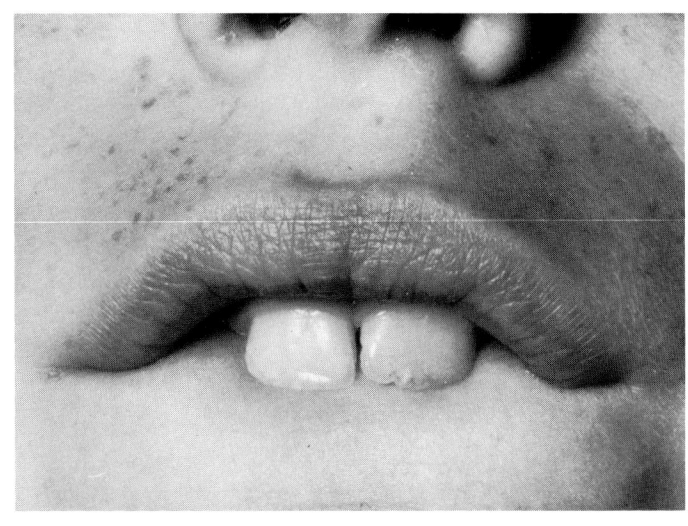

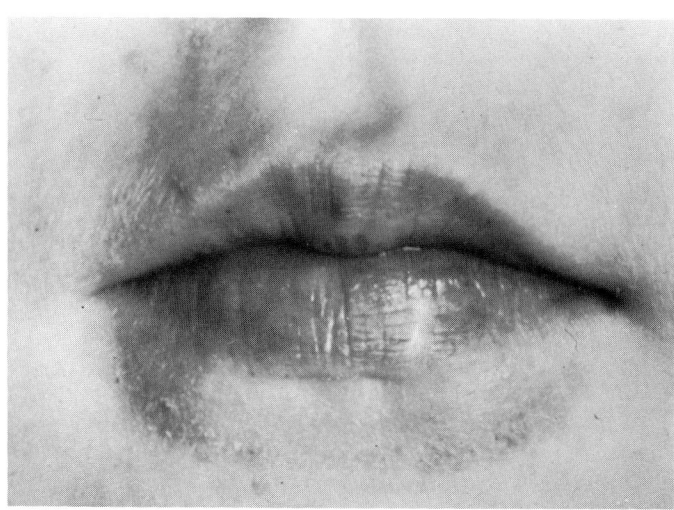

Figure 2-13 Patient with chapped lower lip (see Figure 2-14).

ORAL DIAGNOSIS 31

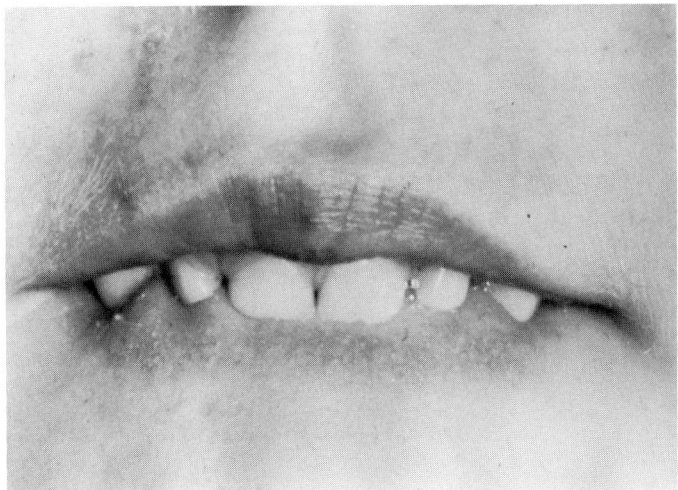

Figure 2-14 Chronic lip-sucking and lip-chewing.

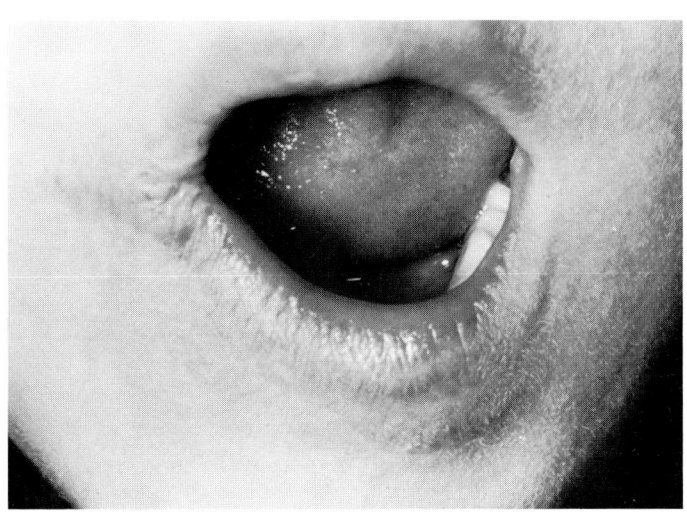

Figure 2-15 Dryness of the commissure of the lips on the right side. May be caused by a licking habit.

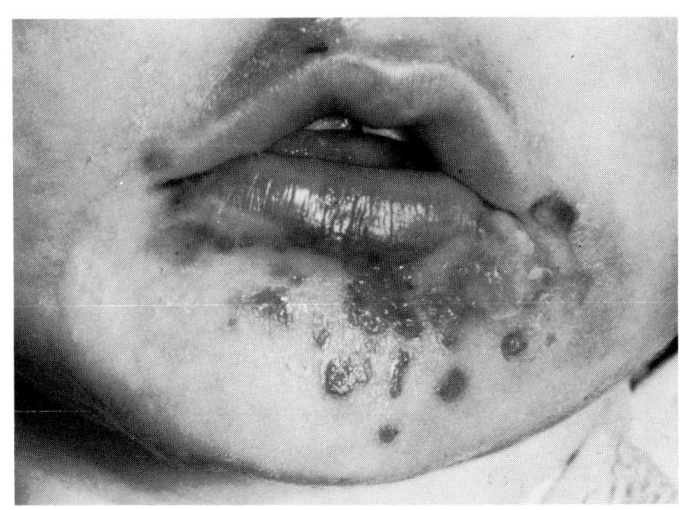

Figure 2-16 Primary herpetic gingivostomatitis on the lower face. This is a very painful condition and the patient usually does not wish to eat or drink. Treatment consists mainly of preventing dehydration and secondary infection. Hospitalization may be necessary if dehydration does occur. The lesions heal within 7 to 14 days without causing scars.

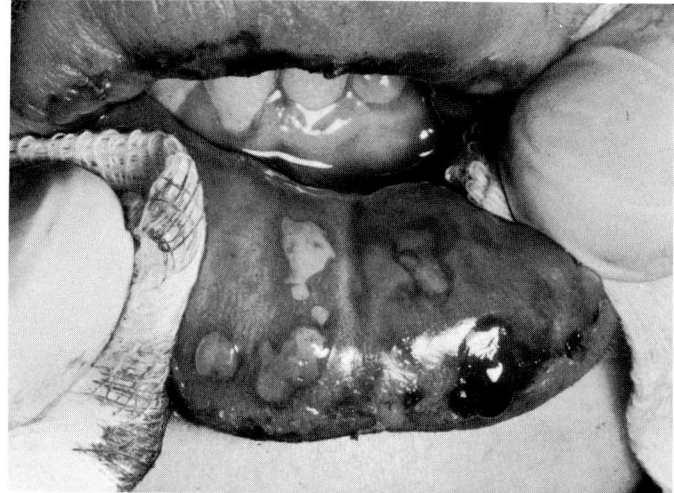

Figure 2-17 Primary herpetic gingivostomatitis of the lower lip and oral mucosa. Same patient as presented in Figure 2-16.

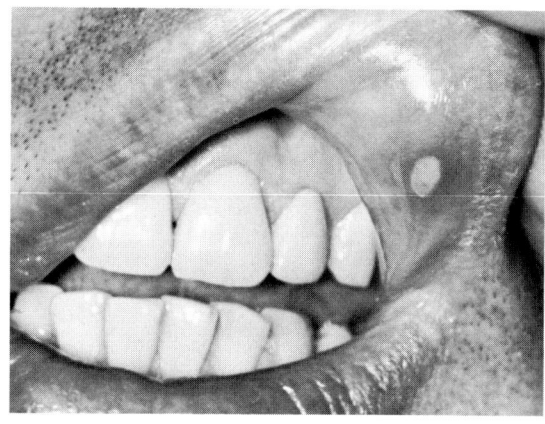

Figure 2-18 Canker sore (recurrent aphthous ulcer) of the oral mucosa of the upper lip. Treatment is palliative; these lesions heal within 7 to 14 days and cause no scars.

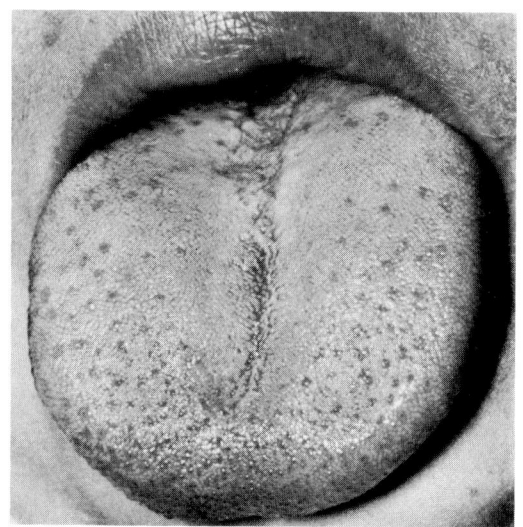

Figure 2-19 Tongue extended to allow examiner to test mobility.

ORAL DIAGNOSIS 33

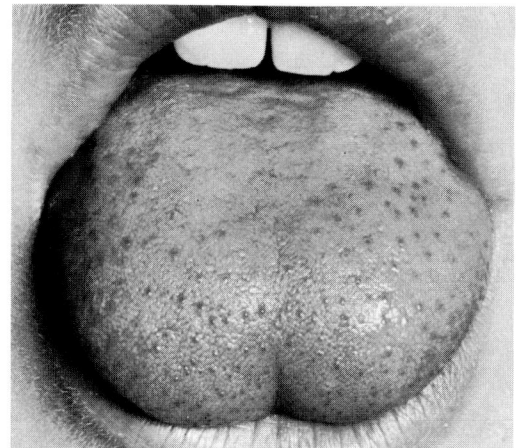

Figure 2-20 Mobility of tongue inhibited because of ankyloglossia.

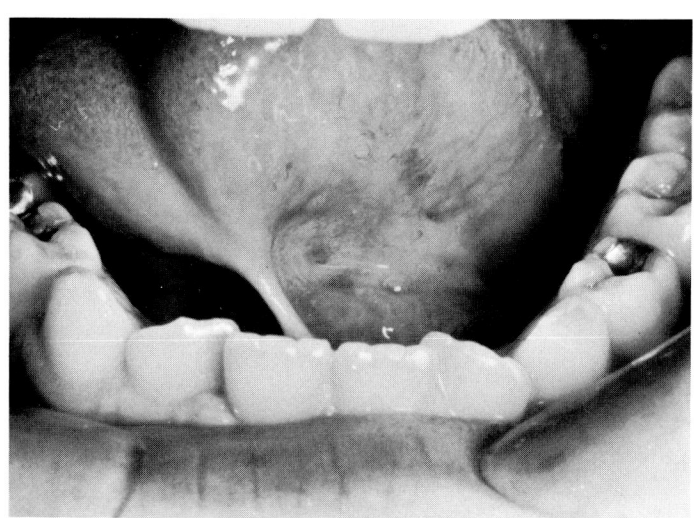

Figure 2-21 Lingual frenum of patient with ankyloglossia.

Figure 2-22 Geographic tongue. These lesions usually disappear spontaneously; however, recurrences are not uncommon. Always inspect the superior, inferior, and lateral surfaces of the tongue.

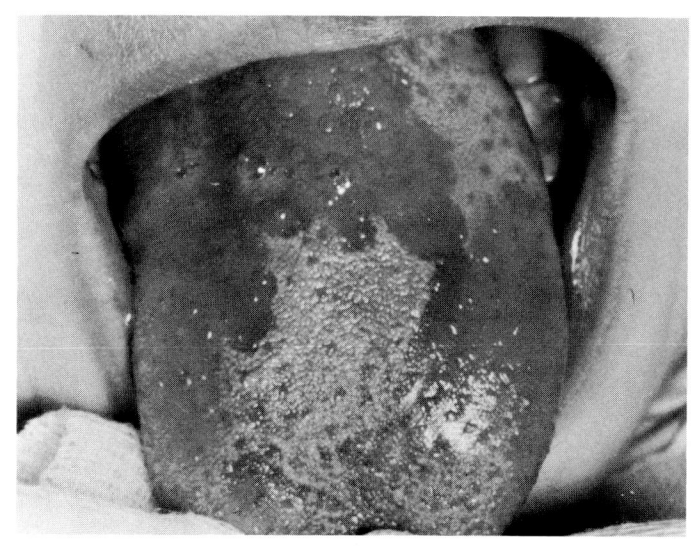

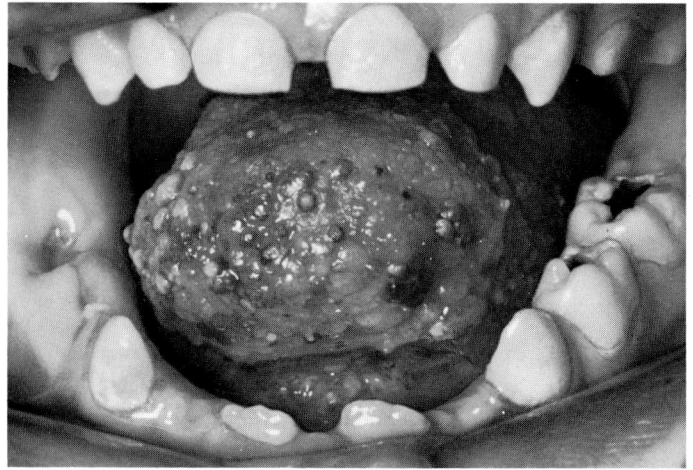

Figure 2-23 Cavernous hemangioma of the tongue in a young child.

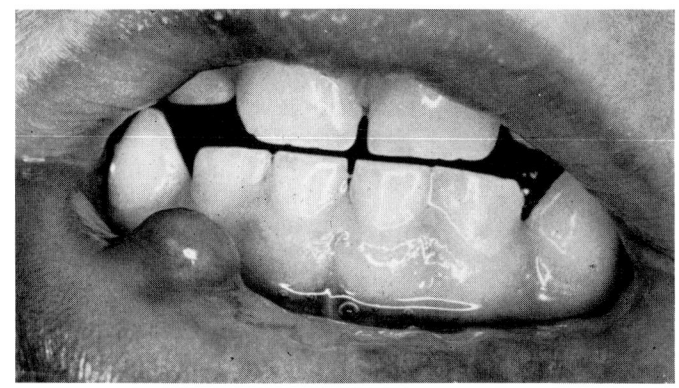

Figure 2-24 Mucocele caused by retention of mucin in the tissue following injury to the lip. (From Kerr, D. A., and Ash, M. M.: *Oral Pathology*, 2nd ed., Lea & Febiger, Philadelphia, 1965, p. 121.)

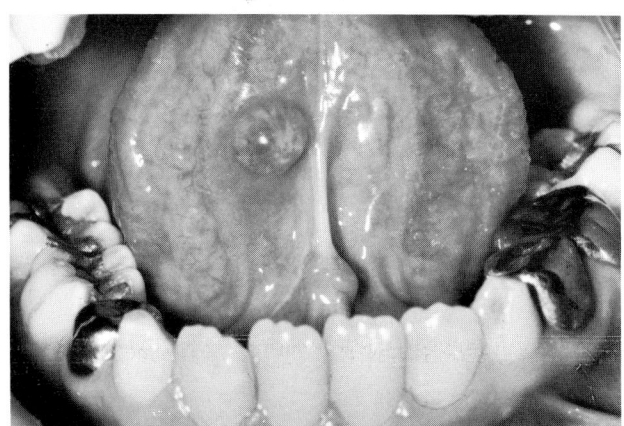

Figure 2-25 Inspection of floor of the mouth. Note capillary hemangioma on the inferior surface of the tongue next to the lingual frenum.

ORAL DIAGNOSIS

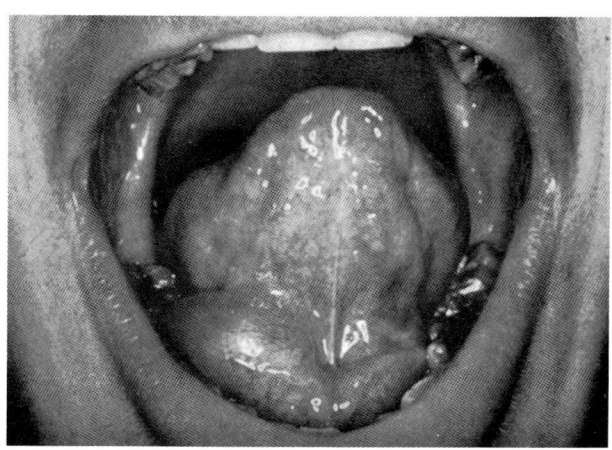

Figure 2-26 Ranula in the floor of the mouth. (From Krueger, G. O.: *Oral Surgery*, 2nd ed., C. V. Mosby Co., St. Louis, 1961, p. 271.)

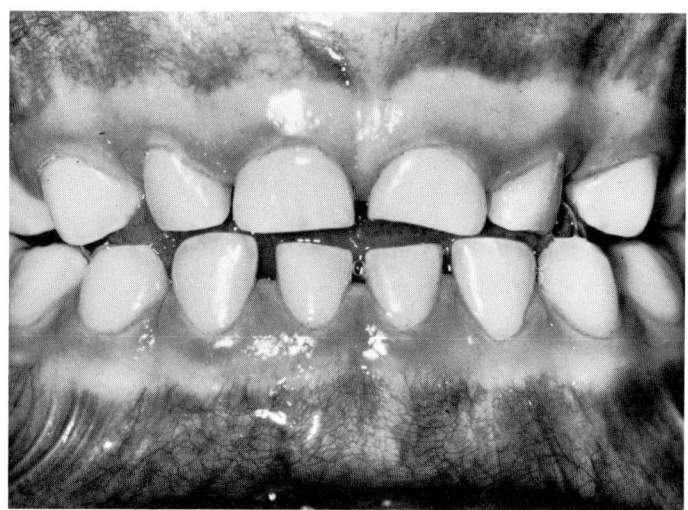

Figure 2-27 A 5-year-old child with marginal gingivitis.

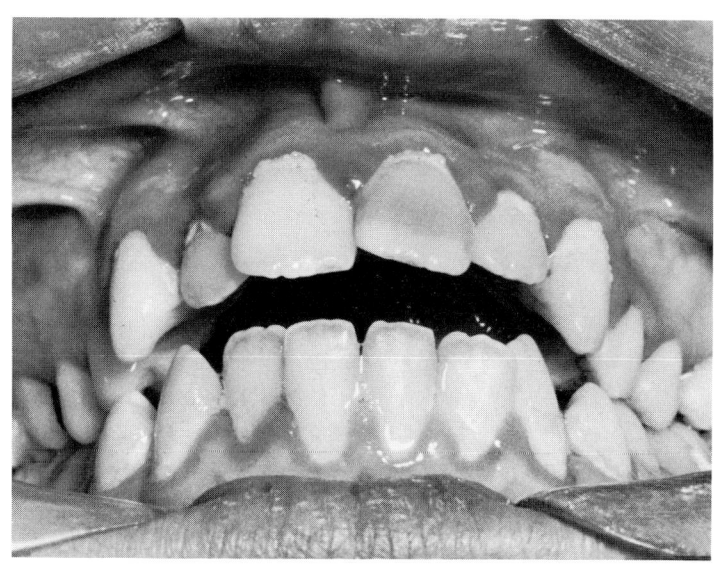

Figure 2-28 Teenager with gingivitis caused by accumulation of debris and materia alba around the teeth. Patient practiced poor oral hygiene. Gingival hemorrhage occurs easily on contact. Treatment consists of thorough prophylaxis, followed by home care.

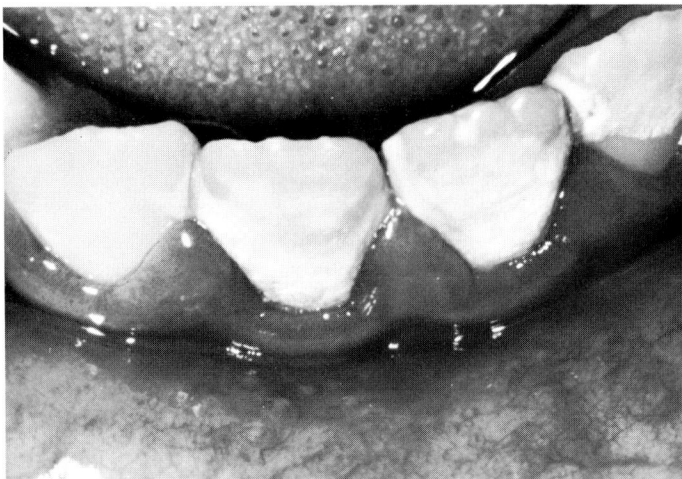

Figure 2-29 A 7-year-old child with heavy deposits of calculus on the labial surfaces of the mandibular permanent incisors. Note gingivitis. Calculus is the most common cause of gingivitis and must be removed. It is unusual for heavy deposits of calculus to develop in children under 12 years of age.

Figure 2-30 An 8-year-old child with calculus on the lingual surfaces of the mandibular permanent incisors. This is usually the first site of calculus accumulation.

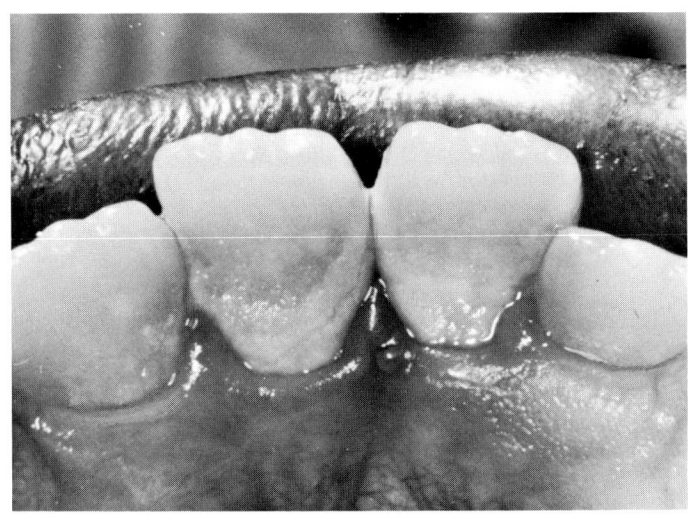

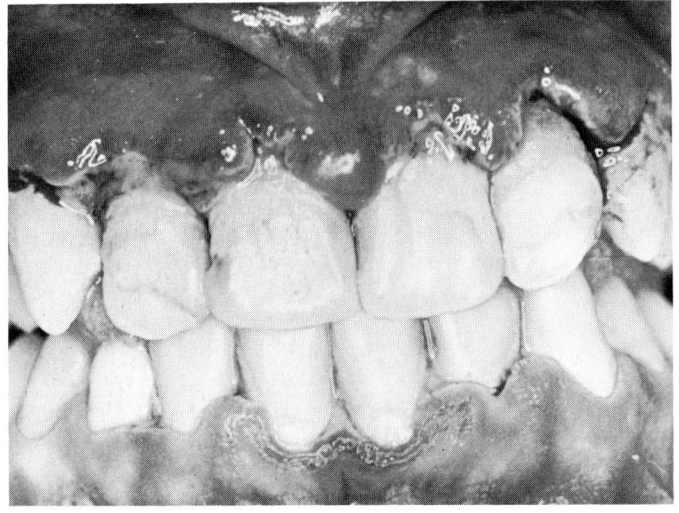

Figure 2-31 Necrotizing ulcerative gingivitis. It is seldom seen in children under 10 years of age. Interdental papillae often have a crater, with areas of sloughing tissue over the red, edematous gingiva. Initial treatment is a prophylaxis to remove the local irritants, followed by diligent home care of the involved area. Antibiotics are used only to treat secondary infections. (Courtesy Department of Oral Biology, School of Dentistry, University of Washington.)

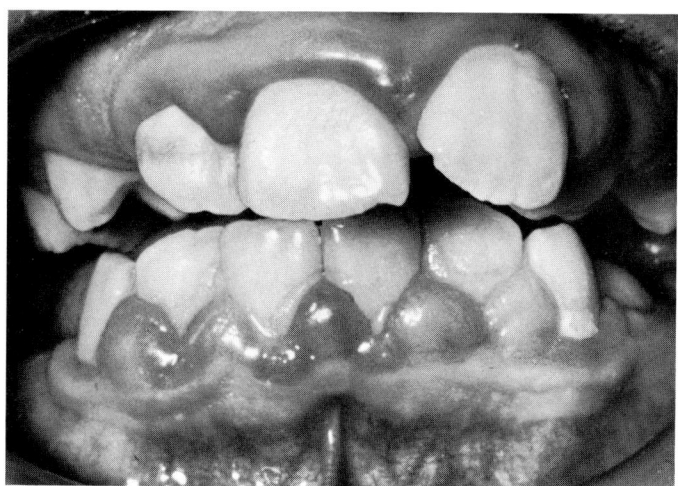

Figure 2-32 Pubertal gingivitis. Tissues are soft and bleed easily. The condition is associated with a hormonal imbalance during puberty and normally disappears when hormonal balance is restored. The importance of good oral hygiene should be stressed to teenagers.

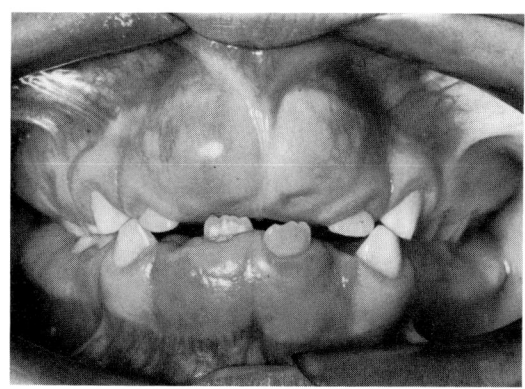

Figure 2-33 Idiopathic gingival fibromatosis (hereditary gingival fibromatosis). This is a familial defect similar in appearance to Dilantin hyperplasia; however, it occurs in individuals with no history of having received Dilantin therapy. Although gingivoplasty improves the condition, the overgrowth of connective tissue tends to recur.

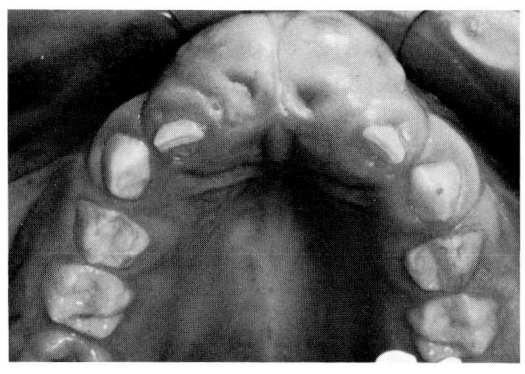

Figure 2-34 Idiopathic gingival fibromatosis of the maxillary arch (same patient as seen in Figure 2-33).

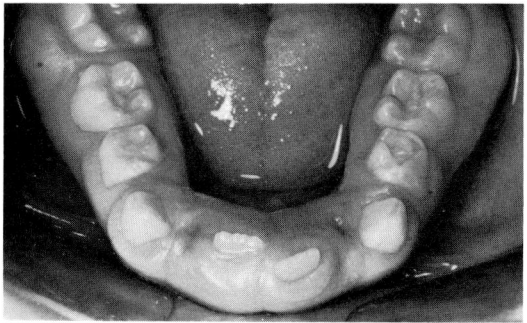 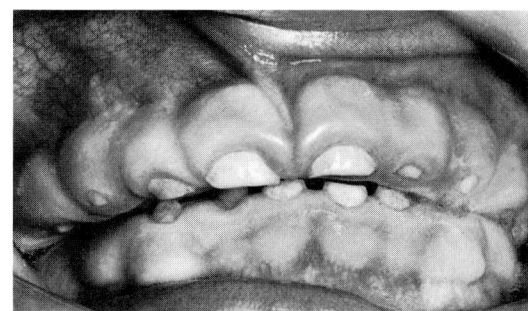

Figure 2-35 **Figure 2-36**

Figure 2-35 Idiopathic gingival fibromatosis of the mandibular arch (same patient as seen in Figures 2-33 and 2-34).

Figure 2-36 Idiopathic fibromatosis in a preschool child.

Figure 2-37 Dilantin hyperplasia in a teenager. Gingivoplasty is the treatment of choice; however, following removal of the tissue the gingiva will become hyperplastic once again if the patient continues to ingest Dilantin. *Careful* oral hygiene will retard this tendency (see Figure 2-38).

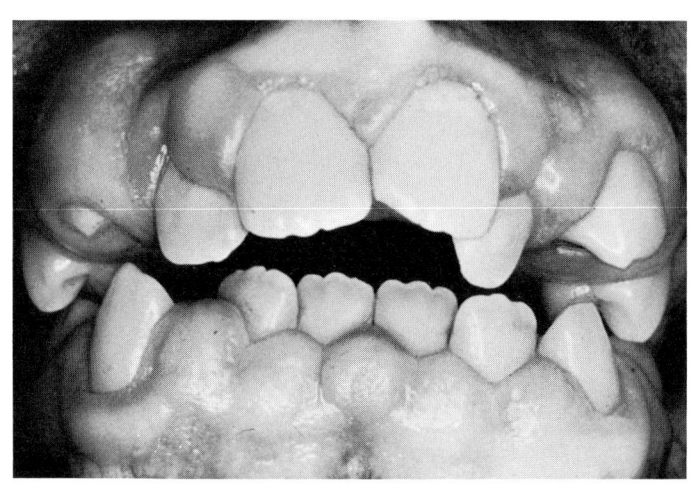

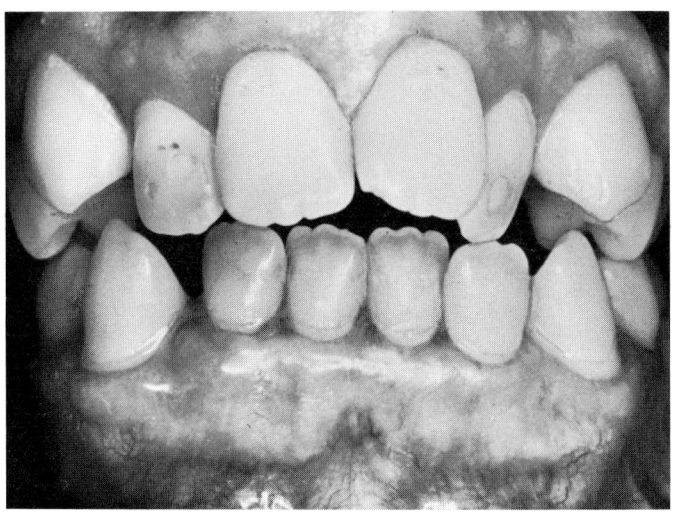

Figure 2-38 Teenager with Dilantin hyperplasia following gingivoplasty (same patient as seen in Figure 2-37).

ORAL DIAGNOSIS

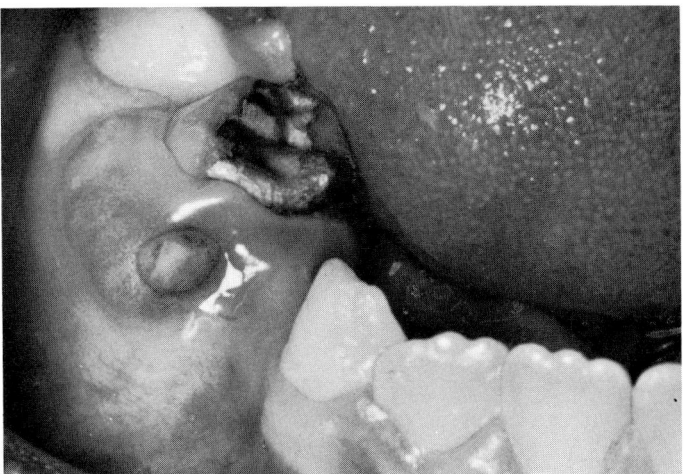

Figure 2-39 Periapical abscess of mandibular right primary second molar. In many cases this condition is not painful and consequently may be present for a long period of time. Tooth was extracted.

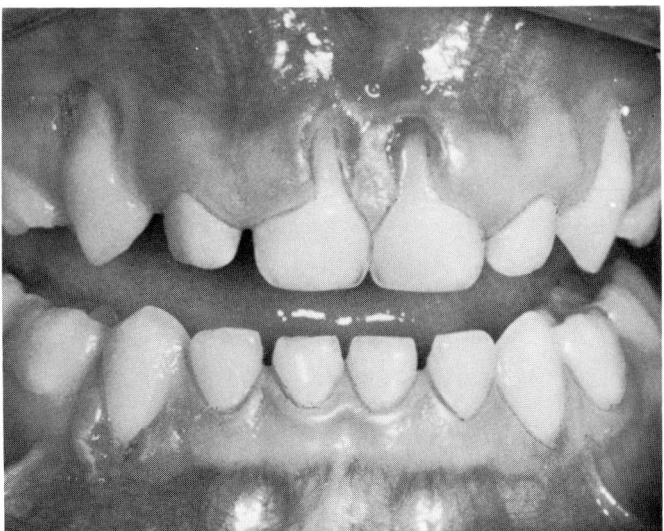

Figure 2-40 Localized gingival recession resulting from a habit of picking at the tissue with the fingernail. Note tissue around maxillary primary centrals and cuspids and the mandibular right primary cuspid.

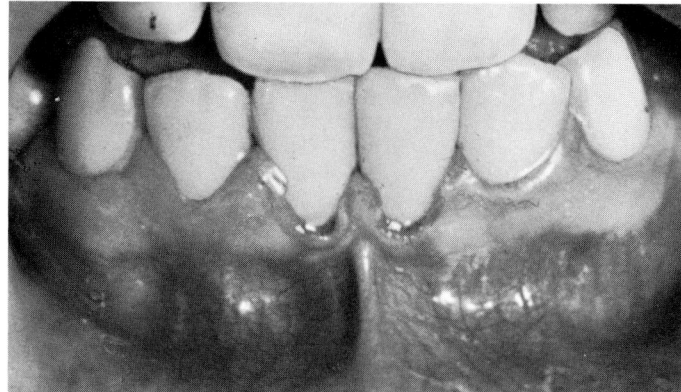

Figure 2-41 Loss of integrity (stripping) of gingival margin around the mandibular permanent central incisors. Numerous factors compound this periodontal problem (occlusal trauma, area of food impaction, frenum attachment, and encroachment on the alveolar mucosa). Periodontal treatment is definitely indicated, otherwise stripping will continue.

Figure 2-42 Patient has a habit of picking at the labial gingiva with a fingernail. A careful history is required to determine the true cause of this habit.

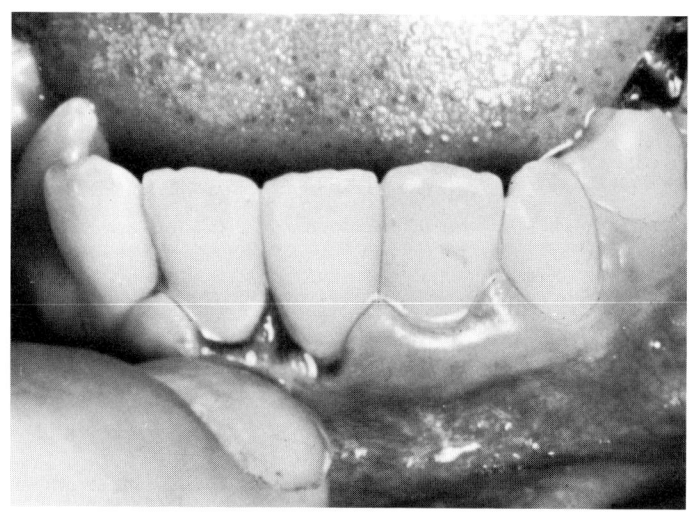

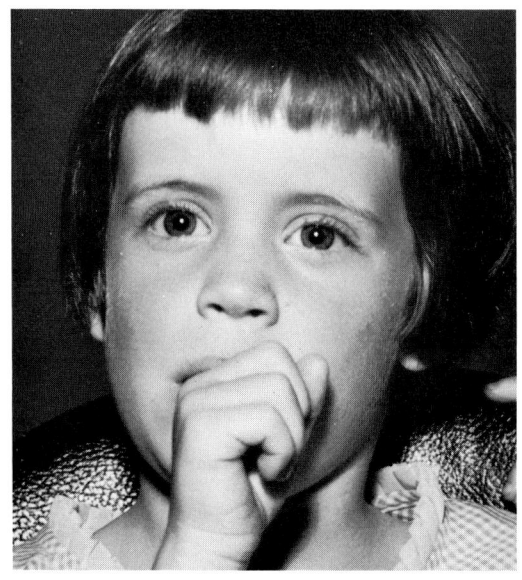

Figure 2-43 A 5-year-old child with an anterior open bite caused by a finger-sucking habit.

ORAL DIAGNOSIS 41

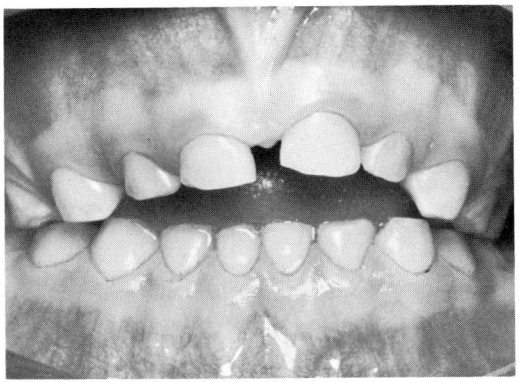

Figure 1-44 Finger-sucking habit in a pre-school child caused an anterior open bite.

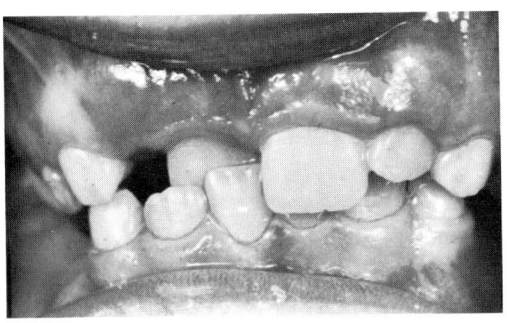

Figure 2-45 An 8-year-old child with an anterior crossbite.

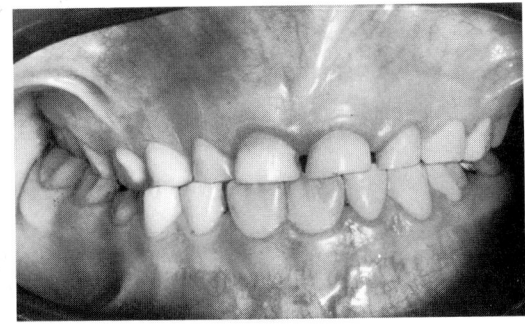

Figure 2-46 A 6½-year-old child with a posterior crossbite.

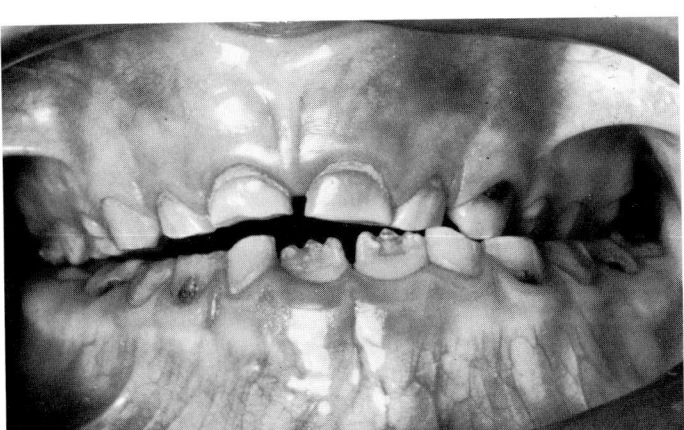

Figure 2-47 Tetracycline staining of primary dentition in a 6-year-old child. Before the dentist examines the teeth for caries and prepares radiographs, he should check the color, shape, structure, size, and number of teeth. (See Chapter 3, Anomalies.)

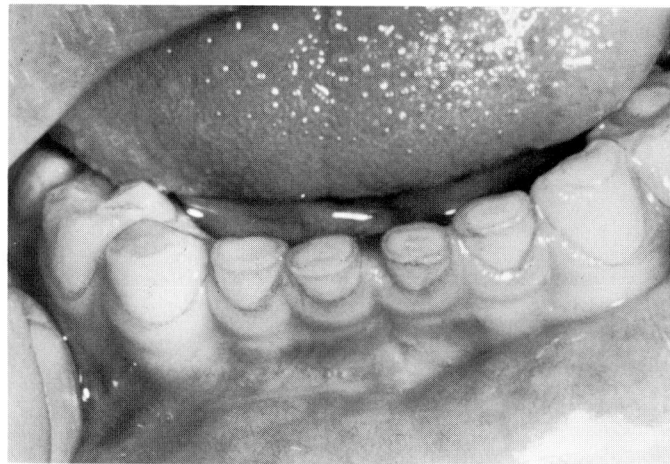

Figure 2-48 A 5½-year-old child with the habit of bruxism. Note extreme abrasion of the primary incisors.

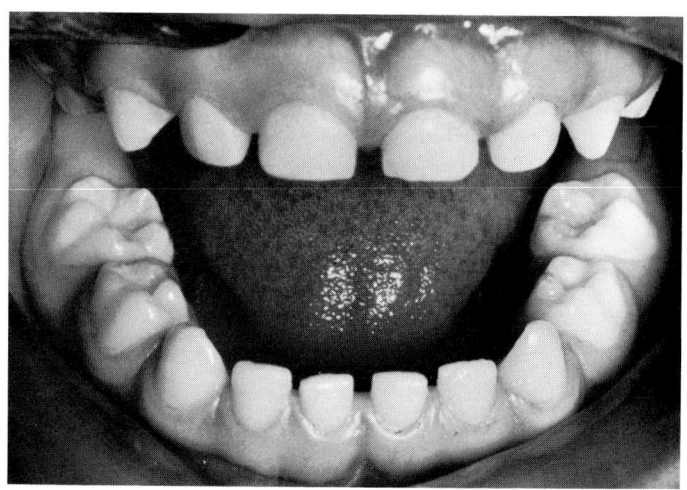

Figure 2-49 A 5-year-old child with a favorable dentition, ready to be examined for dental caries. A good set of radiographs, adequate light and air, dental floss, and a sharp explorer are necessary to determine areas of caries.

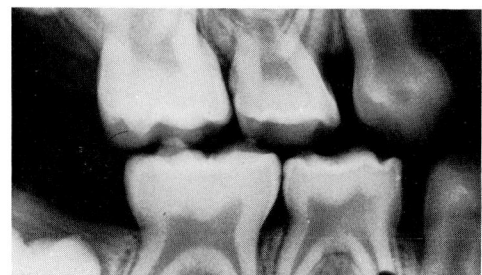 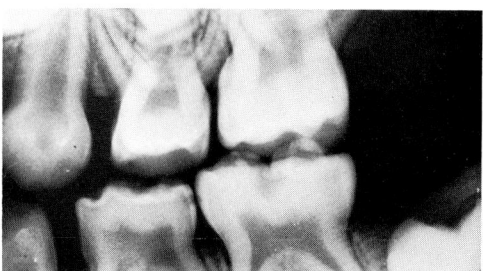

Figure 2-50 Patient J. D., bitewings of a 4-year-old child showing areas of initial caries on the proximal surfaces of maxillary and mandibular primary molars. Parent disregarded advice of the dentist to restore the involved teeth, and chose to postpone treatment. See Figure 2-51 for bitewings of same child 12 months later.

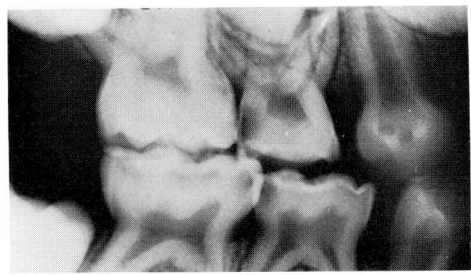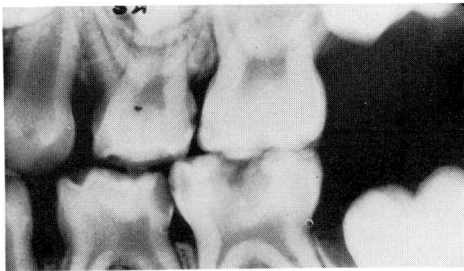

Figure 2-51 Patient J.D., 12 months after first examination. Note the extent of the carious involvement of the mandibular left primary second molar. This series of bitewings illustrates well the rapid progress of dental caries in the primary dentition and points out the need for early restoration.

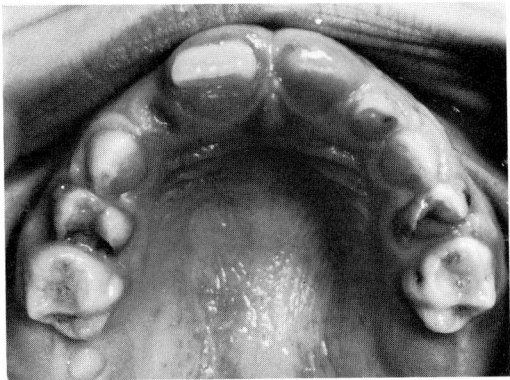

Figure 2-52 Loss of arch length caused by extensive caries of the disto-occlusal surfaces of the maxillary right and left primary first molars. Note how the primary second molars have drifted mesially. Had the primary first molars been restored to natural contour, this would not have occurred.

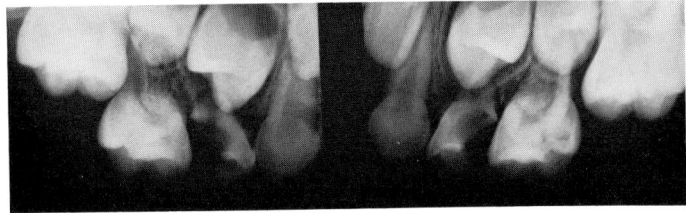

Figure 2-53 Radiographs showing mesial migration of maxillary right and left second primary molars into carious area of the primary first molars. Note the reduced space in which the bicuspids may erupt.

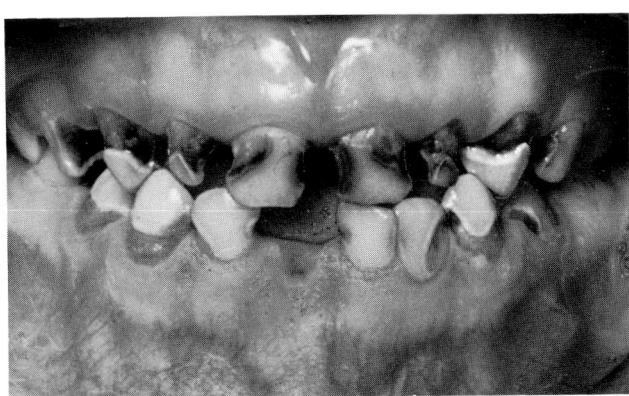

Figure 2-54 Rampant caries in a 5-year-old child.

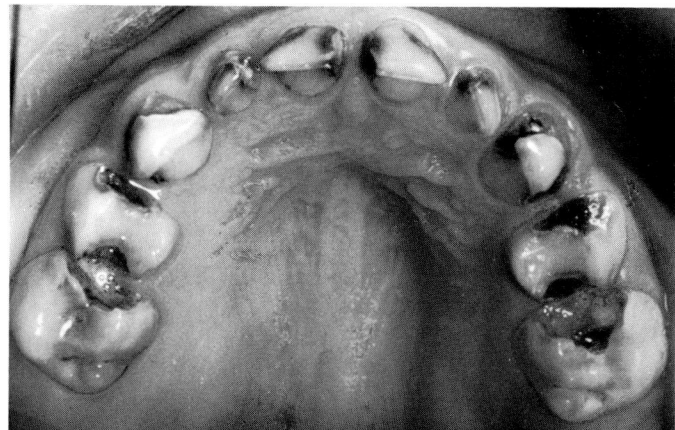

Figure 2-55 Maxillary arch, same patient as seen in Figure 2-54.

Figure 2-56 Gingival caries in a 7½-year-old child.

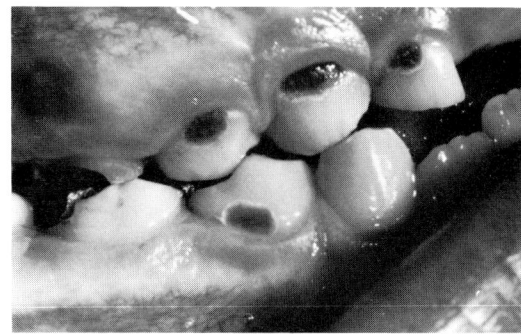

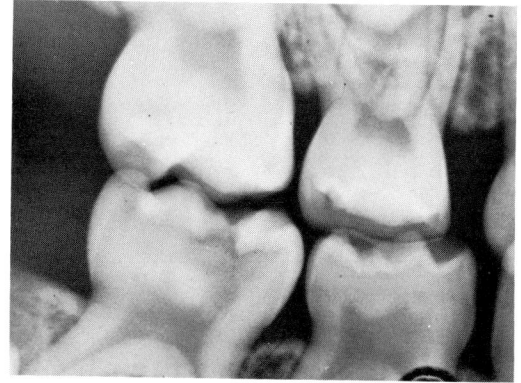

Figure 2-57 Caries of an occlusal pit in a mandibular primary second molar. Lesions like this may be overlooked clinically because of the small size of the external opening. Although there are no other areas of caries, the condition has progressed until it is now involving a pulp horn. When inspecting radiographs, it is important to look at all susceptible surfaces and not just the involved proximal surfaces.

Figure 2-58 Rampant caries of the primary dentition. Note the fistula over the maxillary left central incisor.

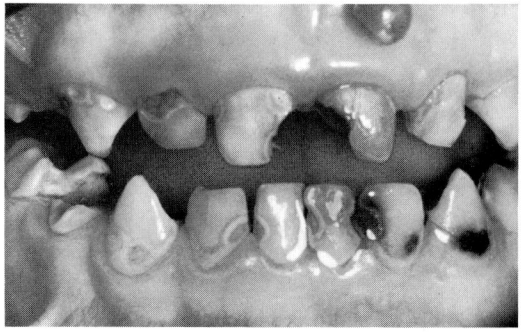

ORAL DIAGNOSIS 45

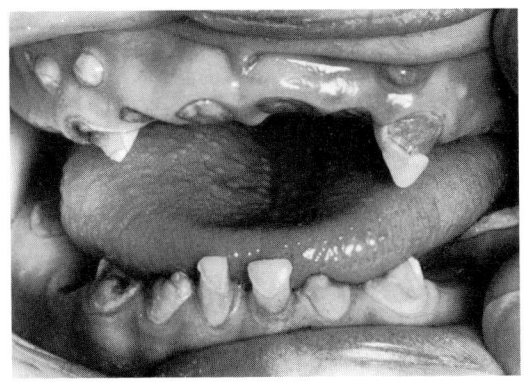

Figure 2-59 Rampant caries of the primary dentition. Teeth were extracted and dentures were made for this child.

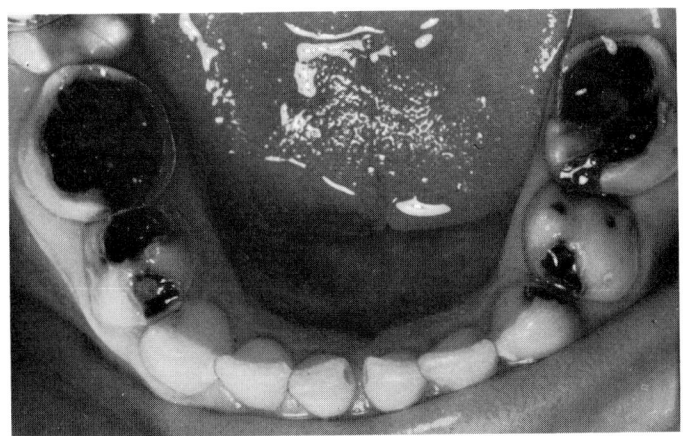

Figure 2-60 A 6-year-old child with arrested caries of the primary molars. There were no pulpal exposures (the dentin was stained and hard) and the teeth were restored with stainless steel crowns.

Figure 2-61 A 10-year-old child with extensive occlusal caries of the mandibular permanent first molars. These teeth often are lost because of the rapid progress of occlusal caries. Early restoration is important.

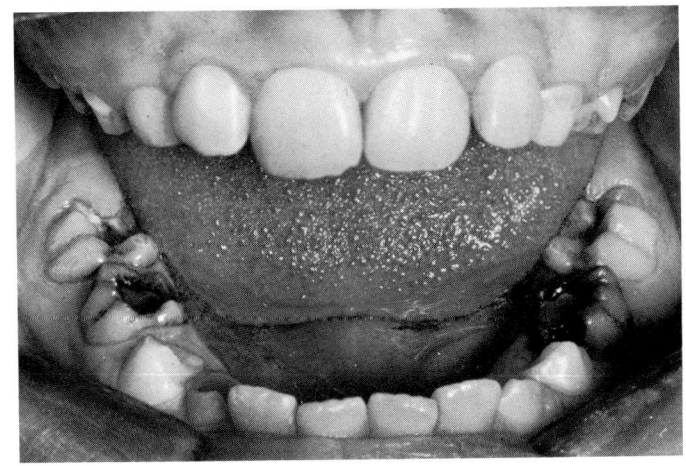

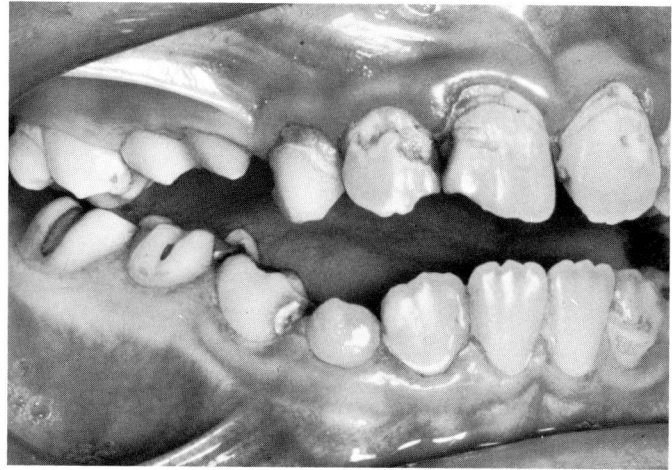

Figure 2-62 A 10-year-old child with extensive gingival caries of the maxillary permanent incisors resulting partly from very poor hygiene. Note edematous gingival tissue.

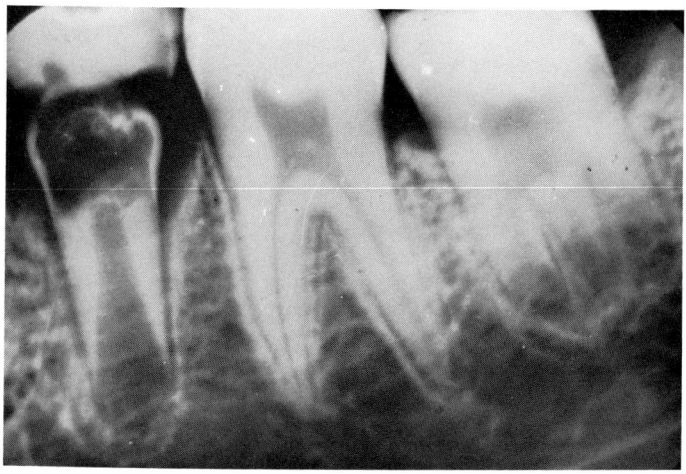

Figure 2-63 Idiopathic internal resorption of a mandibular second bicuspid. These teeth may be saved if early treatment is initiated. (See Figure 2-64 for illustration of treatment of a case of idiopathic internal resorption.)

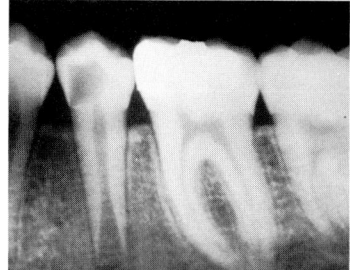 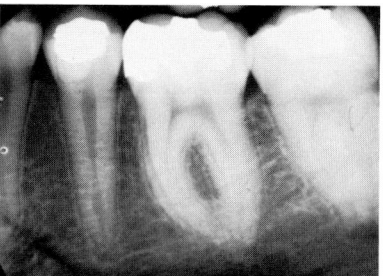

Figure 2-64 Idiopathic internal resorption of a mandibular second bicuspid. A, Preoperative radiograph. B, Postoperative radiographs following pulpotomy done with calcium hydroxide paste in the area of internal resorption. The tooth was then restored with zinc phosphate cement base and an amalgam restoration. Note continued root development.

ORAL DIAGNOSIS 47

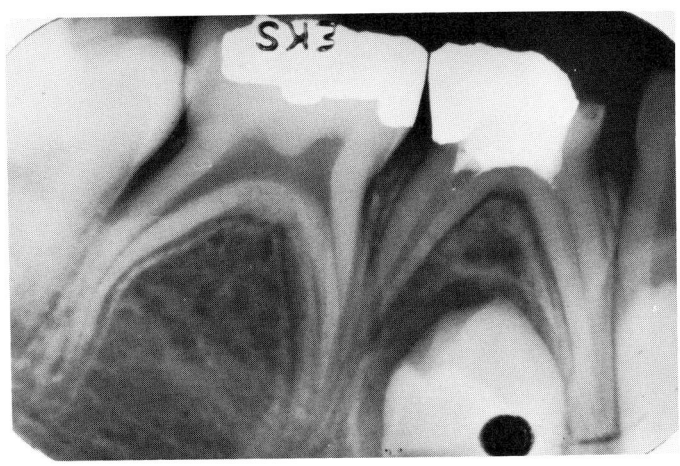

Figure 2-65 Periapical radiograph of the mandibular primary first molar following pulpotomy done with formocresol. (See Figures 2-66 and 2-67.)

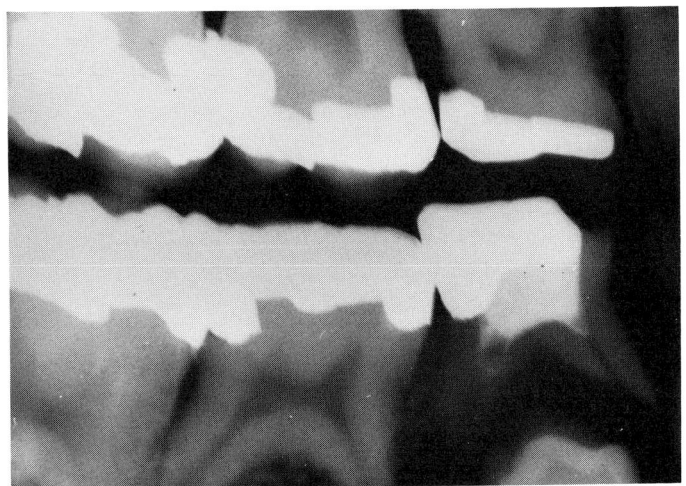

Figure 2-66 Bitewing radiograph taken 12 months after pulpotomy with formocresol. Note the radiolucent area under the mandibular primary first molar (indicative of a pulpotomy failure). The dentist then took a periapical radiograph of the involved area. (See Figure 2-67.)

Figure 2-67 Periapical view of the involved area. The mandibular first and second primary molars were extracted and the pathologist diagnosed the condition as a dentigerous cyst. This case illustrates the necessity for taking adequate radiographs.

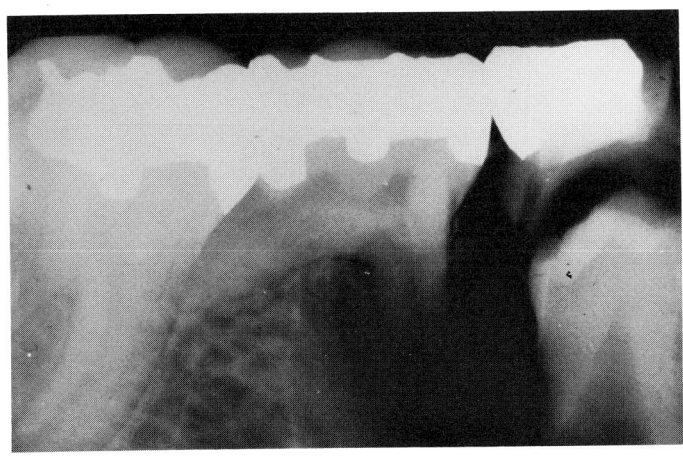

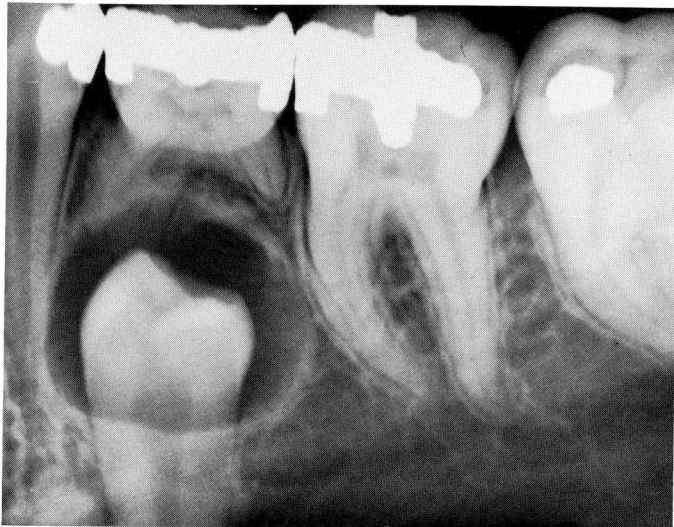

Figure 2-68 A questionable radiolucent area around a mandibular second bicuspid. Early establishment of a diagnosis and treatment are important to prevent further damage. The pathologist diagnosed this condition as a dentigerous cyst.

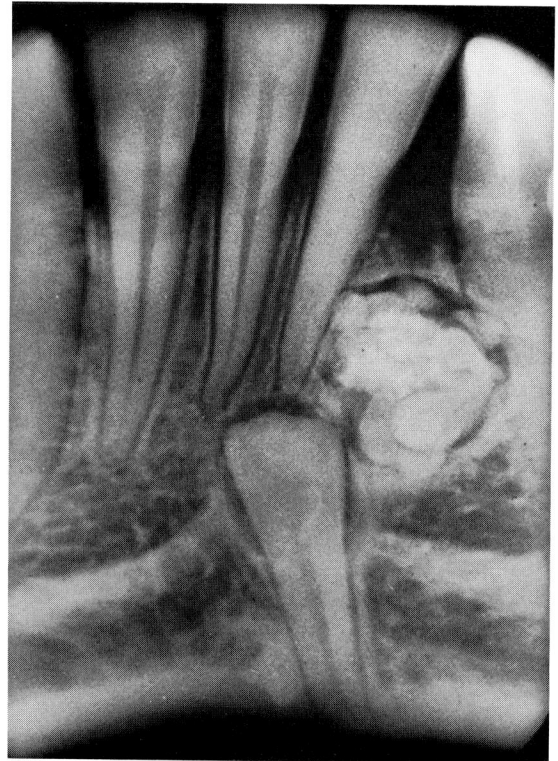

Figure 2-69 An odontoma which obstructed eruption of the mandibular lateral incisor.

ORAL DIAGNOSIS 49

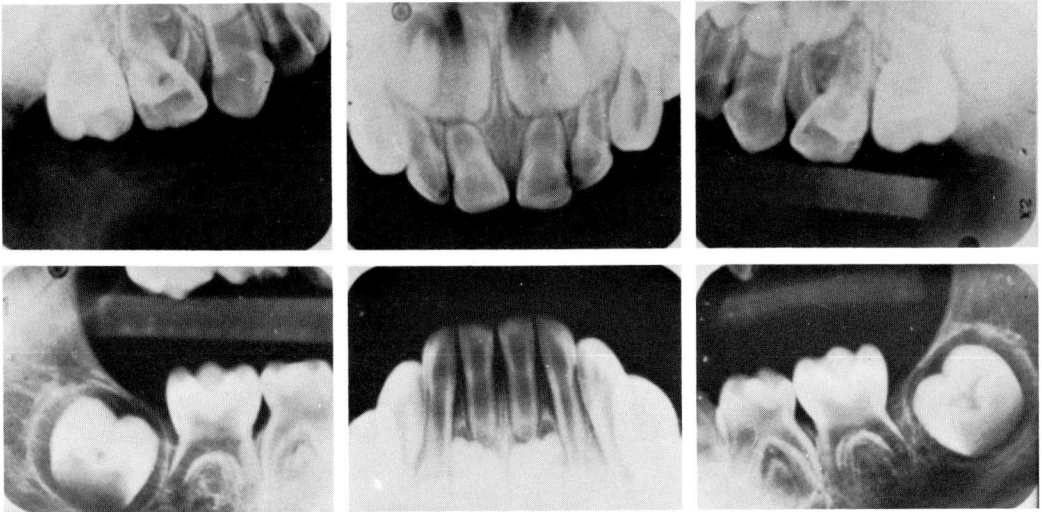

Figure 2-70 Radiographs of a 3-year-old boy with vitamin D-resistant rickets. Note large size of pulp chambers. These cases require prophylactic placement of steel crowns to prevent enamel wear and subsequent dentin exposure and pulpal abscess. (Courtesy Dr. William Tracy, University of Oregon Dental School.)

ANOMALIES OF THE DENTITION

Chapter 3

A majority of the bizarre and unusual anomalies of human teeth become evident during the childhood years. In these cases the dentist who treats the family is usually first called on to make the diagnosis and perform whatever immediate treatment may be required. Too often hereditary conditions are incorrectly diagnosed and dismissed as the result of "fever" or "faulty nutrition." Parents may thus feel unnecessarily guilty about circumstances over which they have no control whatsoever. It is a source of satisfaction to the practitioner to be able to pinpoint the nature of a particular anomaly and it is the purpose of this chapter to enable him to do so.

A classification of anomalies of the dentition is of value to the clinician seeking information useful in making a diagnosis. The six chief categories listed below are further subdivided in the section just preceding their detailed description.

I. Anomalies of number of teeth
II. Anomalies of shape of teeth
III. Anomalies of color of teeth
IV. Anomalies of structure and texture of teeth
V. Anomalies of eruption and exfoliation of teeth
VI. Anomalies of position of teeth

Anomalies of Number of Teeth

Supernumerary teeth result from aberrations in the initiation or proliferation period of the life cycle of the tooth. The best available evidence points to genetic factors as being responsible for this anomaly. Several large-scale studies have been reported on the incidence of supernumerary teeth in children, and although there is some variation in data, there is agreement that the anomaly is much more prevalent in the permanent dentition than in the primary. Published reports on the prevalence of supernumeraries in the primary dentition range from a low figure of 0.3 per cent[7] to a high of 1.8 per cent.[5] The majority of these teeth are located in the maxillary or mandibular incisor region and are of normal shape. No reliable evidence exists for any sex differences in the primary dentition in regard to prevalence of supernumerary teeth.

The incidence of supernumerary teeth in the permanent dentition in children under 14 years of age has been reported by different investigators as ranging from 2 to 3 per cent. Grahnen[7] in a study of Swedish children reported a figure of 3.1 per cent, and Castaldi[4] in a similar study of Canadian children reported 3.1 per cent. Clayton[5] in a group of American children found an incidence of 2.7 per cent. It is of interest that both Castaldi and Clayton found a significantly higher number of supernumeraries in boys than in girls. The majority of these teeth are located in the maxillary incisor region (mesiodens) with a smaller percentage in the bicuspid region and are generally conical or of unusual shape. An observation of importance to the diagnostician is that in cleidocranial dysostosis, a familial and dominant hereditary syndrome involving missing clavicles, there are usually a number of supernumerary teeth.

Teeth that are congenitally or developmentally missing cause many problems for the practicing dentist. Early recognition depends upon careful clinical examination and adequate radiographic surveys. As with supernumerary teeth, missing teeth represent a fault or aberration in either the initiation or proliferation stage of the life cycle of the tooth. There is ample evidence in the literature that the chief causative factor is heredity, and there are well-documented reports of pedigrees through several generations. In rare instances, bone disease, tumors, or radiation may result in lack of tooth formation.

Missing teeth occur less frequently in the primary dentition than in the permanent. Since the primary tooth bud gives rise to the anlage of the succedaneous tooth it follows that the absence of the primary tooth should mean the absence of the permanent tooth also. This is not always the case, however. Studies of the incidence of missing primary teeth in different population groups show considerable variation but in all instances primary teeth are missing less frequently than permanent. Menczer[8] reported 0.09 per cent missing primary teeth in a group of American preschool children, while Grahnen[7] reported 0.4 per cent in a comparable group of Swedish children. Both investigators found the maxillary primary lateral incisor most commonly missing.

In the permanent dentition the incidence of hypodontia, exclusive of third molars, was found to be 3.8 per cent in the Evanston[1] dental caries study. The group studied comprised over 13,000 children aged 12 to 14 years. In Grahnen's comparable survey[7] of 1,006 Swedish school children aged 11 to 14 years, the incidence of missing teeth was 6.1 per cent. In all studies in which radiographs have been employed there is agreement that in children the most commonly missing tooth is the mandibular second bicuspid, followed by the maxillary lateral incisor, and finally by the maxillary second bicuspid. Grahnen[6] feels, on the basis of family studies, that the so-called peg lateral is actually a modified manifestation of hypodontia.

Certain characteristic syndromes have long been observed to be associated with multiple missing teeth. In hereditary anhidrotic ectodermal dysplasia there is usually oligodontia or anodontia. This condition chiefly affects males. It has been classified as a sex-linked recessive trait. In Down's syndrome (mongolism), Brown and Cunningham[3] reported that as high as 43 per cent of affected children exhibited missing teeth, usually the maxillary lateral incisors.

The clinical management of cases involving missing teeth can be decided only on an individual basis. In some instances no treatment may be indicated, while in others orthodontic correction plus prostheses may be required.

I. ANOMALIES OF NUMBER

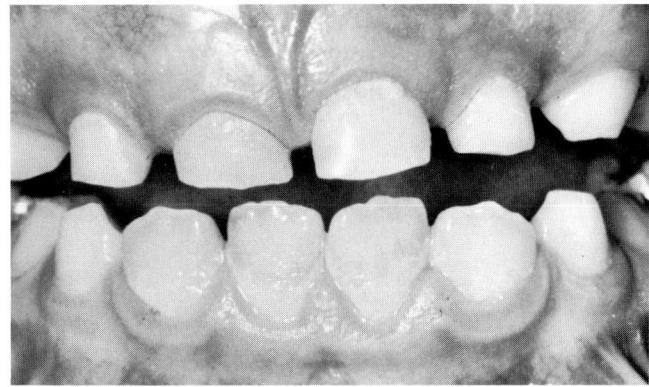

Figure 3-1 Intraoral view of a 7-year-old child with a supernumerary tooth in the area of the developing maxillary right permanent central incisor. At this age, the anomaly will be detected only by radiographic survey.

ANOMALIES OF THE DENTITION

I. ANOMALIES OF NUMBER *Continued*

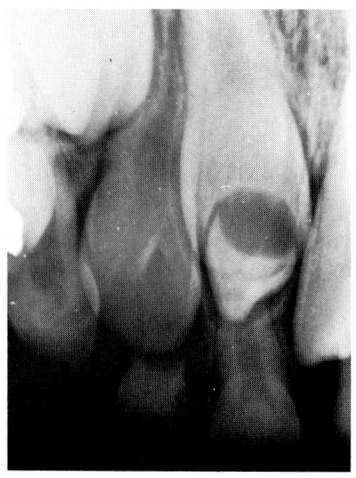

Figure 3-2 Radiograph of patient seen in Figure 3-1. Note supernumerary tooth in area of right permanent central incisor. If supernumerary teeth are not extracted they usually cause eruption to be delayed or cause deflection in the normal path of eruption of the neighboring developing permanent tooth or teeth.

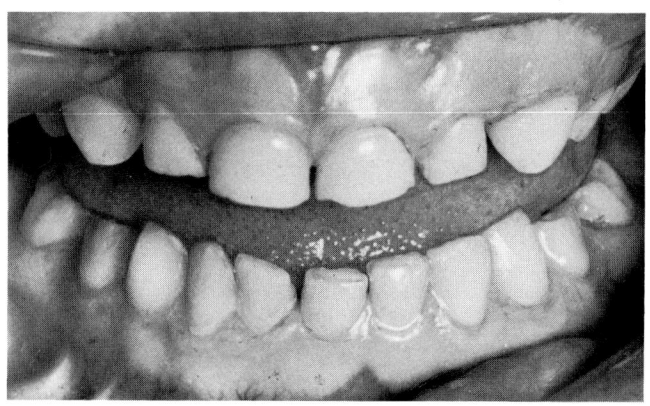

Figure 3-3 Supernumerary mandibular primary incisor.

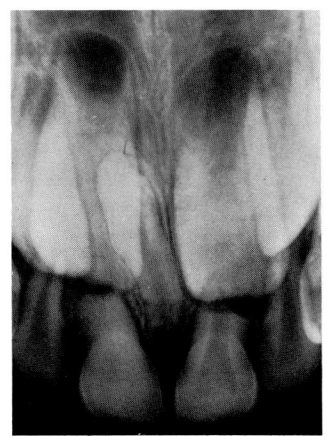

Figure 3-4 Midline supernumerary (mesiodens) in a 5-year-old child. Extraction of the mesiodens is the treatment of choice.

I. ANOMALIES OF NUMBER Continued

Figure 3-5 Two supernumerary teeth in area of maxillary permanent central incisor in an 8½-year-old child. Note how the supernumeraries caused delayed eruption of the permanent central incisors. Both maxillary permanent lateral incisors have erupted. Immediate extraction of the supernumeraries is indicated.

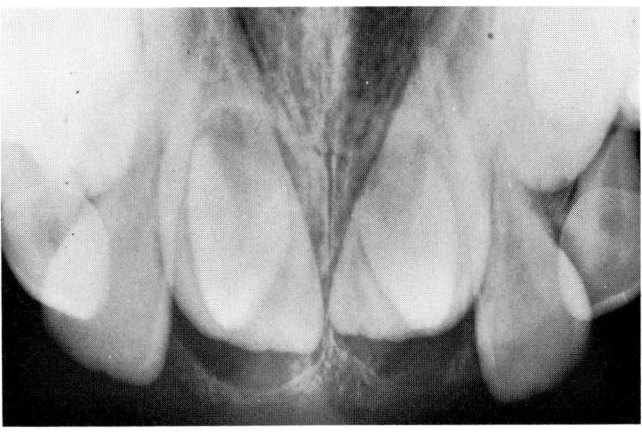

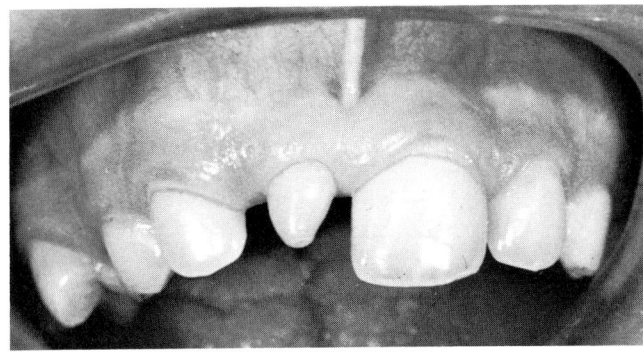

Figure 3-6 Erupted midline supernumerary (mesiodens).

Figure 3-7 Midline supernumerary (mesiodens). Radiograph of patient seen in Figure 3-6. Note that eruption of maxillary right permanent central incisor is retarded. Immediate extraction of the supernumerary is necessary for the incisor to erupt. Even then, it is likely that the incisor will erupt in a poor position. Minor orthodontic treatment is frequently necessary to align a permanent incisor whose eruption has been retarded because of a supernumerary tooth.

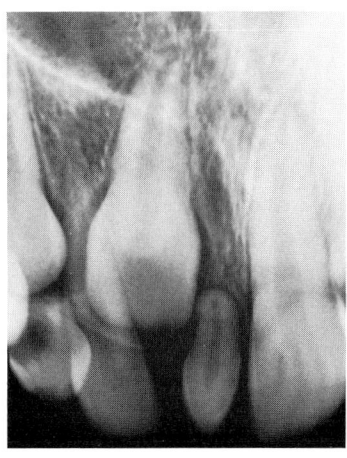

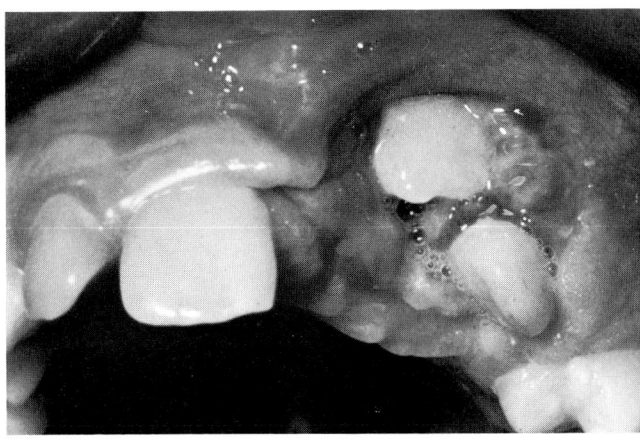

Figure 3-8 An erupting permanent maxillary left central incisor following removal of a supernumerary tooth in the area. Eruption is frequently slow in these cases.

I. ANOMALIES OF NUMBER Continued

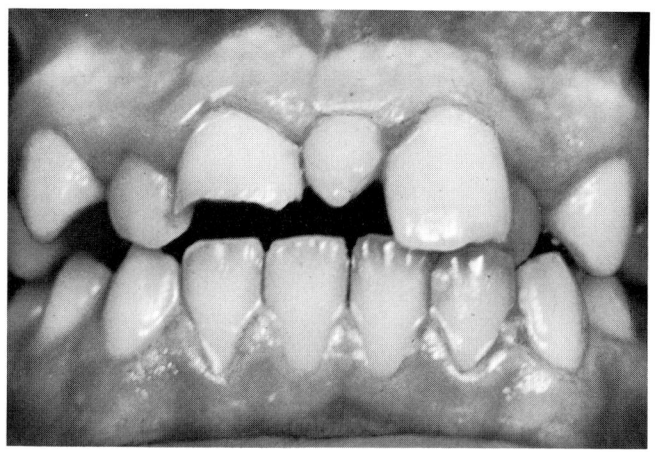

Figure 3-9 Midline supernumerary (mesiodens). Note crowding in area of maxillary permanent lateral incisors. The supernumerary must be extracted.

Figure 3-10 Midline supernumerary (mesiodens). Note that the maxillary right permanent central incisor has rotated. It was most likely deflected from its normal path of eruption by the mesiodens. The mesiodens should be extracted.

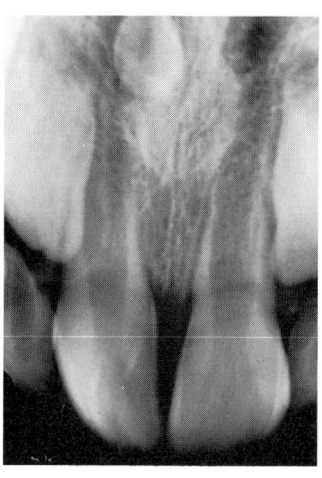

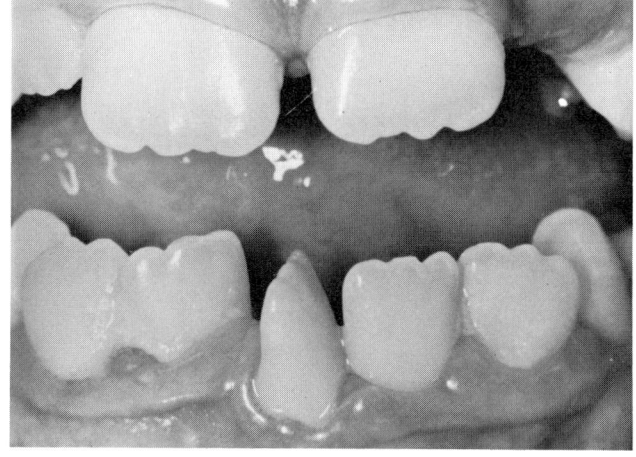

Figure 3-11 Midline supernumerary (mesiodens) of the mandibular arch. Mesiodens usually occur in the maxillary arch. Note crowding of the mandibular permanent incisors. Extraction of the mesiodens is treatment of choice.

Figure 3-12 Developing supernumerary teeth in area of mandibular cuspid and bicuspid. Extraction of supernumeraries is treatment of choice.

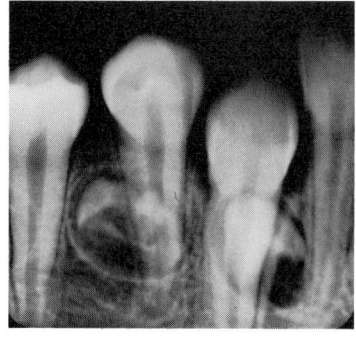

I. ANOMALIES OF NUMBER *Continued*

Figure 3-13 A 9-year-old girl with cleidocranial dysostosis. Note how patient can closely approximate the right and left shoulder (a diagnostic sign). These individuals usually have supernumerary teeth and eruption of their permanent dentition is retarded.

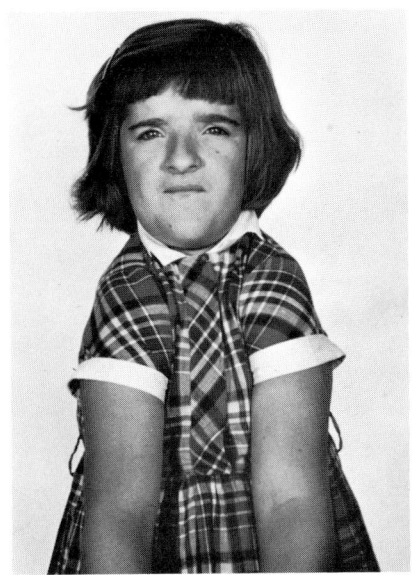

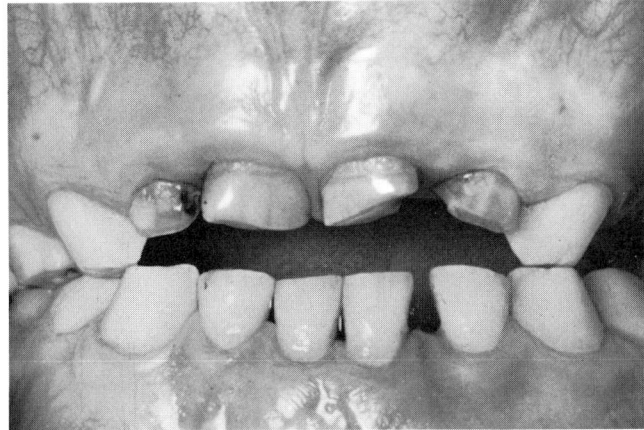

Figure 3-14 Intraoral view of the 9-year-old girl shown in Figure 3-13. Note that eruption of maxillary and mandibular incisors is retarded.

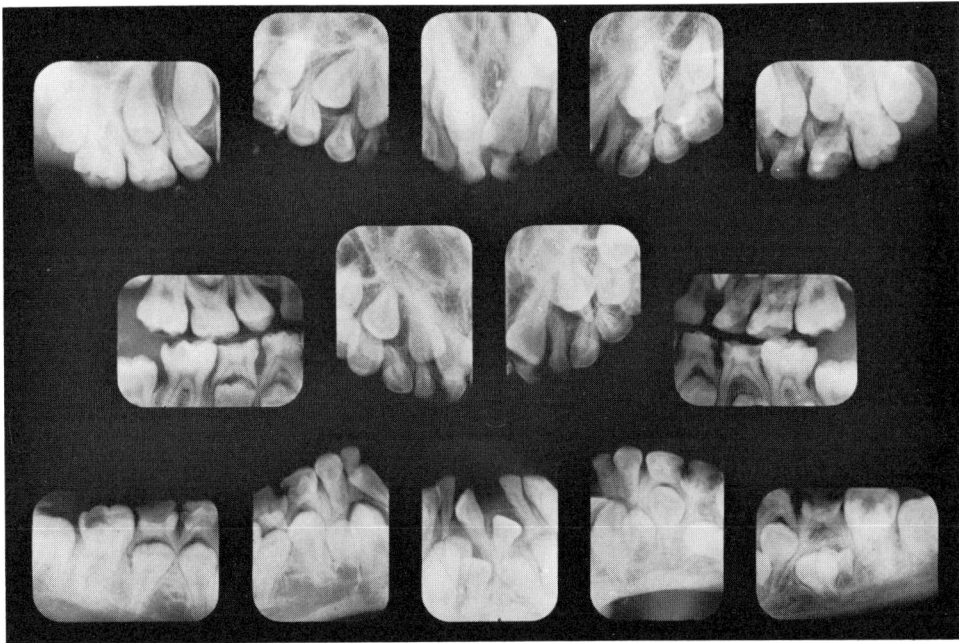

Figure 3-15 Full-mouth radiographs of a 9-year-old girl with cleidocranial dysostosis. Note that eruption of permanent teeth is retarded, and there are supernumeraries in the upper and lower left quadrants.

I. ANOMALIES OF NUMBER Continued

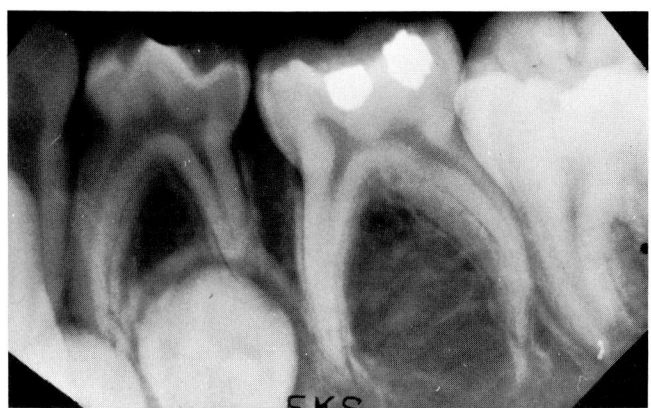

Figure 3-16 Mandibular second bicuspid is missing. Next to the third molar, this tooth is the one most frequently missing in the human dentition.

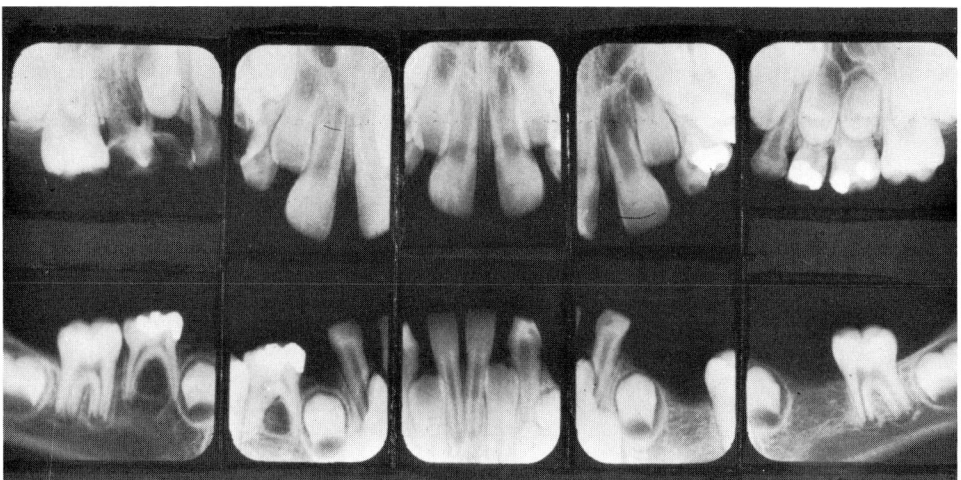

Figure 3-17 Full-mouth radiographs of a 7-year-old boy in whom the mandibular second bicuspids and the maxillary right second bicuspid are missing.

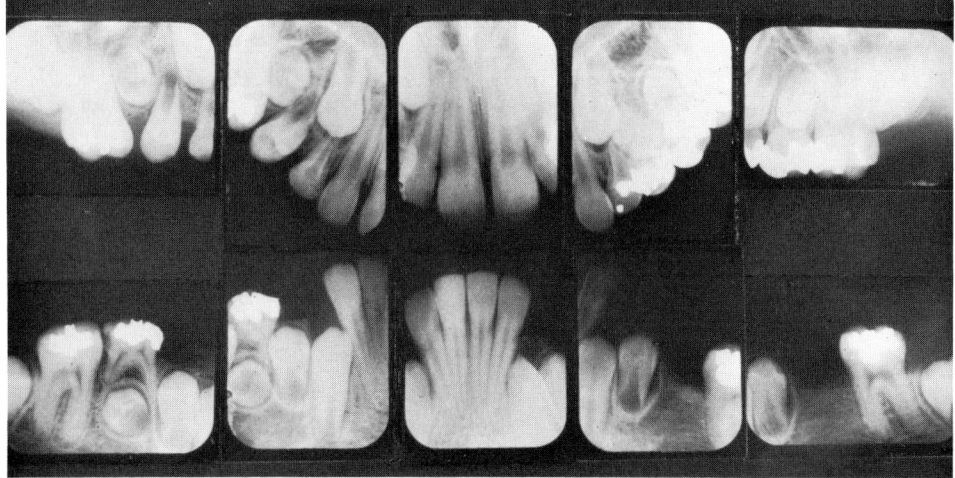

Figure 3-18 Same boy as seen in Figure 3-17, 2 years later. Note development of right maxillary and mandibular second bicuspids. During the preschool years it is unwise to prognosticate about failure of development of the bicuspids.

I. ANOMALIES OF NUMBER Continued

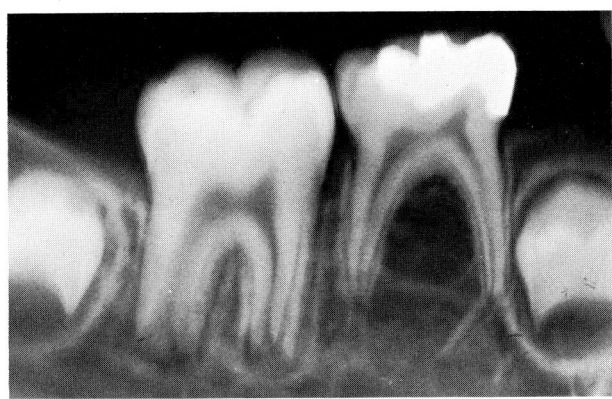

Figure 3-19 Periapical view of mandibular right bicuspid area in boy shown in Figure 3-17. It appears that second bicuspid is missing.

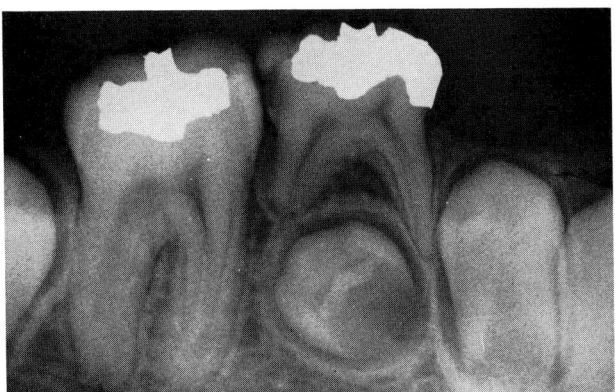

Figure 3-20 Same area as seen in Figure 13-19, 2 years later. Note development of second bicuspid crown.

Figure 3-21 Same patient. Periapical view of maxillary right bicuspid. Second bicuspid apparently is missing.

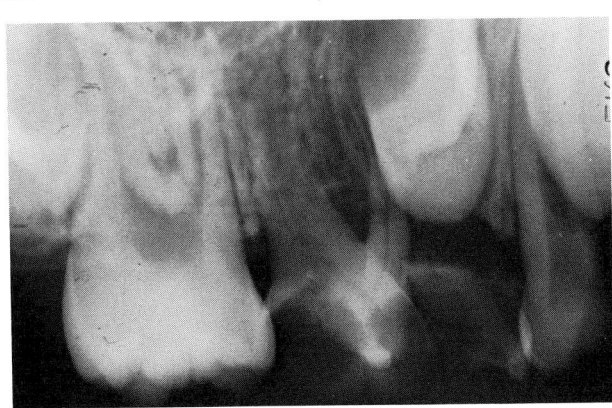

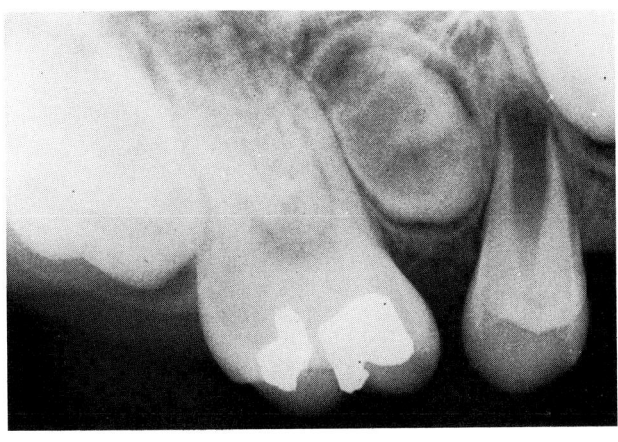

Figure 3-22 Same area seen in Figure 13-21, 2 years later. Note development of second bicuspid crown.

I. ANOMALIES OF NUMBER Continued

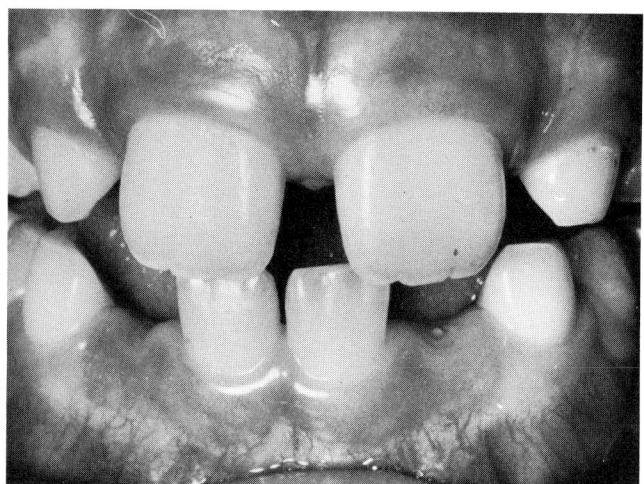

Figure 3-23 A 7½-year-old child in whom maxillary permanent lateral incisors were developmentally missing. Next to the third molars and mandibular second bicuspids, these permanent teeth are the ones most often developmentally missing.

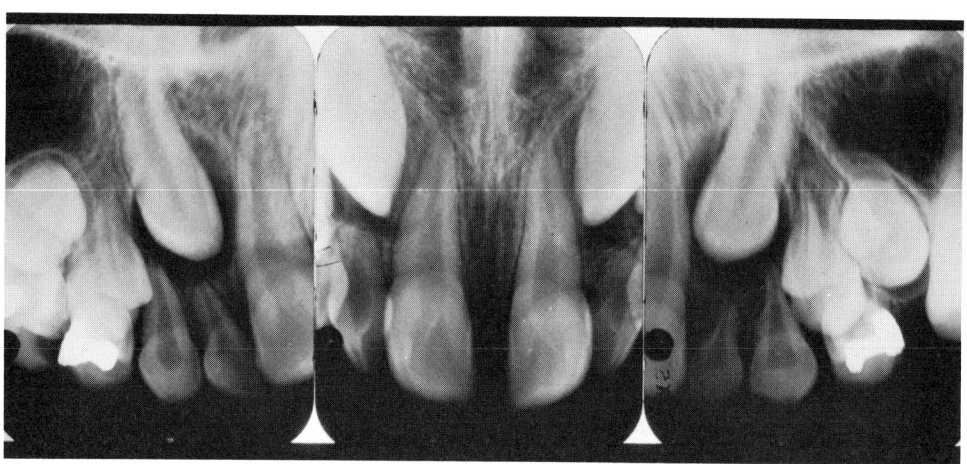

Figure 3-24 Radiograph of 9-year-old child showing developmentally missing maxillary permanent lateral incisors.

Figure 3-25 Extraoral view of a child in whom maxillary permanent lateral incisors are developmentally missing. The wide diastema is often an indication that lateral incisors are missing.

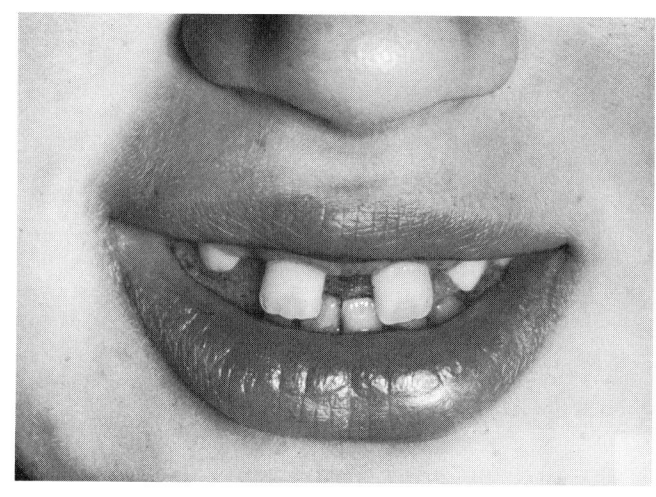

I. ANOMALIES OF NUMBER Continued

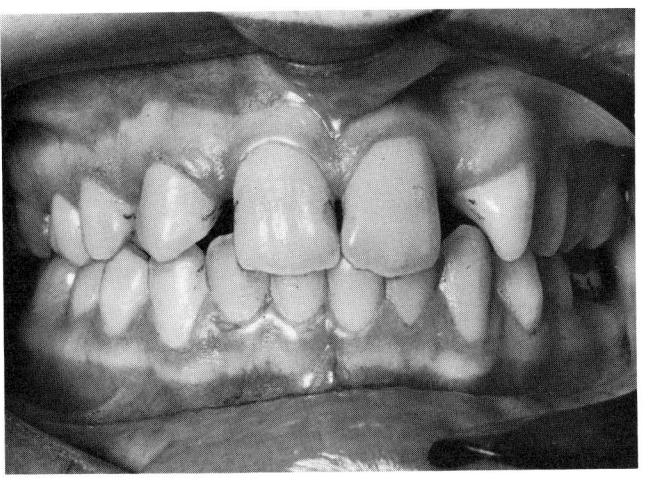

Figure 3-26 Adult with developmentally missing maxillary lateral incisors.

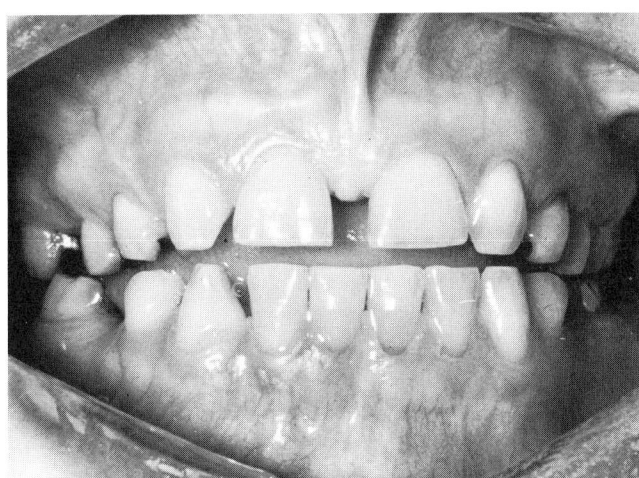

Figure 3-27 Adult with developmentally missing maxillary lateral incisors. Note how maxillary cuspids have been recontoured (incisal edges) to more closely resemble lateral incisors for esthetic improvement.

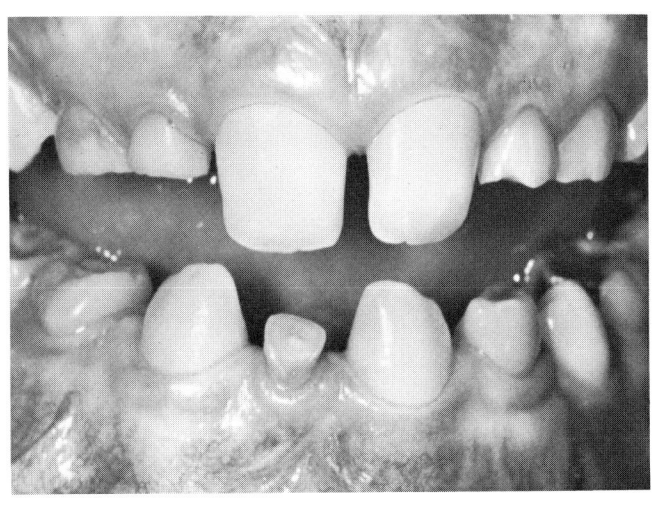

Figure 3-28 Child with some missing permanent incisors. There is no history of hereditary ectodermal dysplasia.

I. ANOMALIES OF NUMBER Continued

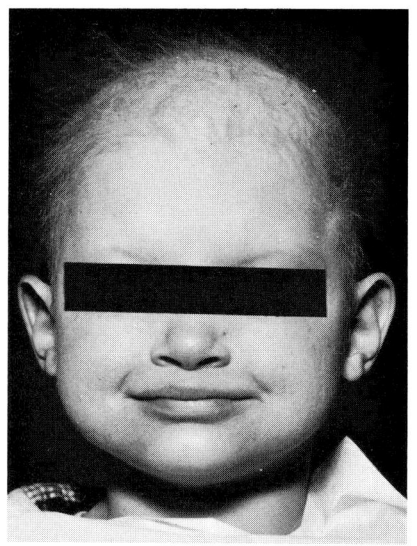

Figure 3-29 Facial view of boy with hereditary anhidrotic ectodermal dysplasia. This condition is a sex-linked recessive trait which affects mainly males. It is characterized by lack of sweat glands, sparse hair, dry skin, and absence of teeth.

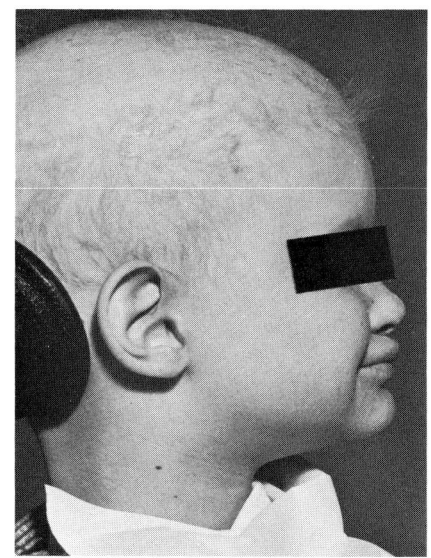

Figure 3-30 Same boy as shown in Figure 3-29. Note saddle nose, prominent lips, sparse hair, and lack of eyebrows, all typical of ectodermal dysplasia.

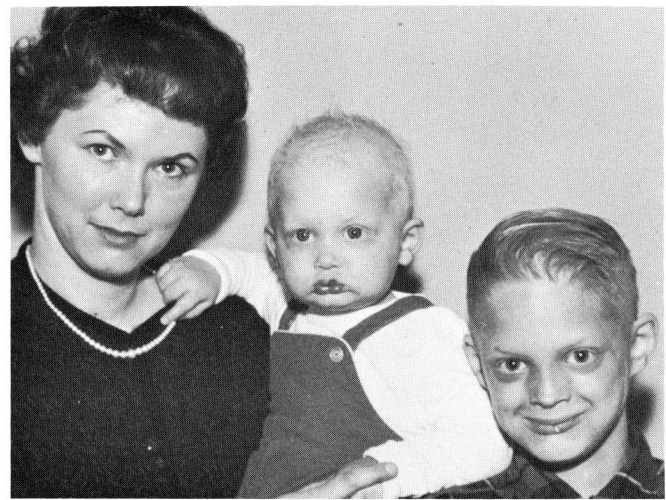

Figure 3-31 Two male children in family have ectodermal dysplasia. Mother shows no manifestations of this condition. Older boy has normal hair distribution.

I. ANOMALIES OF NUMBER Continued

Figure 3-32 Boy, age 3 years, with anhidrotic ectodermal dysplasia. Conical teeth are characteristic and usually require modification for reasons of appearance.

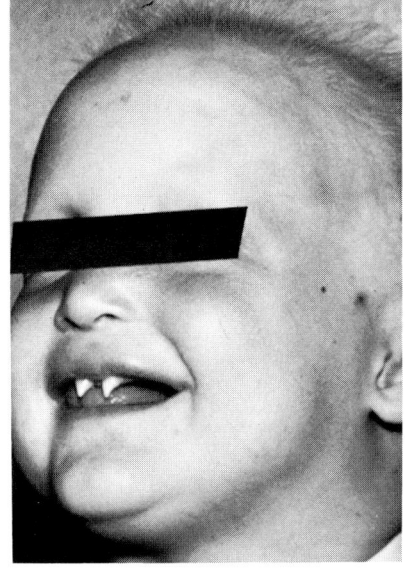

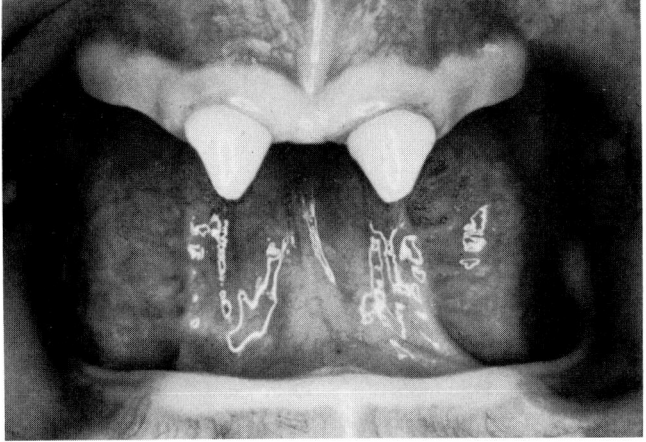

Figure 3-33 Same child as seen in Figure 3-32. Lack of alveolar bone development is due to absence of teeth.

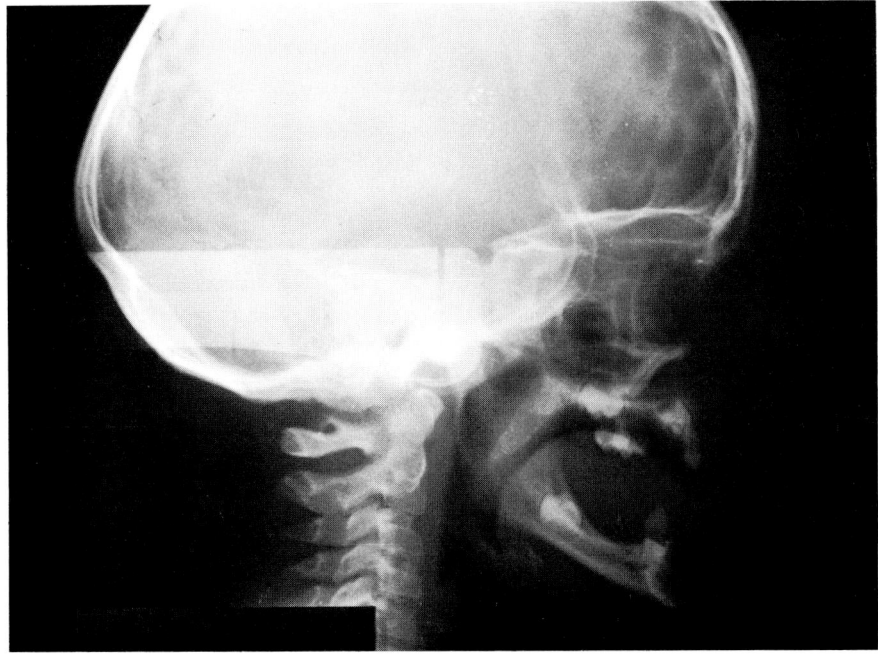

Figure 3-34 Cephalometric radiograph of a child with ectodermal dysplasia showing lack of tooth development. Although alveolar bone is deficient in these cases, basal bone or skeletal bone development proceeds normally.

I. ANOMALIES OF NUMBER Continued

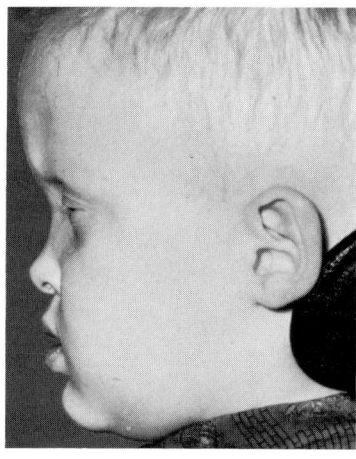

Figure 3-35 Four-year old boy with anhidrotic ectodermal dysplasia. Note characteristic facial appearance in profile.

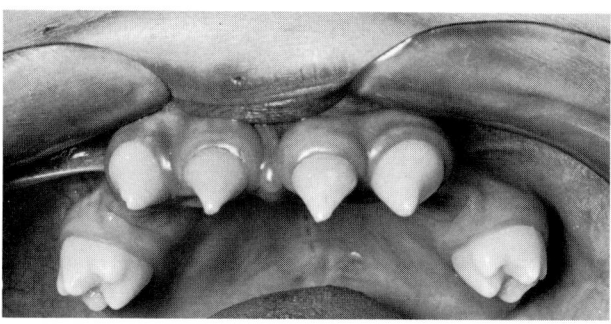

Figure 3-36 Maxillary arch of boy shown in Figure 3-35. Note conical shape of primary incisors, a typical finding. Alveolar bone development is lacking because of absence of permanent teeth.

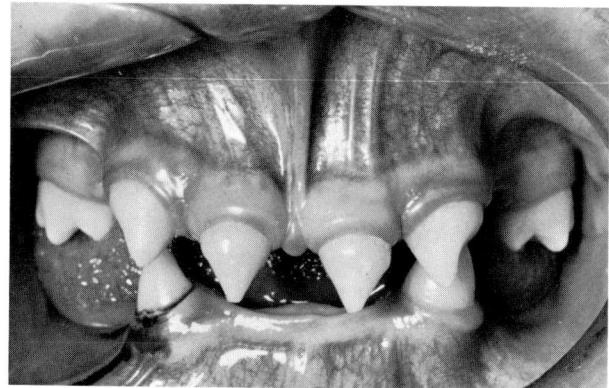

Figure 3-37 Anterior intraoral view of boy seen in Figure 3-35. Note lack of ridge in area posterior to lower canines. (See Chapter 12 for description of prosthetic treatment of this patient.)

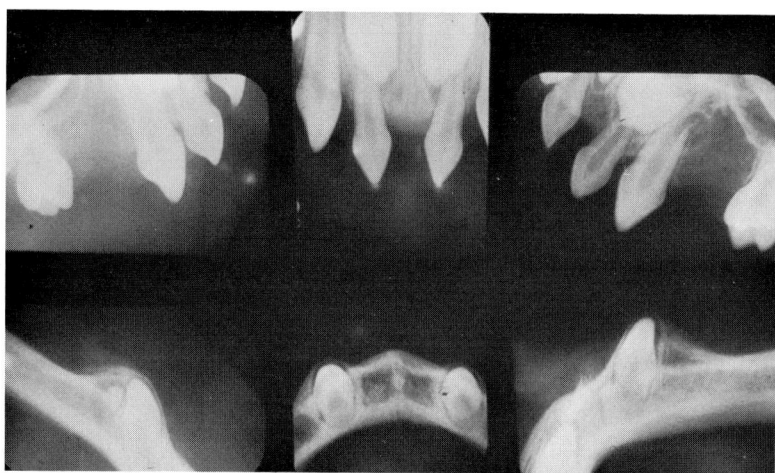

Figure 3-38 Radiographs of boy seen in Figure 3-35. Note lack of primary as well as permanent teeth. This patient was fitted with a lower denture and upper partial denture after the upper teeth were modified.

Anomalies of Shape of Teeth

Variations in crown and root configuration of teeth may be of a hereditary nature or may result from disease or trauma. Frequently these anomalies are limited to one or two teeth. In making a diagnosis the radiograph is a necessity, and in most cases the patient's history will also be of value. Few studies have been reported on the incidence of these conditions. Grahnen[7] in a survey of 1,006 children aged 11 to 14 years, found that 1.7 per cent exhibited peg lateral incisors in the upper arch. He found fused or geminated teeth in 0.5 per cent of a group of 3 to 5-year-old children. Clayton[5] reported that 0.47 per cent of a group of children aged 3 to 12 years had geminated or fused teeth, a figure that compares closely with Grahnen's. The occurrence of fused or geminated teeth in the permanent dentition is much less common than in the primary dentition. A classification of anomalies of shape of teeth is of value in reaching a diagnosis.

CLASSIFICATION

- A. Gemination
- B. Fusion
- C. Dilaceration
- D. Concrescence
- E. Hutchinson's incisor*
- F. Mulberry molar*
- G. Peg lateral
- H. Exaggerated cingulum
- I. Supernumerary cusps
- J. Claw-shaped incisors
- K. Taurodontism
- L. Dens-in-dente
- M. Macrodontia
- N. Microdontia†
- O. Hypoplastic defects and generalized malformations resulting from trauma, exanthematous disease, and genetic syndromes.‡

---

*Associated disease complex, congenital syphilis.
†Associated genetic syndrome, primordial dwarfism.
‡See Chapter 3, Anomalies of Structure and Texture, Chapter 13, Trauma to Primary Teeth, and Chapter 14, Trauma to Permanent Teeth.

II. ANOMALIES OF SHAPE

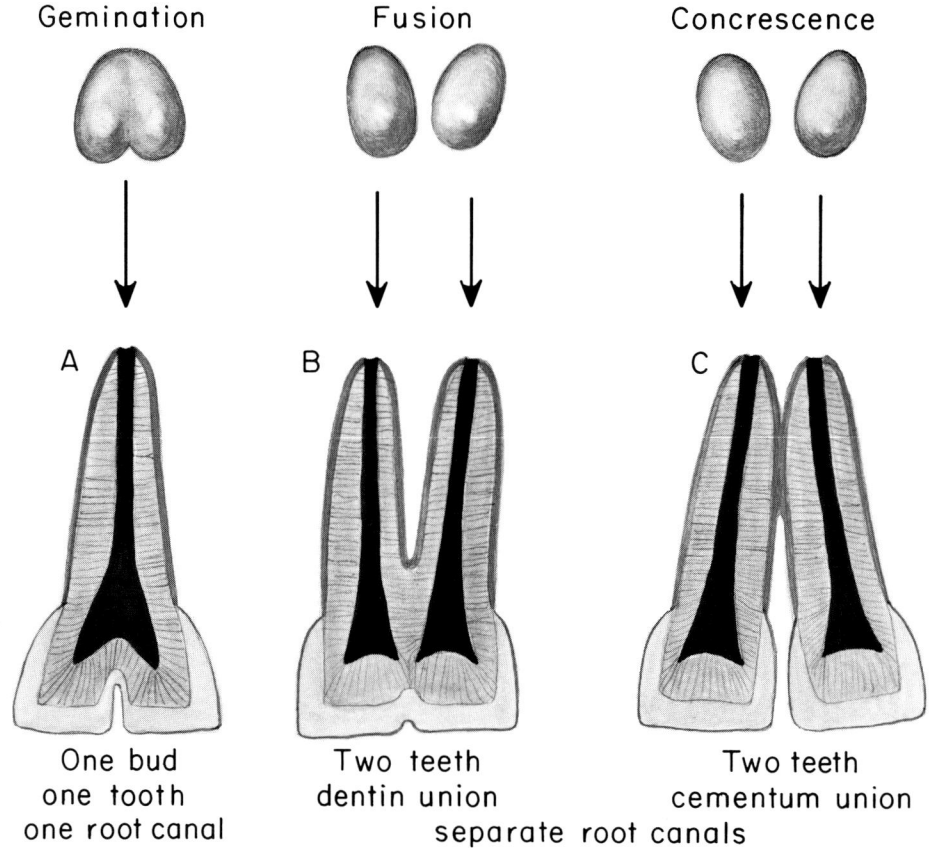

Figure 3-39 Diagrammatic illustration of gemination, fusion, and concrescence. (Modified from Tannenbaum, K. A., and Alling, E. E.: Anomalous tooth development: case report of gemination and twinning. Oral Surg. Oral Med. Oral Path. *16*:883-887, July, 1963.)

II. ANOMALIES OF SHAPE Continued

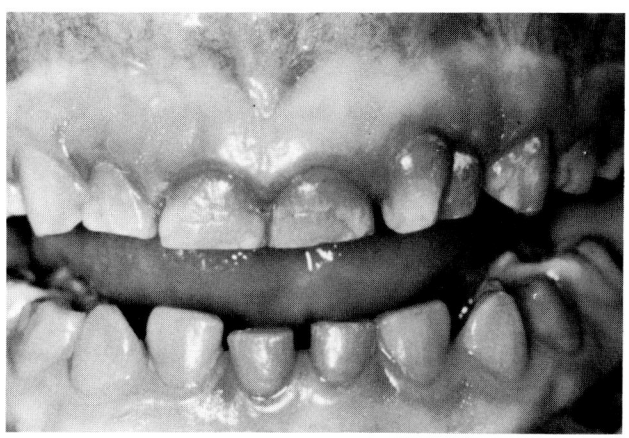

Figure 3-40 Gemination of a maxillary left primary lateral incisor.

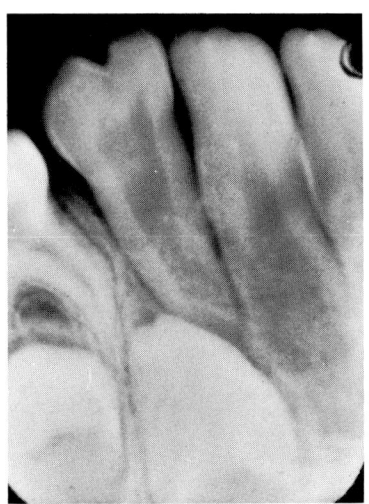

Figure 3-41 Radiograph of geminated mandibular primary cuspid.

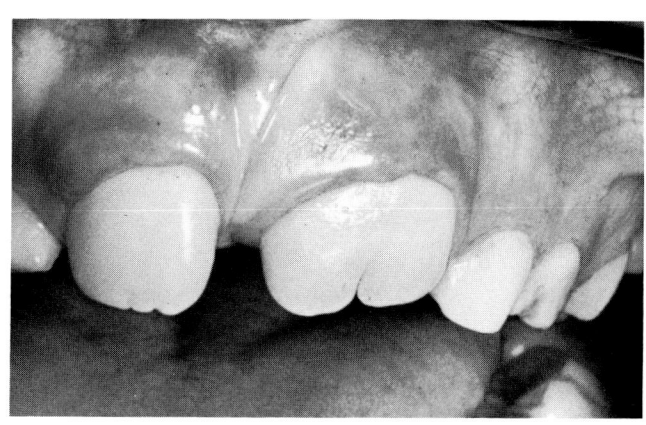

Figure 3-42 Gemination of the maxillary left permanent central incisor.

II. ANOMALIES OF SHAPE Continued

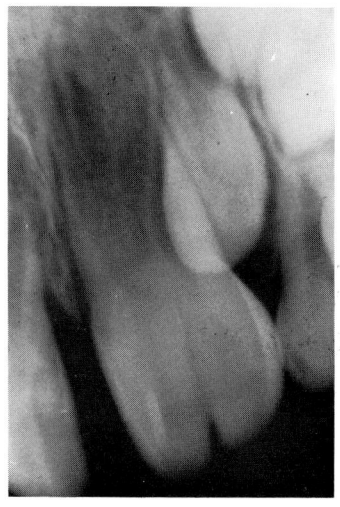

Figure 3-43 Radiograph of the geminated left permanent maxillary central incisor shown in Figure 3-42. Note presence of one pulp chamber and pulp canal.

Figure 3-44 Fusion of the mandibular primary right cuspid and lateral incisor.

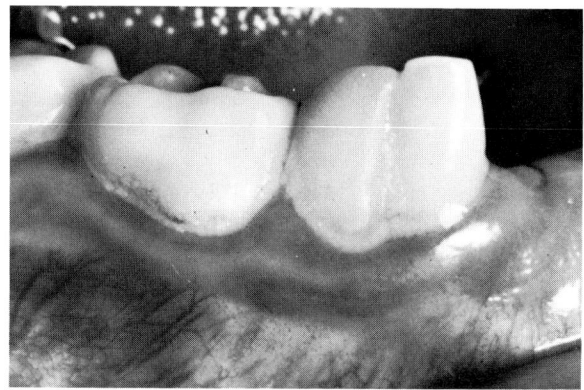

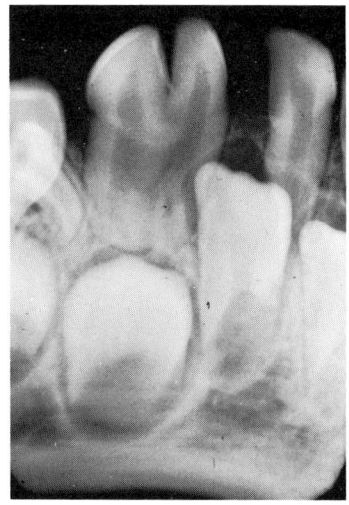

Figure 3-45 Radiograph of fused mandibular right cuspid and lateral incisor. Note presence of separate pulp chambers and pulp canals.

II. ANOMALIES OF SHAPE Continued

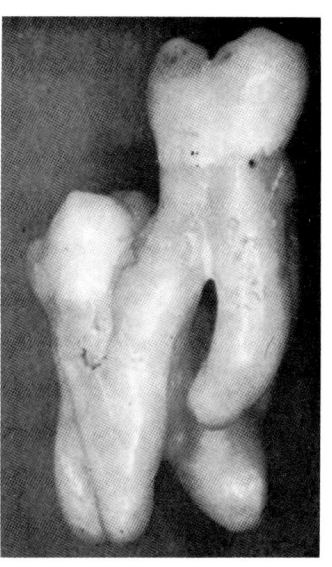

Figure 3-46   Concrescence. Fusion of molar roots by cementum. (From Kerr, D. A., and Ash, M. M., *Oral Pathology*, 2nd ed., Lea & Febiger, Philadelphia, 1965, p. 55).

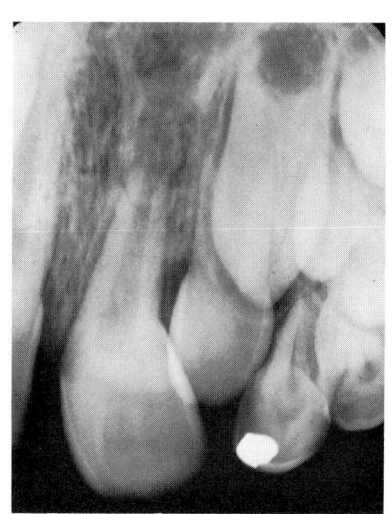

Figure 3-47   Dilaceration of the maxillary left permanent central incisor.

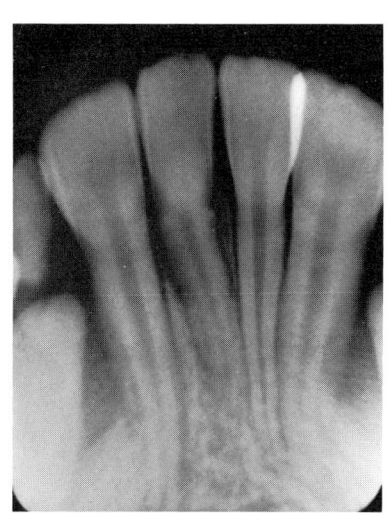

Figure 3-48   Dilaceration of the mandibular right permanent central incisor.

II. ANOMALIES OF SHAPE Continued

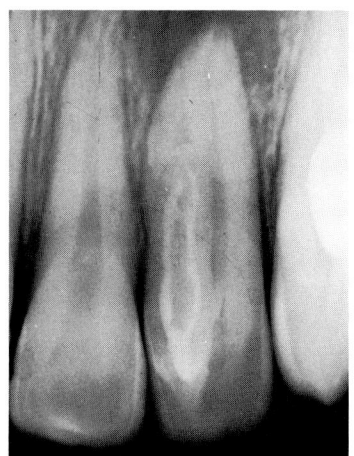

Figure 3-49 Dens-in-dente of the maxillary left permanent central incisor.

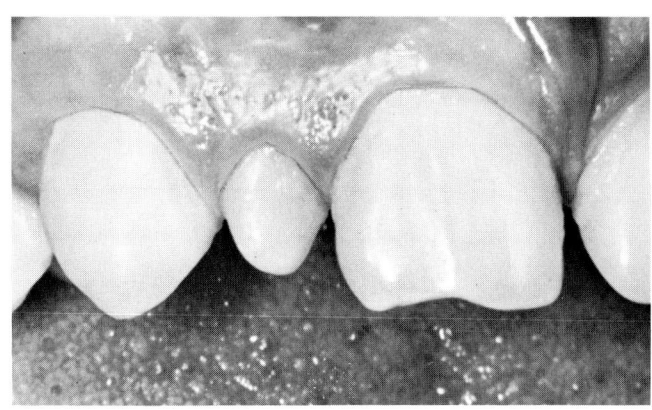

Figure 3-50 Peg-shaped maxillary right permanent lateral incisor.

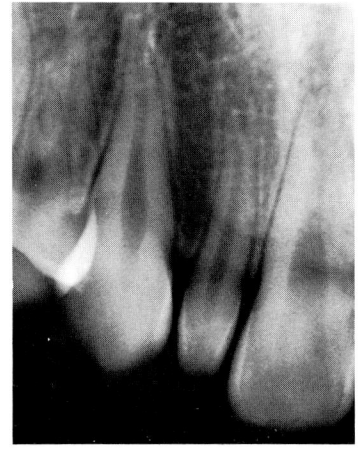

Figure 3-51 Radiograph of peg-shaped lateral incisor illustrated in Figure 3-50.

Figure 3-52 Maxillary central incisors with exaggerated cingula.

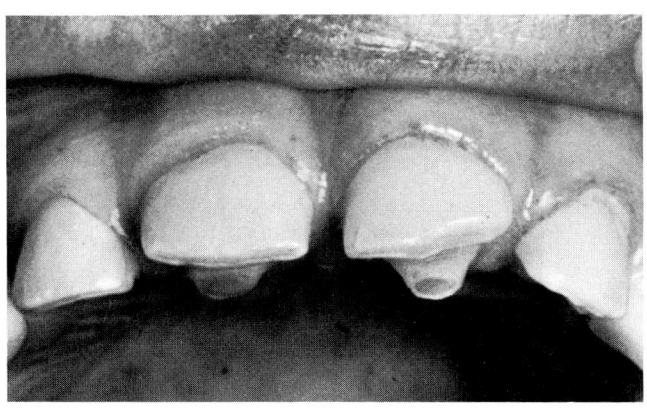

ANOMALIES OF THE DENTITION

II. ANOMALIES OF SHAPE Continued

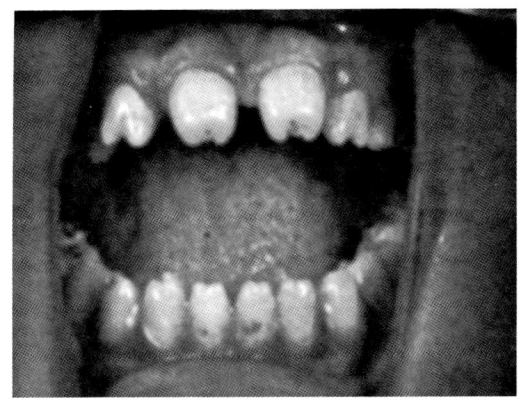

Figure 3-53 Hutchinson's incisors. These may be the end-result of congenital syphilis. (From Kerr, D. A. and Ash, M. M.: *Oral Pathology*, 2nd ed., Lea & Febiger, Philadelphia, 1965 p. 52.)

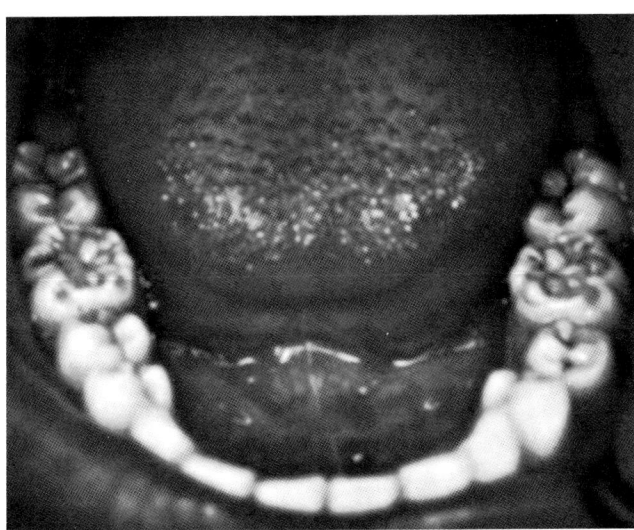

Figure 3-54 Mulberry molars. Typical shape associated with congenital syphilis. (From Colby, R. A., Kerr, D. A., and Robinson, H. B. G.: *Color Atlas of Oral Pathology*, 2nd ed., J. B. Lippincott Co., Philadelphia, 1961, p. 48.)

Figure 3-55 Taurodontism of a mandibular left first primary molar. Note the unusual root configuration, in which there is an increased height of the pulp chamber and less constriction at the cementoenamel junction. Taurodontism may be associated with Klinefelter's syndrome. (Courtesy Dr. Lloyd B. Austin.)

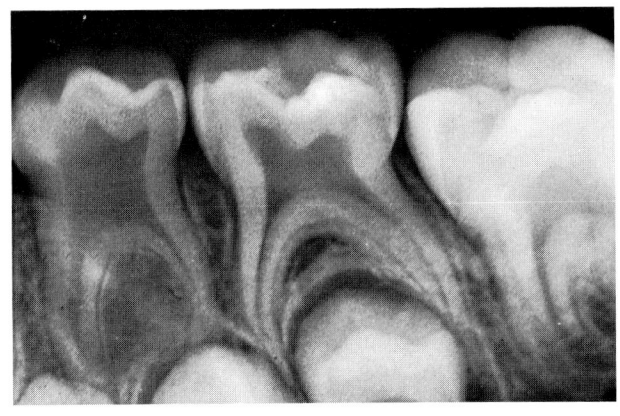

Anomalies of Color of Teeth

Often the first evidence of variation from normal in the human dentition is an observable difference in the color of the teeth. Some of these variations are apparent only to the trained eye, others are so obvious that they are a cause of great concern to parent and child alike. In recent years the widespread use of tetracyclines has added a new category of intrinsic discoloration of teeth, emphasizing again the role of the dentition as a permanent record of the life cycle of the individual.

While a series of color photographs of dental anomalies would be instructive, it should be pointed out that color is never a reliable diagnostic criterion in itself. Clinical examination, patient history, and radiographs are always essential in making a final diagnosis. The first consideration is whether the color or stain in a particular case is intrinsic or extrinsic. Prophylaxis utilizing pumice should be done to remove green stains or yellow pigmentation caused by vitamin syrups or tobacco. If the color is intrinsic it will be necessary to consider its distribution, and the patient's history, place of residence, early illnesses, and family background.

Classification

1. Yellow teeth: tetracycline staining, pigmentation due to premature birth, amelogenesis imperfecta.
2. Brown teeth: tetracycline staining, amelogenesis imperfecta, dentinogenesis imperfecta, pigmentation due to premature birth, cystic fibrosis, porphyria.
3. Blue to blue-green teeth: erythroblastosis fetalis.
4. White or cream-colored opaque teeth; amelogenesis imperfecta.
5. Teeth with specific white areas: fluorosis, snow-capped teeth, idiopathic opacities.
6. Reddish-brown teeth: porphyria.
7. Gray-brown teeth: dentinogenesis imperfecta.
8. Miscellaneous discolorations due to extrinsic staining from foods, drugs, tobacco, or other agents.

Note: Examples of amelogenesis imperfecta and dentinogenesis imperfecta will be found in the next section under Anomalies of Structure and Texture of Teeth.

ANOMALIES OF THE DENTITION

III. ANOMALIES OF COLOR

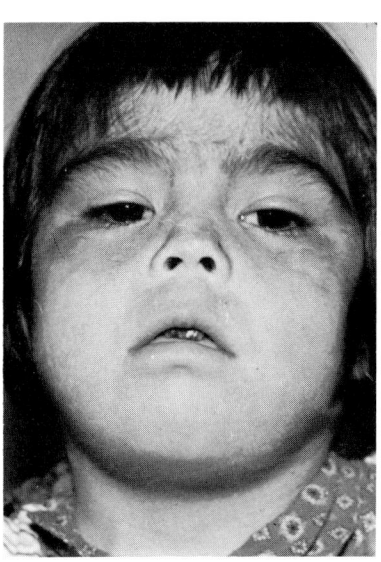

Figure 3-56 Full-face view of 6-year-old girl with hereditary porphyria, a rare metabolic error resulting in failure of conversion of porphyrins. Urine is a burgundy red color and there is discoloration of teeth and bones. (Figures 3-57 to 3-62 are illustrations of same patient.)

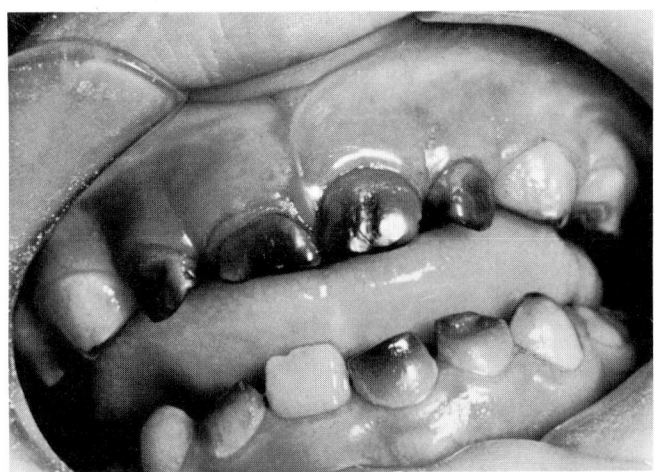

Figure 3-57 Intraoral view. Note discolored primary incisors, which are reddish-brown and fluoresce under ultraviolet light: these features are characteristic of tissues containing porphyrins.

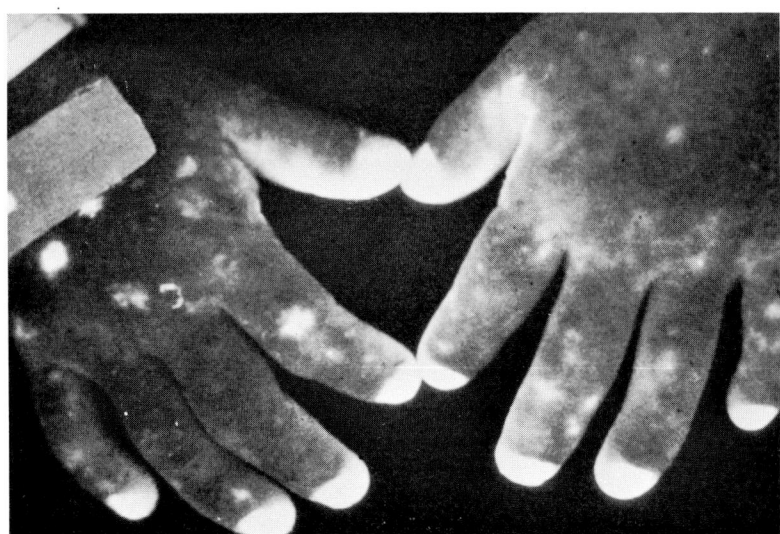

Figure 3-58 Note fluorescence of fingernails under ultraviolet light.

74 ANOMALIES OF THE DENTITION

III. ANOMALIES OF COLOR *Continued*

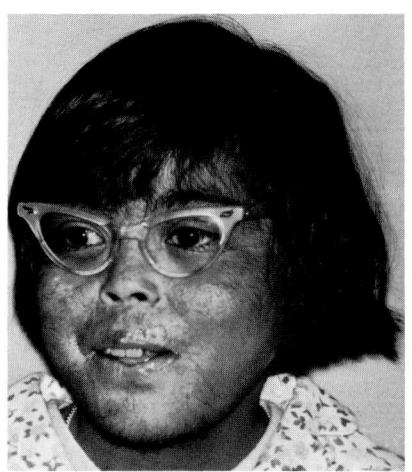

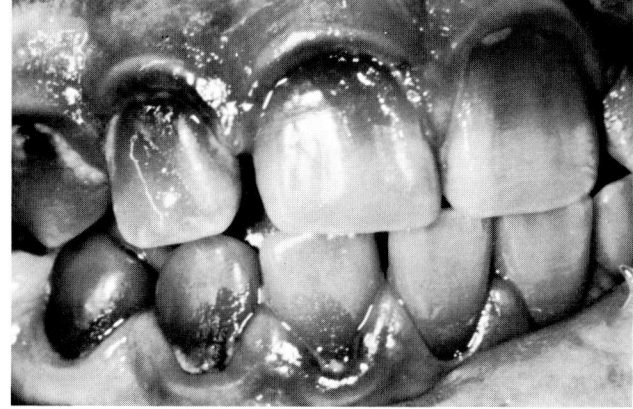

Figure 3-59 Patient at 14 years of age. Note abundant facial hair, a characteristic of this condition.

Figure 3-60 Patient at 14 years of age. Intraoral view. Note dark brown pigmentation.

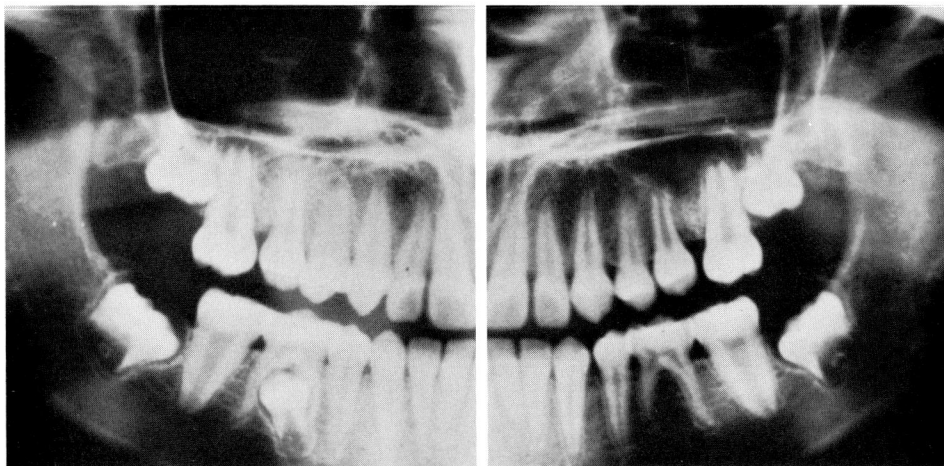

Figure 3-61 Panoramic radiograph. Teeth appear normal. Note that bicuspid is missing in lower left quadrant.

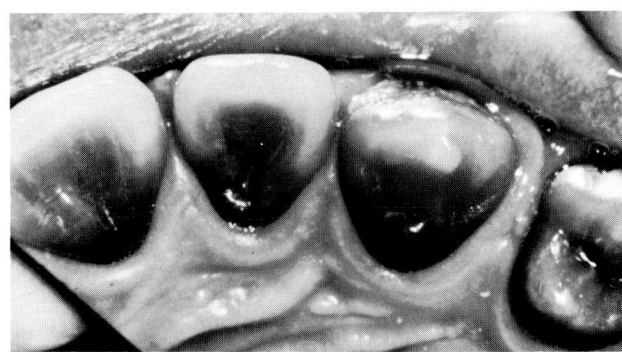

Figure 3-62 Lingual view of maxillary permanent teeth. Note dark brown color.

III. ANOMALIES OF COLOR Continued

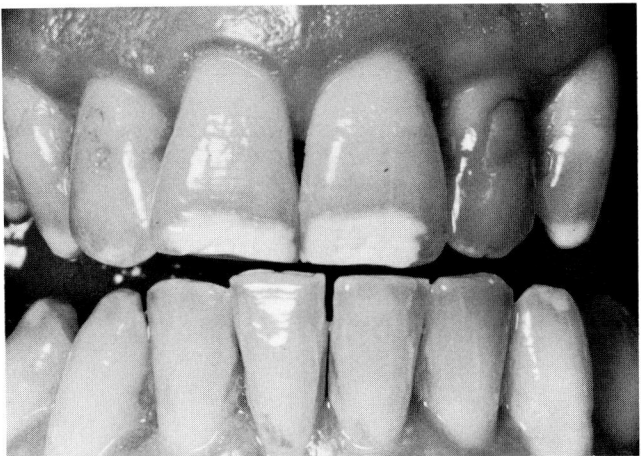

Figure 3-63 Hereditary snow-capped teeth. In this patient, white areas appear on maxillary anteriors only.

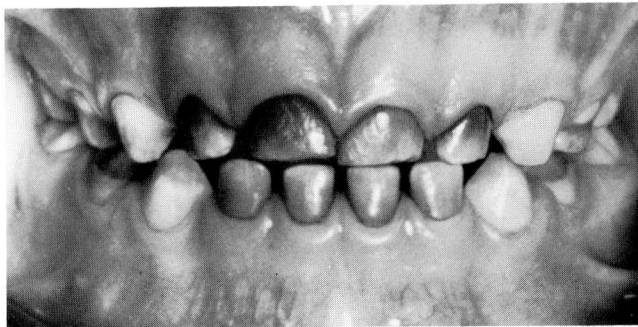

Figure 3-64 Erythroblastosis fetalis (hemolytic disease of the newborn). Primary teeth undergoing calcification up to time of baby's birth exhibit characteristic blue-green color because of absorption of bile pigments by dentin.

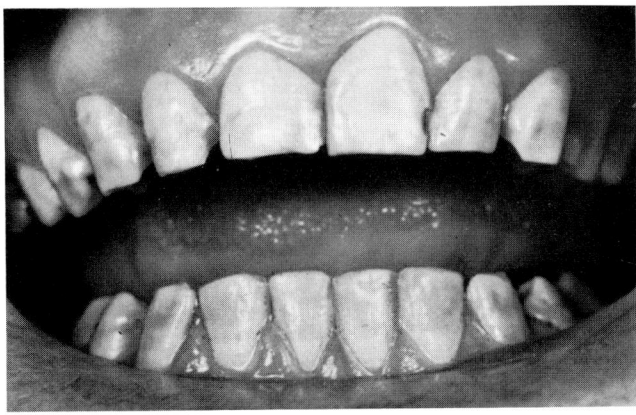

Figure 3-65 Fluorosis. A mottled appearance, with brownish areas, is characteristic of moderate fluorosis.

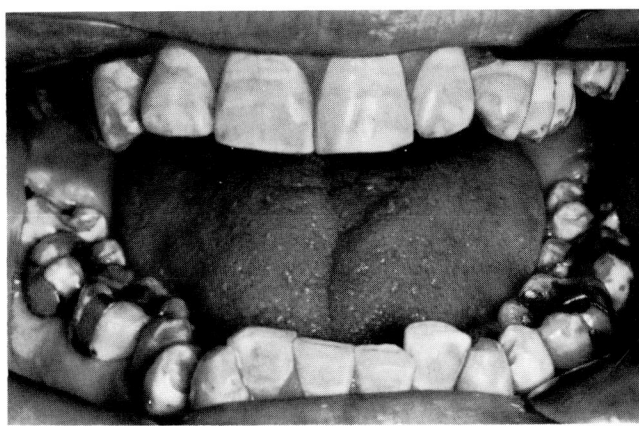

Figure 3-66 Fluorosis. There are brownish areas on these teeth, but a very mild fluorosis would be characterized by frosty white tips on cusps and incisal edges.

III. ANOMALIES OF COLOR *Continued*

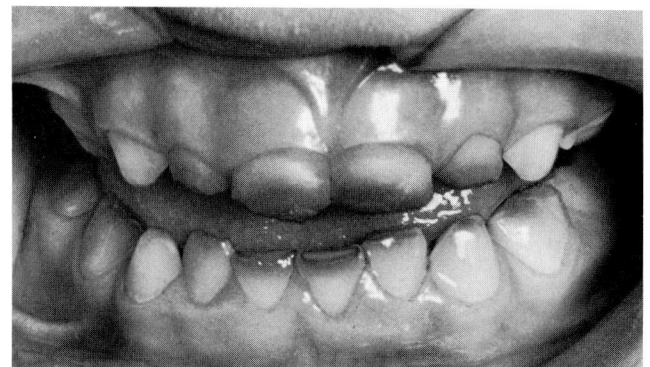

Figure 3-67 A five-year-old child with yellow staining and hypoplasia in the primary teeth as a result of jaundice associated with premature birth.

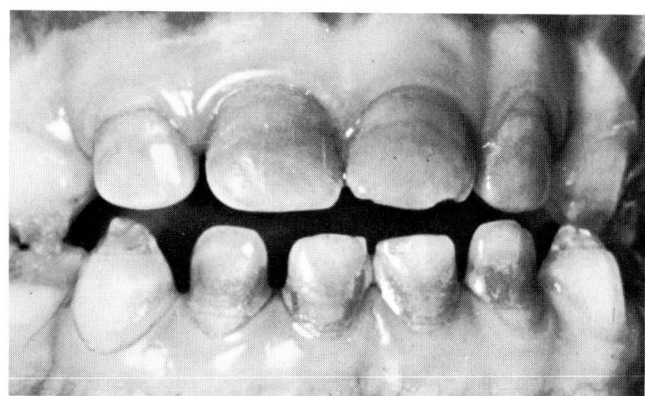

Figure 3-68 Tetracycline staining. Instead of the typical white color of primary teeth, a yellow pigmentation was seen in this case.

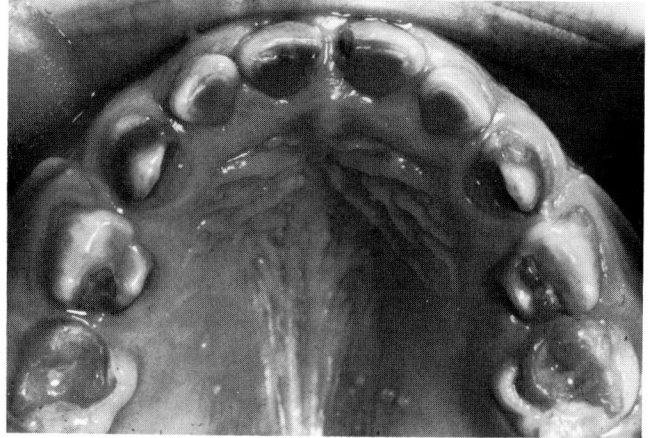

Figure 3-69 Tetracycline staining. This degree of pigmentation is due to continued medication with tetracyclines.

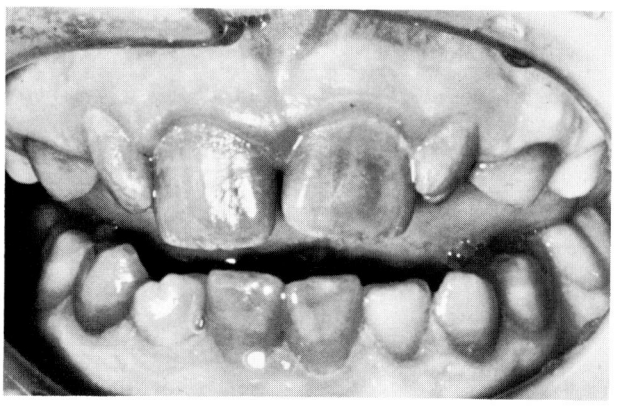

Figure 3-70 Cystic fibrosis. Brown-gray discoloration of teeth may be due to continuous antibiotic therapy or to the disease process itself, or both.

Anomalies of Structure and Texture of Teeth

In this category are included the hereditary syndromes, such as amelogenesis imperfecta and dentinogenesis imperfecta, as well as the miscellaneous factors that may affect enamel or dentin formation. It should be pointed out that there are conflicting reports in the literature concerning the genetic analysis of these syndromes; consequently, in order to make a diagnosis all aspects of the anomaly should be considered.

CLASSIFICATION

I. Hereditary Syndromes
    A. Enamel—amelogenesis imperfecta
        1. Hereditary enamel hypocalcification (three subdivisions)
        2. Hereditary enamel hypoplasia (four subdivisions)
    B. Dentin
        1. Dentinogenesis imperfecta
        2. Dentin dysplasia
        3. Shell teeth
II. Other Manifestations of Anomalous Structure and Texture
    A. Fluorosis
    B. Porphyria
    C. Hypophosphatasia
    D. Hypoplasia due to febrile disease
    E. Hypoplasia due to trauma
    F. Hypoplasia due to radiation
    G. Hypoplasia due to vitamin deficiency
    H. Hypoplasia due to hypothyroidism
    I. Hypoplasia due to pseudohypoparathyroidism
    J. Hypoplasia due to vitamin D-resistant rickets
    K. Hypoplasia due to premature birth and neonatal factors

TABLE 3-1. AMELOGENESIS IMPERFECTA*

	HEREDITARY ENAMEL HYPOPLASIA (FAULT OF APPOSITION-MATRIX FORMATION)				HEREDITARY ENAMEL HYPOCALCIFICATION (FAULT OF CALCIFICATION-MATURATION)		
	Type 1	Type 2	Type 3	Type 4	Type 1	Type 2	Type 3
	Enamel thin but hard; smooth and glossy	Enamel hard but pitted on external surface	Enamel hard but vertically grooved and wrinkled on external surface (Witkop)	Local areas of hypoplasia, lines, or pits, not related to febrile cause	Enamel soft and cheesy; can be easily removed by an instrument	Enamel dull, easily chipped; cuts readily with rotating instrument	Local areas of hypocalcification usually limited to incisal and occlusal "snow-capped" teeth
Color	Glossy yellow to orange-brown	Normal	Normal	Brown in hypoplastic areas only	Yellow to gray-brown	Dull paper white to creamy white	White tips on incisors, cuspids, and bicuspids
Radiographic appearance	Enamel of normal density but reduced in thickness (one-quarter to one-half normal thickness)	Mottled	Mottled	Radiolucency in areas of defects; no other variation	Enamel of same density as dentin but of normal thickness; crowns and roots otherwise normal	Enamel of normal thickness but of same density as dentin; may be a thin layer of normal enamel along dento-enamel junction	Not distinguishable
Genetic characteristics	Autosomal dominant	Unknown	Sex-linked dominant	Autosomal dominant	Autosomal dominant; occurs 1:1 in siblings	Autosomal dominant	Unreported but definitely familial; should be differentiated from mild fluorosis
Histological characteristics	Above normal organic substances in demineralized sections; stage of life cycle-apposition (matrix formation)	Not reported	Not reported	Not reported	Lack of calcification of matrix in ground sections; stage of life cycle calcification	Areas of deficient mineralization may be seen	Unreported

*Overall incidence reported by Witkop, 1:14,000-16,000[10]

TABLE 3-2. HEREDITARY ANOMALIES OF DENTIN

	INCIDENCE	STAGE AFFECTED IN LIFE CYCLE OF TOOTH	COLOR	RADIOGRAPHIC CHARACTERISTICS	HISTOLOGICAL CHARACTERISTICS	GENETIC CHARACTERISTICS	MISCELLANEOUS
Dentinogenesis imperfecta (hereditary opalescent dentin)	1 in 8,000	Histodifferentiation	Blue-gray to brown	Pulp chambers and root canals obliterated in mature teeth; crowns appear more bulbous; enamel (where not abraded) appears of normal thickness and density; roots often appear foreshortened	Dentoenamel junction smooth and unscalloped; reduced number of odontoblasts; dentinal tubules disorganized and may contain pulpal inclusions; interglobular dentin may be abundant; chemical analysis of dentin shows it to be high in water and organic content compared to normal dentin	Simple, dominant nonsex-linked	Teeth abrade rapidly; caries infrequent; may be associated with blue sclera; may be associated with osteogenesis imperfecta
Dentin dysplasia (rootless teeth)	Very rare; 1 in 96,000	Probably histodifferentiation	Normal	Obliteration of pulp chambers and root canals; lack of root formation; large radiolucent areas around roots	No reduction in number of odontoblasts; presence of large collagenous masses interspersed among tubules is characteristic	Autosomal dominant	No tendency to attrition
Shell teeth	Extremely rare	Probably histodifferentiation	Normal	Normal enamel layer with thin layer of dentin and enormous pulp chamber	No odontoblasts; thin layer of irregular dentin; coarse collagen bundles	Unreported	May be a variant of dentinogenesis imperfecta; only case reported by Rushton[9]

IV. ANOMALIES OF STRUCTURE AND TEXTURE

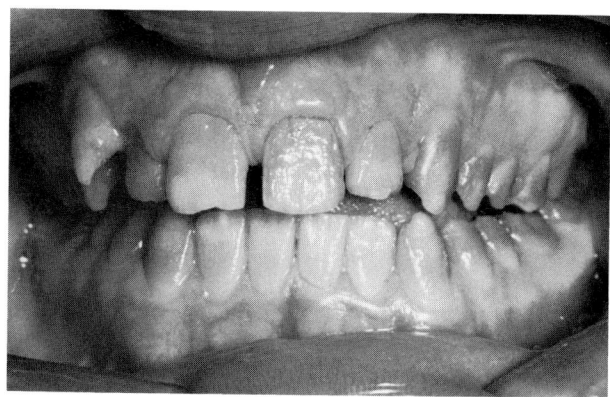

Figure 3-71 Hereditary enamel hypoplasia, smooth hard type, in a 14-year-old boy. The enamel is about one-fourth the usual thickness and has a glossy orange-brown color.

Figure 3-72 Same boy as seen in Figure 3-71, at an earlier age. Radiograph of molar region. Note the thin enamel covering of the crowns and lack of bell shape. Pulp chamber and dentin are normal.

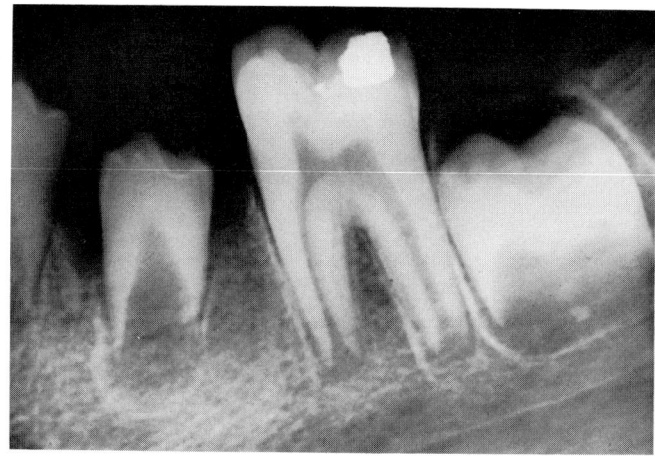

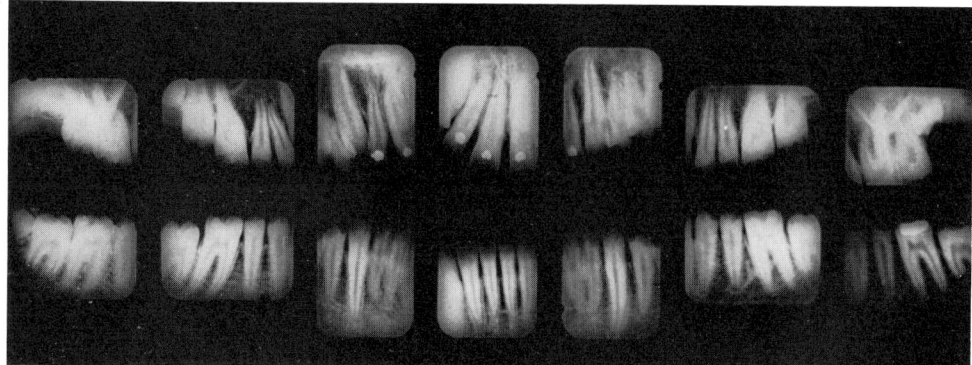

Figure 3-73 Full-mouth radiograph, same patient as illustrated in Figure 3-71. Teeth appear elongated and lacking in contour because of lack of enamel. Treatment consists of providing adequate coverage as teeth abrade.

IV. ANOMALIES OF STRUCTURE AND TEXTURE *Continued*

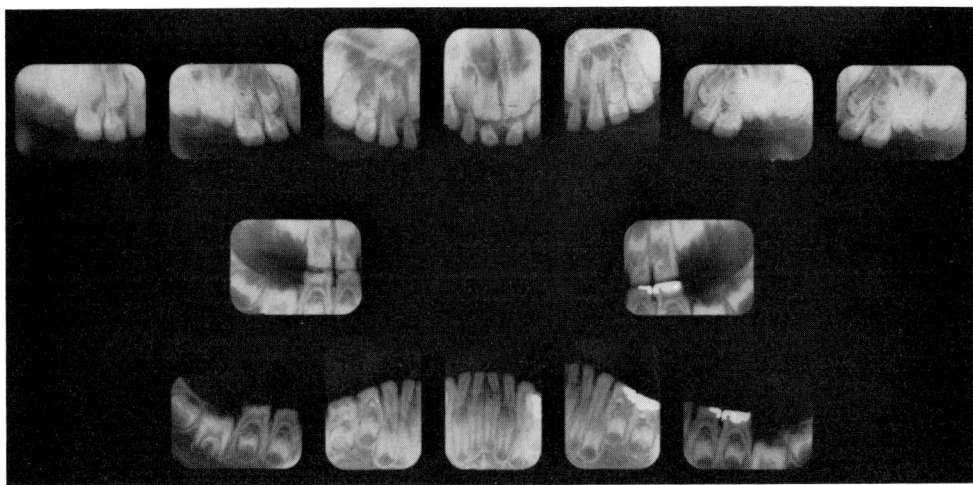

Figure 3-74 Figures 3-74 to 3-76 are full-mouth radiographs which illustrate delay in eruption of permanent teeth in a case of hereditary enamel hypoplasia. Note that the primary dentition exhibits the characteristic thin layer of enamel.

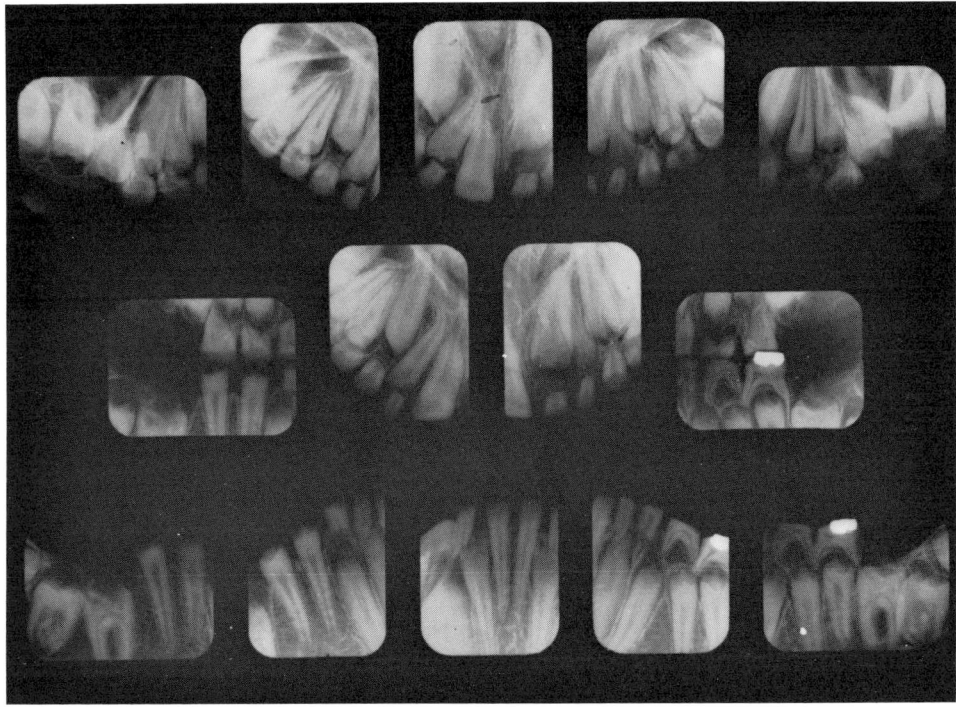

Figure 3-75 Age 12 years. Note lack of eruption of first permanent molars as well as upper incisors.

82 ANOMALIES OF THE DENTITION

IV. ANOMALIES OF STRUCTURE AND TEXTURE Continued

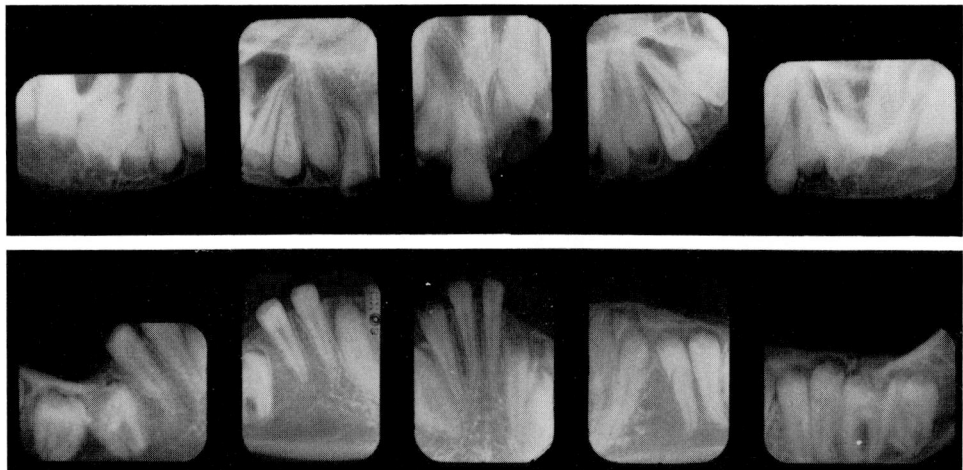

Figure 3-76 Age 14 years, hereditary enamel hypoplasia. Primary teeth were extracted to aid eruption of permanent teeth, but no response is evident at this time. (See Figures 3-74 and 3-75.)

IV. ANOMALIES OF STRUCTURE AND TEXTURE Continued

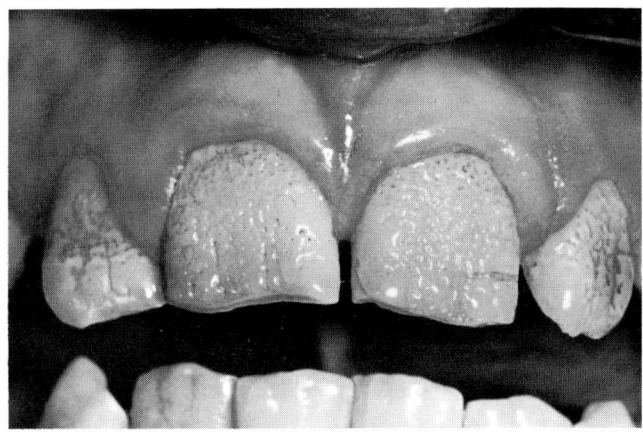

Figure 3-77 Hereditary enamel hypoplasia, hard, pitted type. The enamel is lacking in thickness and is pitted and corrugated.

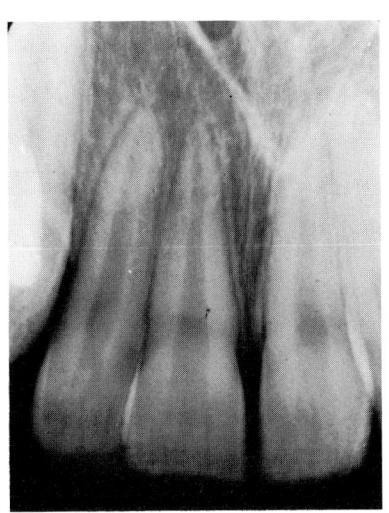

Figure 3-78 Radiograph of maxillary incisors of patient seen in Figure 3-77. Pitted areas appear radiolucent.

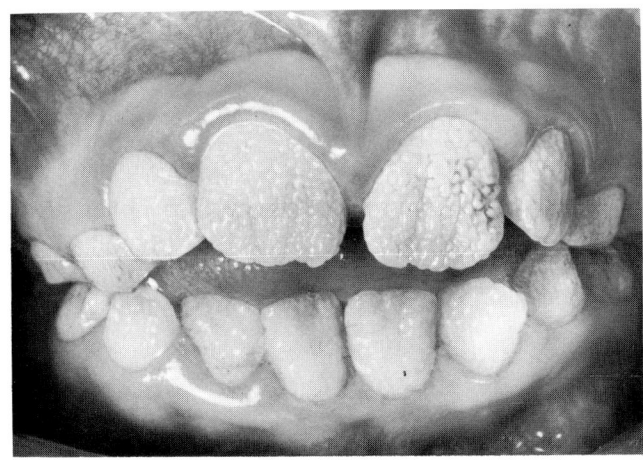

Figure 3-79 Another example of hereditary enamel hypoplasia, hard, pitted type. The color of these teeth is usually close to normal.

IV. ANOMALIES OF STRUCTURE AND TEXTURE *Continued*

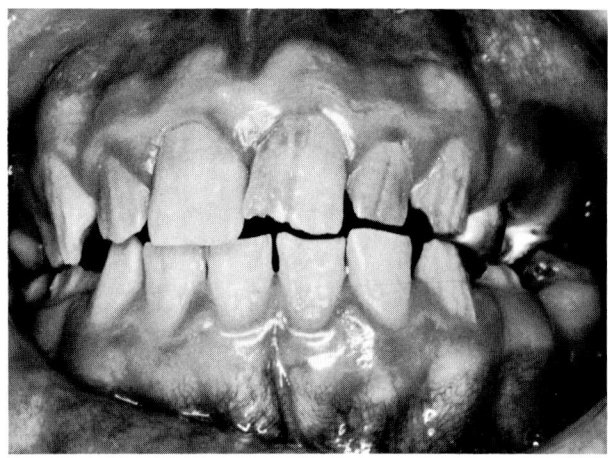

Figure 3-80 Hereditary enamel hypoplasia, with vertical grooving. Enamel layer is lacking in thickness.

Figure 3-81 Hereditary enamel hypoplasia, with horizontal wrinkling and grooving.

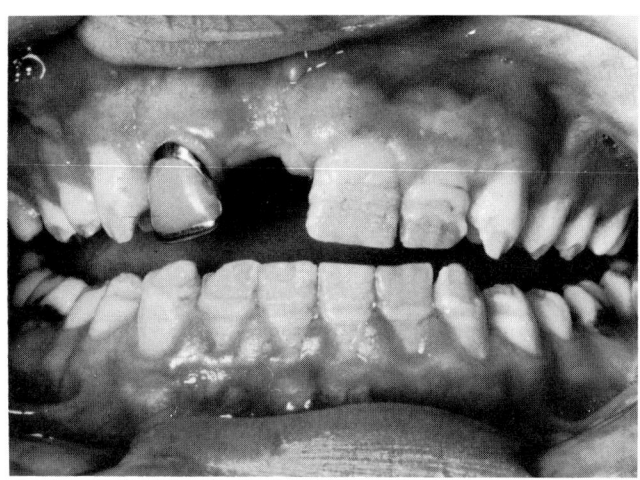

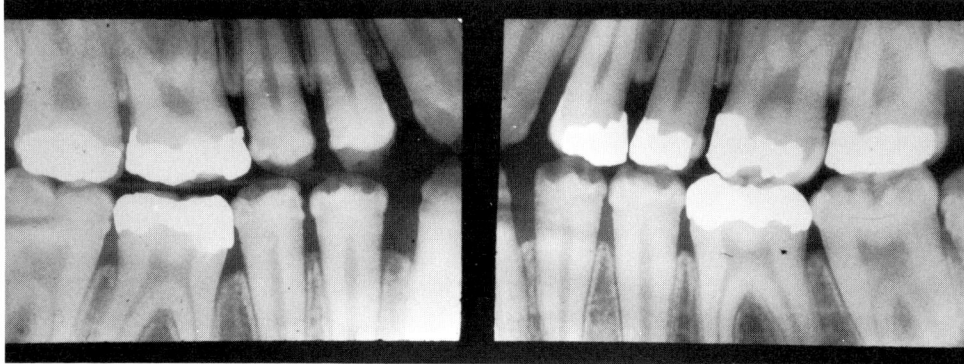

Figure 3-82 Radiographs of patient illustrated in Figure 3-81. Note crinkling and corrugation of crowns of all teeth.

IV. ANOMALIES OF STRUCTURE AND TEXTURE *Continued*

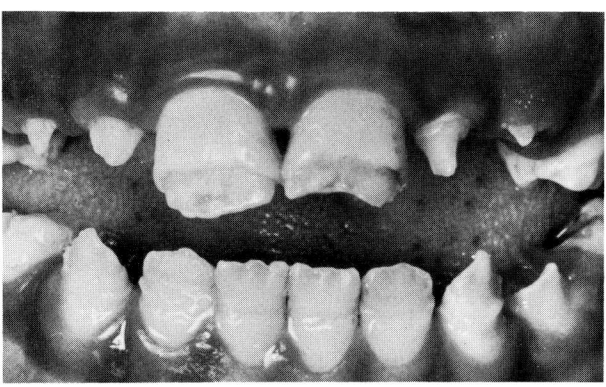

Figure 3-83 Intraoral view of girl with atypical hereditary enamel hypoplasia. The enamel is hard and glossy.

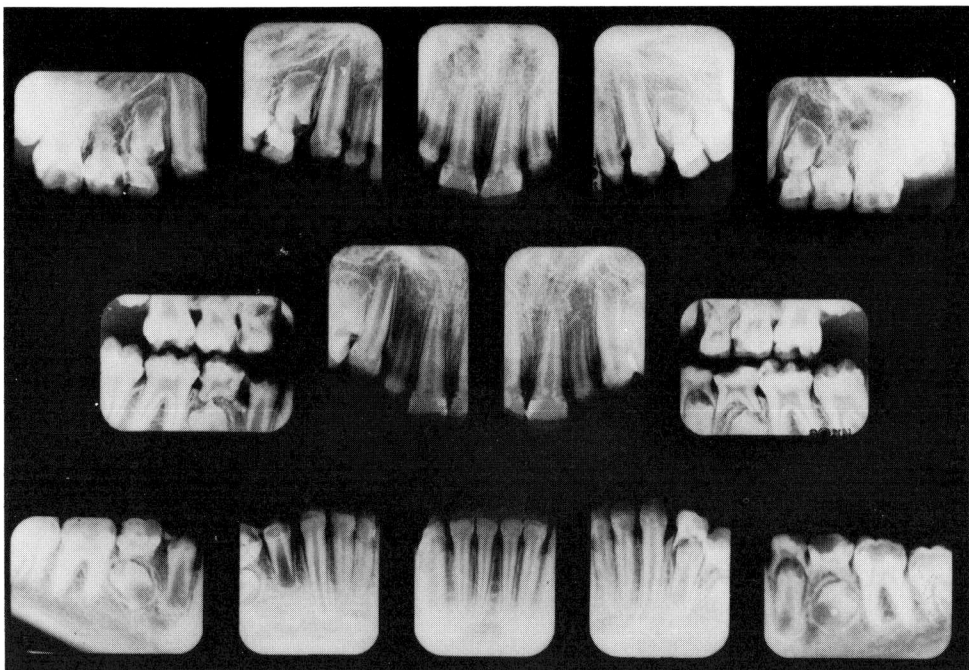

Figure 3-84 Full-mouth radiographs of girl seen in Figure 3-83, showing extent of hypoplasia in all teeth. Pulp canals and dentin appear normal.

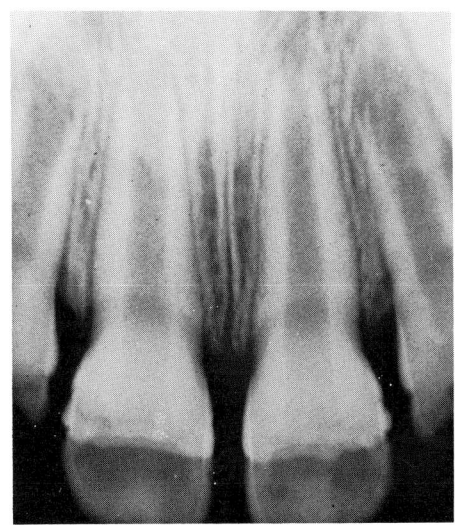

Figure 3-85 Radiographs of maxillary central incisors of girl illustrated in Figure 3-83. Note thin enamel and normal root canals.

IV. ANOMALIES OF STRUCTURE AND TEXTURE *Continued*

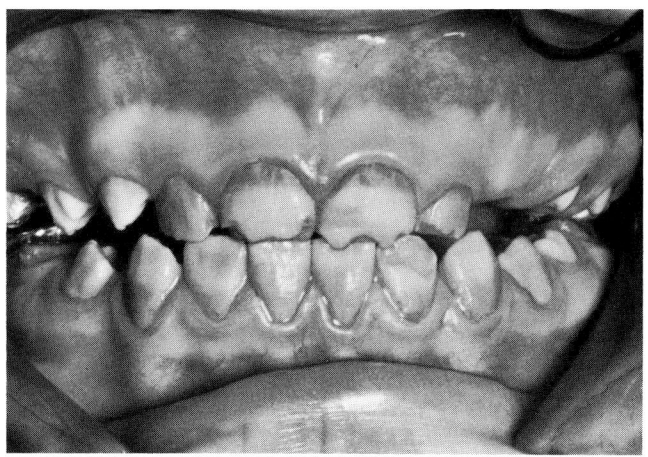

Figure 3-86 Hereditary enamel hypocalcification in an 11-year-old boy. The enamel on these teeth is soft and cheesy, and can be dislodged with an explorer point. These cases require full coverage to prevent wear and loss of contour.

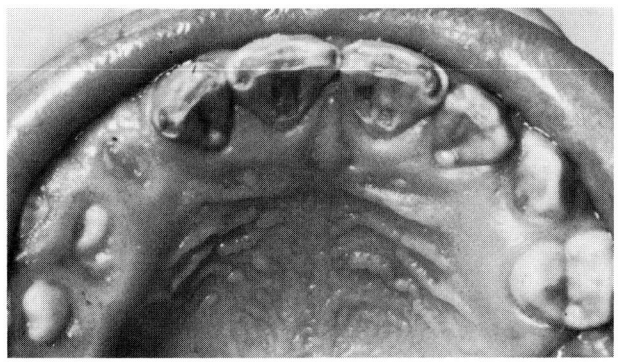

Figure 3-87 Same child as seen in Figure 3-86. Radiographs of these cases show normal pulp chamber morphology, but the enamel is lacking in normal radiopacity.

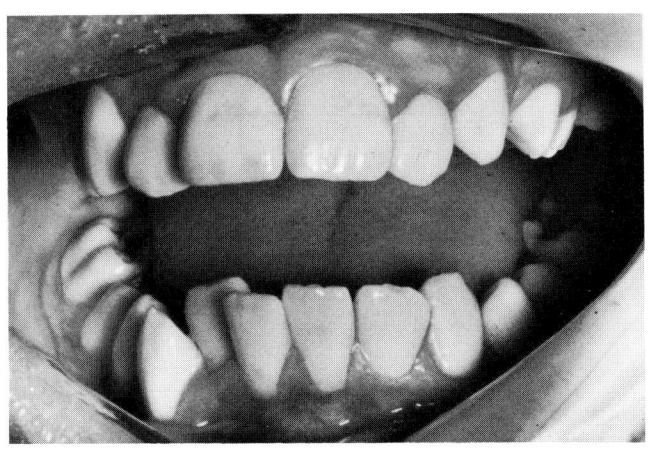

Figure 3-88 Hereditary enamel hypocalcification. In this type the enamel is dull and lusterless, and is easily chipped.

IV. ANOMALIES OF STRUCTURE AND TEXTURE *Continued*

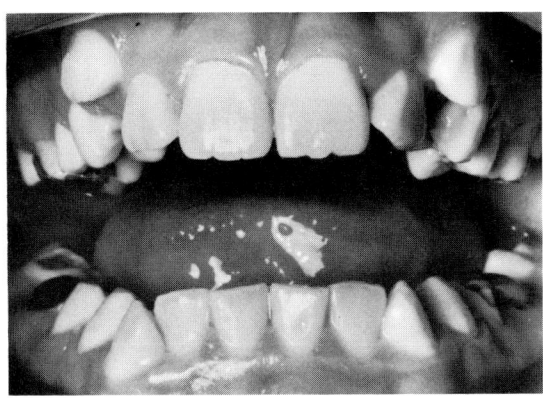

Figure 3-89 Another child exhibiting hereditary enamel hypocalcification. In this case the teeth have a creamy cafe-au-lait color, and are easily abraded.

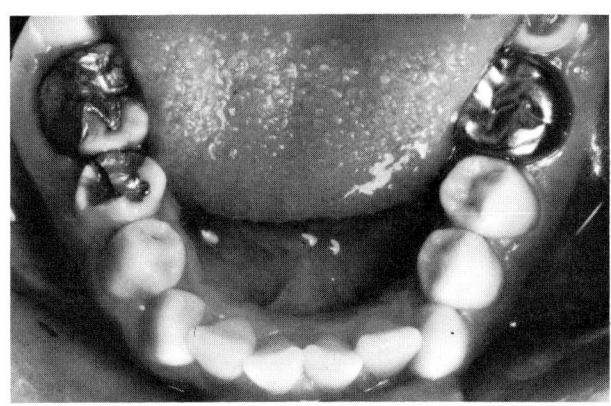

Figure 3-90 Intraoral view of patient illustrated in Figure 3-89. Note chipped enamel around amalgam restoration on the second bicuspid.

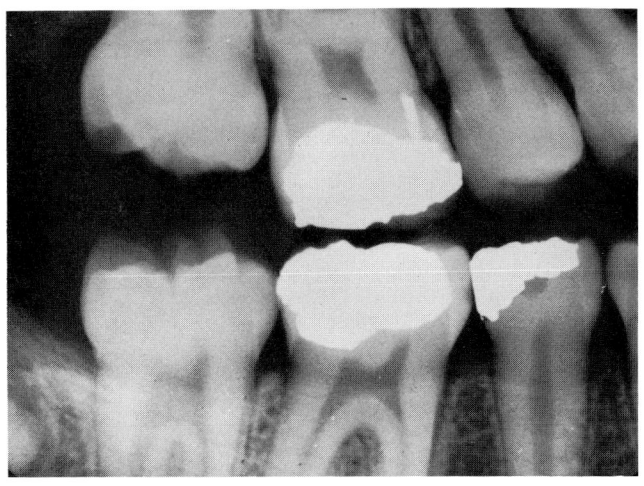

Figure 3-91 Radiograph, right side, in patient illustrated in Figure 3-89. The enamel appears to be of equal density as the dentin. Note the radiopaque line at the dentoenamel junction, particularly on the bicuspids, indicating a zone of more highly calcified enamel.

IV. ANOMALIES OF STRUCTURE AND TEXTURE Continued

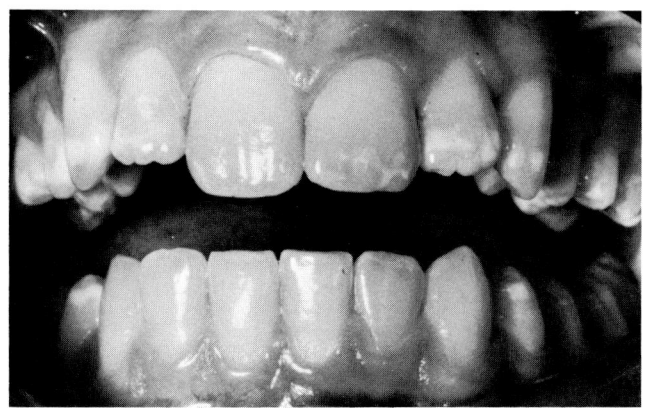

Figure 3-92 Snow-capped teeth, a typical form of hereditary enamel hypocalcification in which there are specific areas near the incisal and occlusal surfaces having a white ground-glass appearance.

Figure 3-93 Snow-capped teeth. The white areas in this case are most prominent on the cuspids and bicuspids. Note that these markings do not conform to defects related to a febrile disease at a specific age.

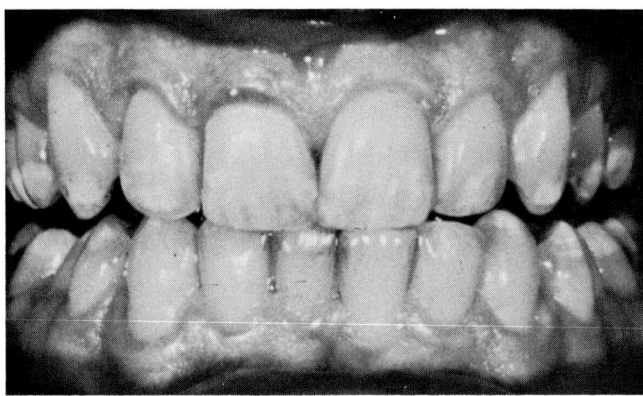

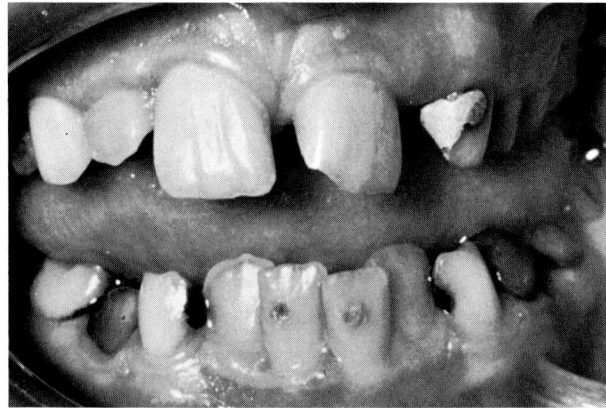

Figure 3-94 Defective enamel on two lower incisors, related to trauma. When child was 2 years of age, he suffered a fall, which caused intrusion of the mandibular primary incisors. This type of hypoplasia is obviously not hereditary.

Figure 3-95 Local hypoplasia on a maxillary incisor in a boy with a history of a facial injury in infancy.

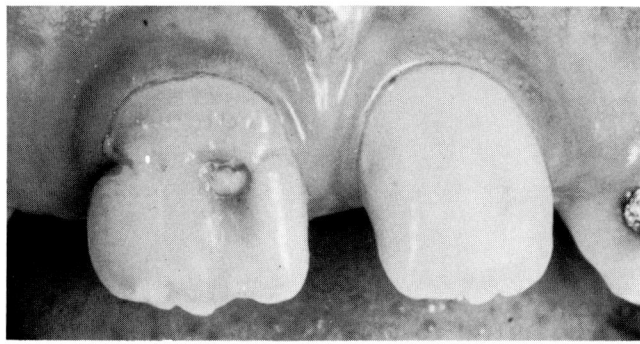

IV. ANOMALIES OF STRUCTURE AND TEXTURE *Continued*

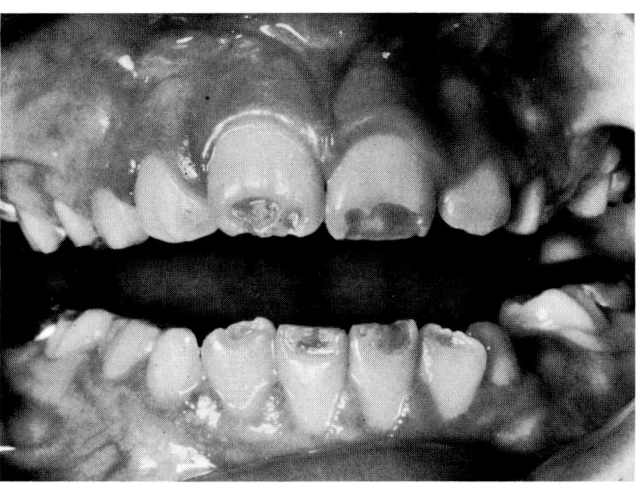

Figure 3-96 Typical enamel hypoplasia related to a history of febrile disease. This child suffered a severe attack of pneumonia at age 8 months. Note that the maxillary lateral incisors are unaffected. This is because these teeth usually do not begin to calcify before 10 to 12 months of age.

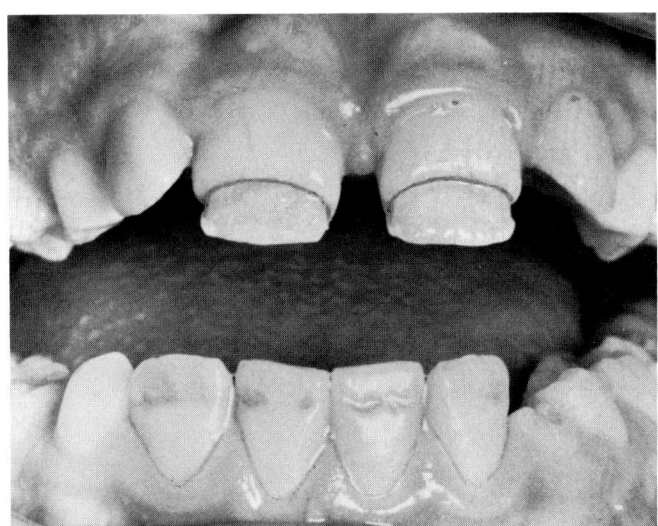

Figure 3-97 Local enamel hypoplasia related to a history of virus infection in infancy. Note that the maxillary laterals are normal, indicating that the disease probably terminated prior to age 10 months.

Figure 3-98 Close-up of mandibular molar region in patient shown in Figure 3-97. Note lack of enamel formation on occlusal of first permanent molar. The second primary molar appears unaffected.

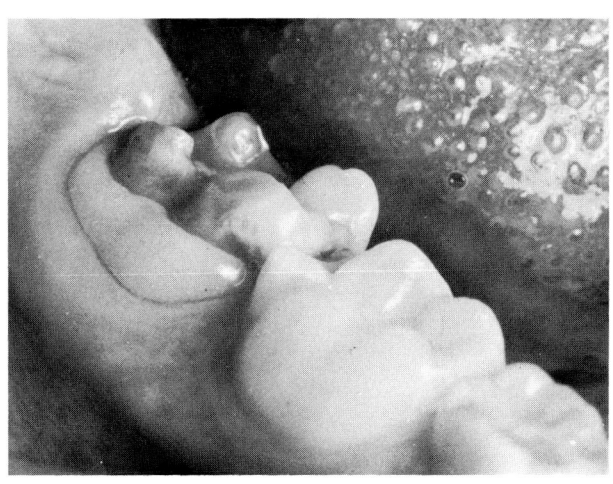

IV. ANOMALIES OF STRUCTURE AND TEXTURE *Continued*

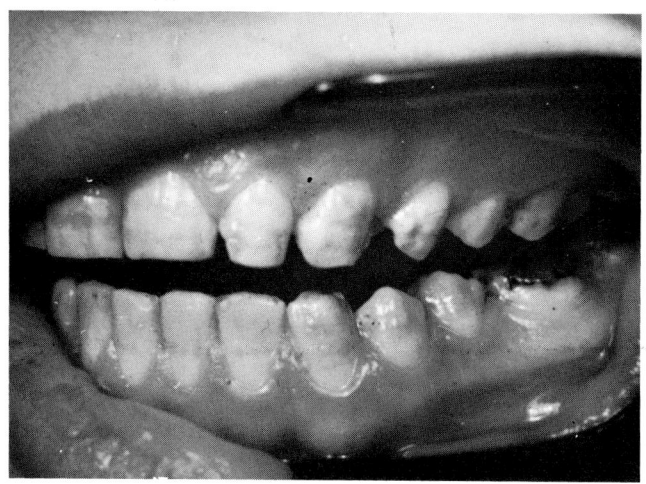

Figure 3-99 Fluorosis or mottled enamel. The effect of high concentrations of fluoride ion is to induce defective calcification in some areas. These in turn undergo distinctive staining giving a characteristic appearance.

Figure 3-100 Enamel hypoplasia in the primary dentition related to maternal disturbances during pregnancy. The areas affected are those that have calcified in the prenatal period.

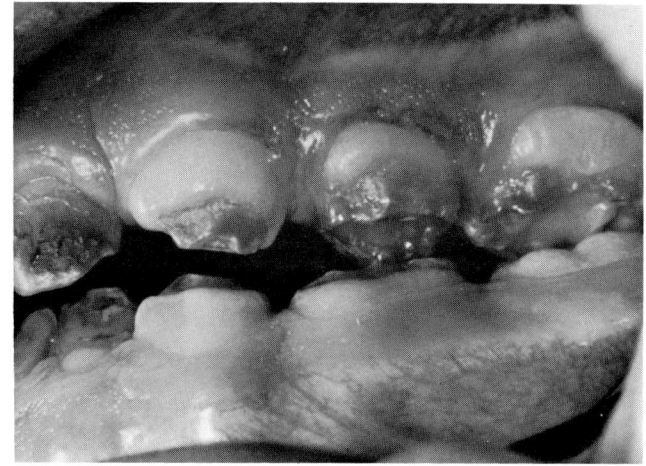

IV. ANOMALIES OF STRUCTURE AND TEXTURE *Continued*

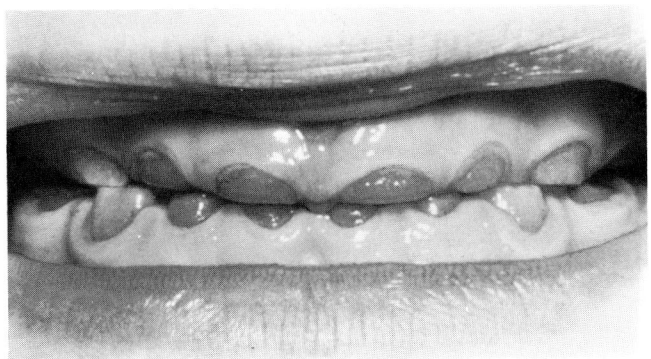

Figure 3-101 Dentinogenesis imperfecta in a 5-year-old girl. An autosomal dominant trait, it is found in the ratio of 1:1 in siblings. Teeth are blue-gray or brown, and abrade rapidly. (For a discussion of treatment, see Chapter 12, Prosthodontics.)

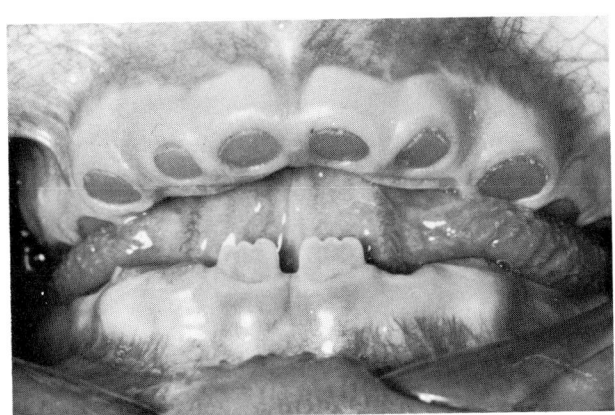

Figure 3-102 Same girl as seen in Figure 3-101. Lower permanent incisors have erupted and maxillary primary teeth are abraded to a marked extent.

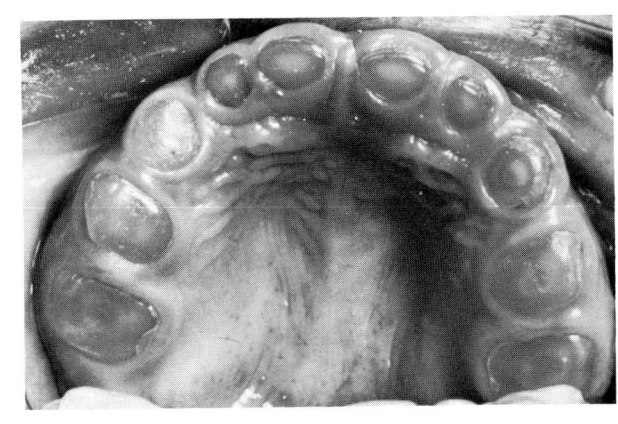

Figure 3-103 Maxillary arch showing extreme abrasion of primary crowns. Frequently these teeth become abscessed as a result of exposure of pulpal horns caused by wear. Full coverage is the treatment of choice.

IV. ANOMALIES OF STRUCTURE AND TEXTURE *Continued*

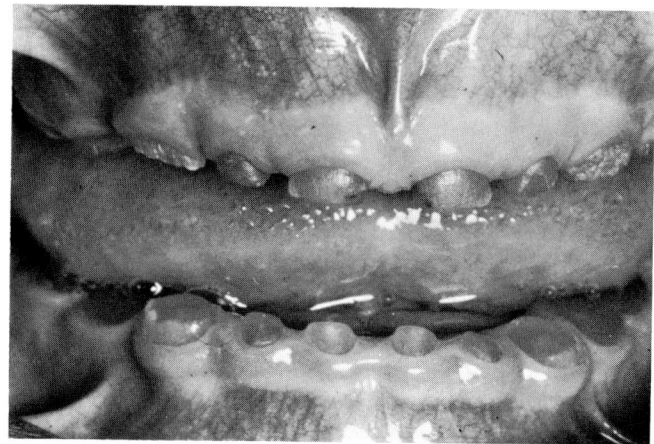

Figure 3-104 Dentinogenesis imperfecta in the primary dentition. Children with this condition may have psychological problems because of their appearance.

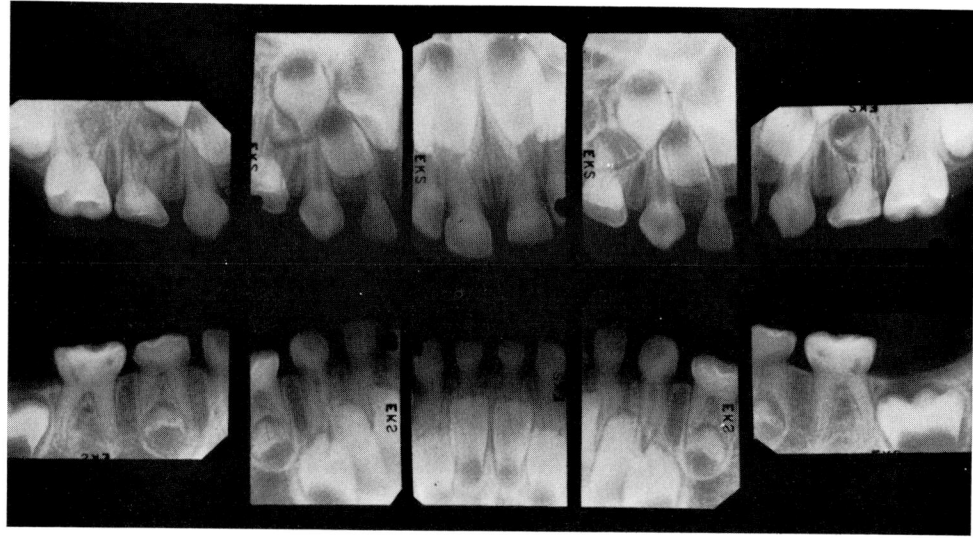

Figure 3-105 Radiographs of a preschool child with dentinogenesis imperfecta. Note obliteration of the pulp chambers with secondary dentin, a characteristic finding. Crowns usually appear more bulbous.

Figure 3-106 Radiograph of an 8-year-old child with dentinogenesis imperfecta. Note that the pulp chamber of the newly erupted permanent molar is not yet completely obliterated, as is the case with the adjacent primary molar.

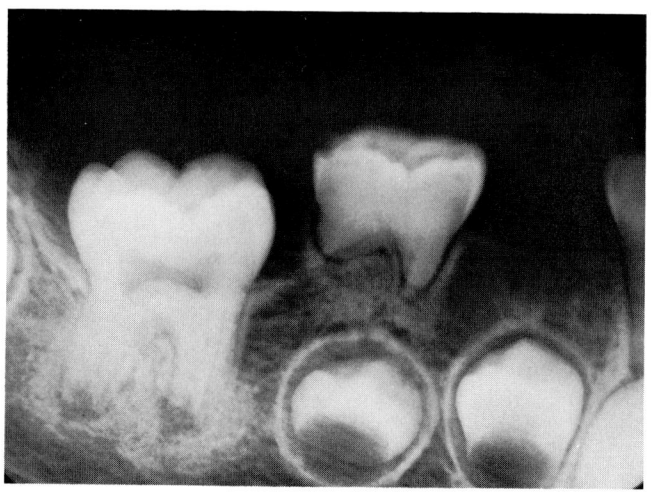

ANOMALIES OF THE DENTITION 93

IV. ANOMALIES OF STRUCTURE AND TEXTURE Continued

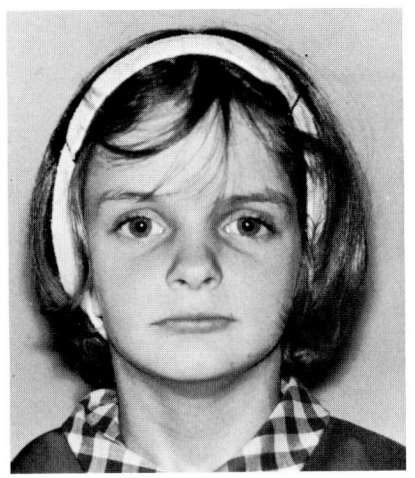

Figure 3-107 Eight-year-old girl with dentinogenesis imperfecta. Note the bite closure because of excessive loss of tooth substance from abrasion.

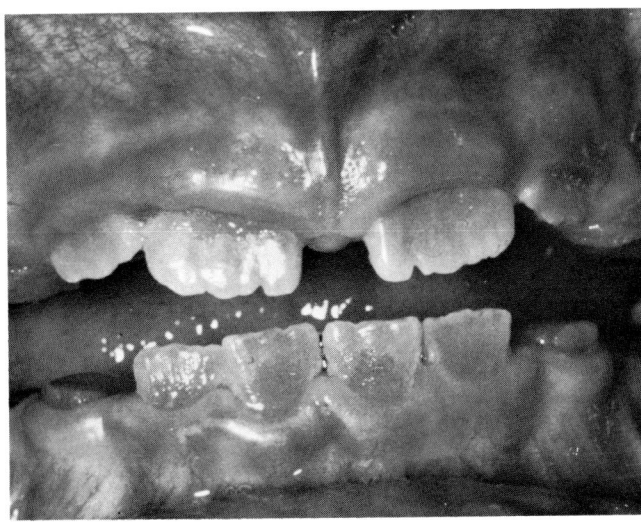

Figure 3-108 Anterior view of teeth of girl seen in Figure 3-107. The teeth have a brownish-gray color. Defects of enamel are sometimes associated with this condition, but the primary defect is one of the dentin.

Figure 3-109 Intraoral view of girl seen in Figure 3-107. Note complete abrasion of posterior teeth.

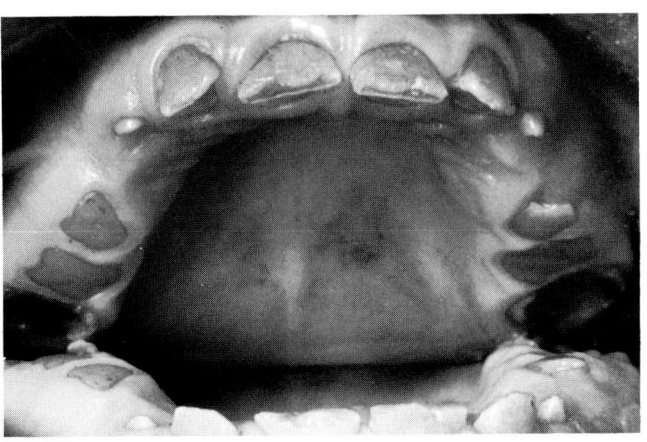

IV. ANOMALIES OF STRUCTURE AND TEXTURE Continued

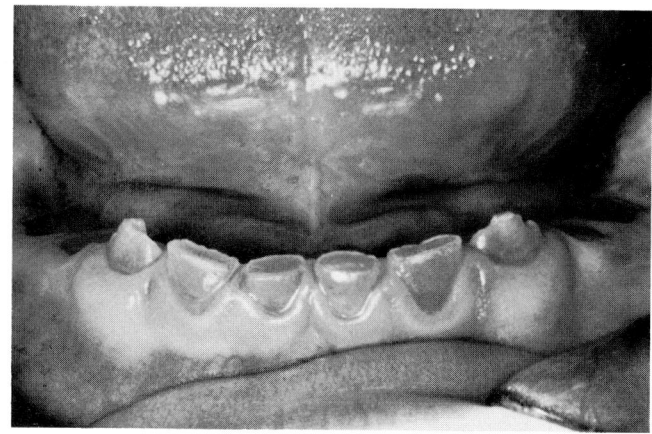

Figure 3-110 Same patient as seen in Figure 3-109. It is often advisable to provide coverage for permanent teeth as soon as they erupt.

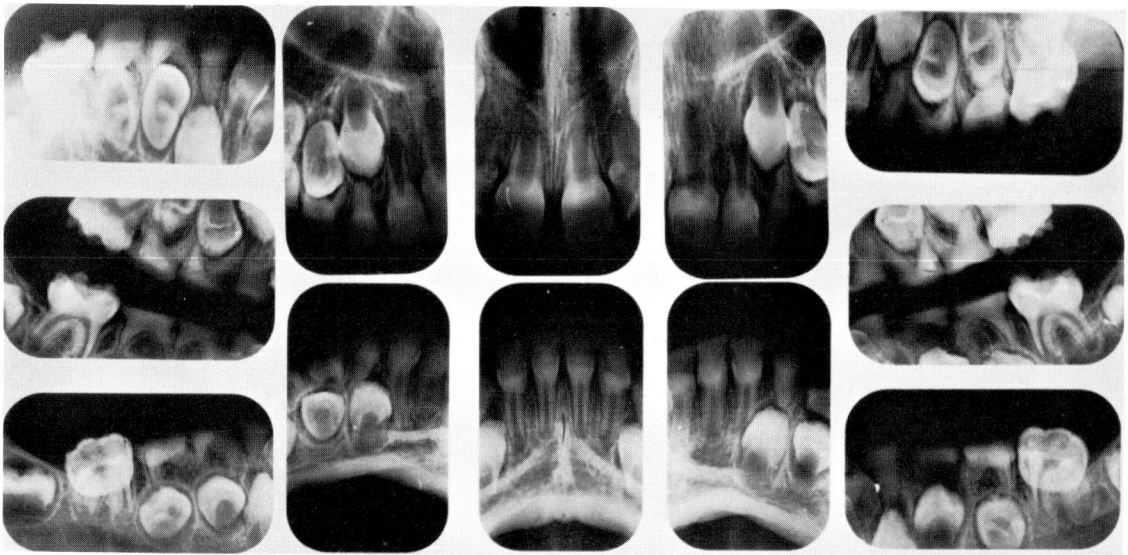

Figure 3-111 Radiographs of 8-year-old girl with dentinogenesis imperfecta. Pulp chambers of primary teeth are completely obliterated. Newly erupted permanent teeth have not as yet undergone significant abrasion, and should be crowned.

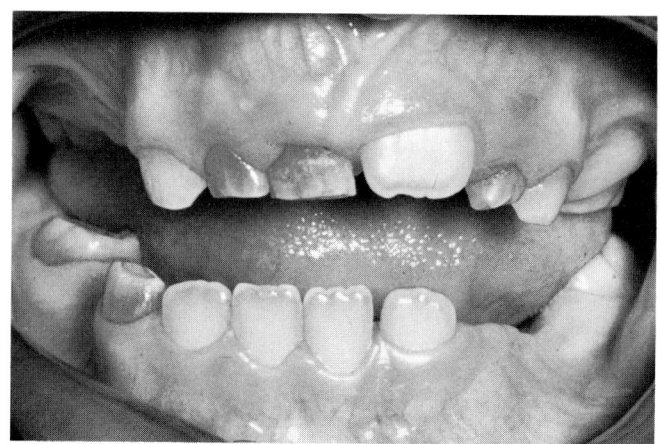

Figure 3-112 An unusual case of dentinogenesis imperfecta in which the primary teeth exhibit the typical color and abrasion pattern but the erupting permanent teeth are normal in appearance.

ANOMALIES OF THE DENTITION 95

IV. ANOMALIES OF STRUCTURE AND TEXTURE *Continued*

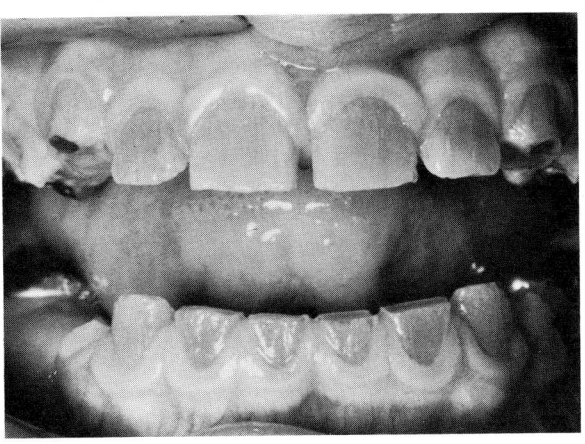

Figure 3-113 A 14-year-old girl with dentinogenesis imperfecta. (See Chapter 12, Prosthodontics, for a discussion of the treatment of this patient.)

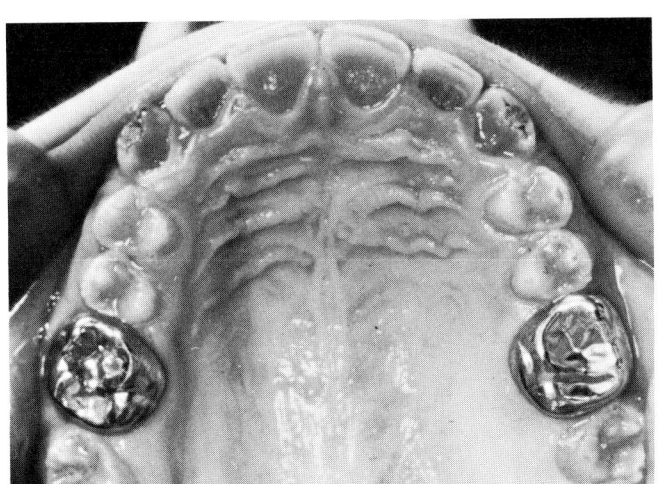

Figure 3-114 Same girl as seen in Figure 3-113. First permanent molars were crowned shortly after eruption to prevent abrasion.

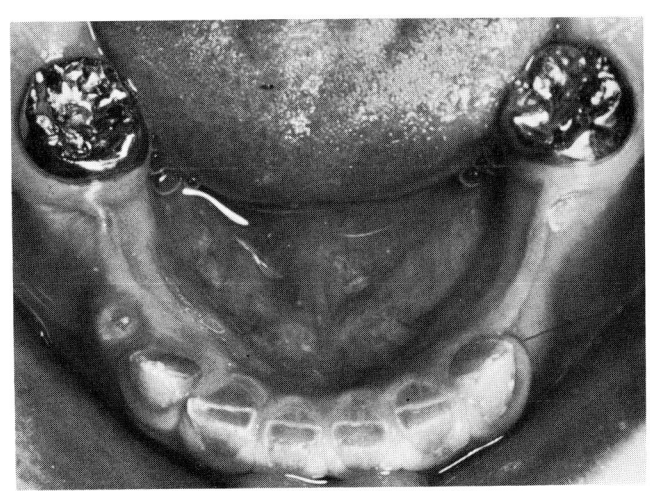

Figure 3-115 Lower arch of girl shown in Figure 3-113. Note wear on lower incisors.

IV. ANOMALIES OF STRUCTURE AND TEXTURE *Continued*

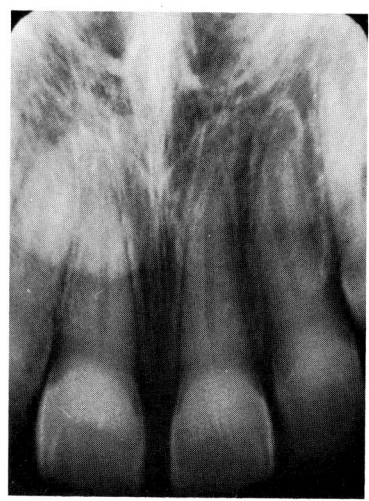

Figure 3-116 Radiographs of anterior teeth of girl with dentinogenesis imperfecta. Note obliteration of pulp chambers with secondary dentin.

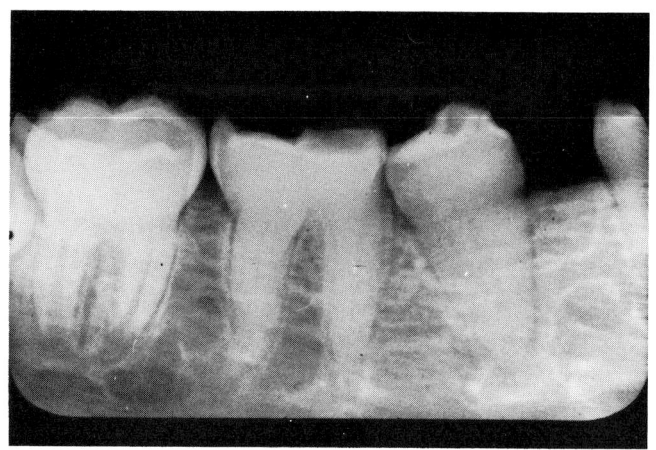

Figure 3-117 Typical radiographic appearance in a case of dentinogenesis imperfecta. Pulp chambers and root canals are obliterated.

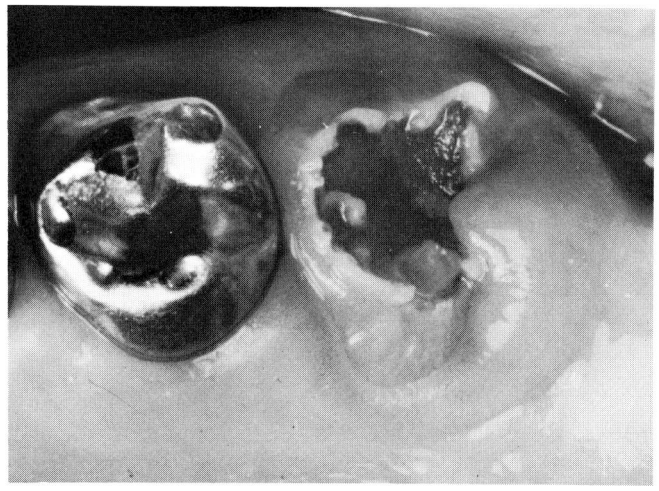

Figure 3-118 Intraoral view of erupting first permanent molar in a child with dentinogenesis imperfecta. Note defective enamel, which is sometimes also seen in this condition. The primary defect is one of the dentin.

IV. ANOMALIES OF STRUCTURE AND TEXTURE *Continued*

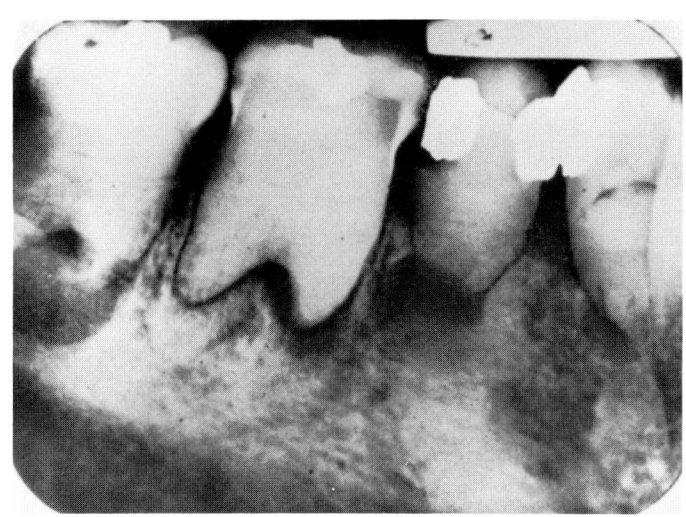

Figure 3-119 Dentinal dysplasia (also termed "rootless teeth"). This anomaly is comparatively rare and is characterized by crowns of normal color, but with pulp chambers obliterated and roots lacking in normal length. Radiolucent areas may be present around these roots. (From Rushton, M. A.: Anomalies of human dentin. Ann. Roy. Coll. Surg. *16*:94, 1955.)

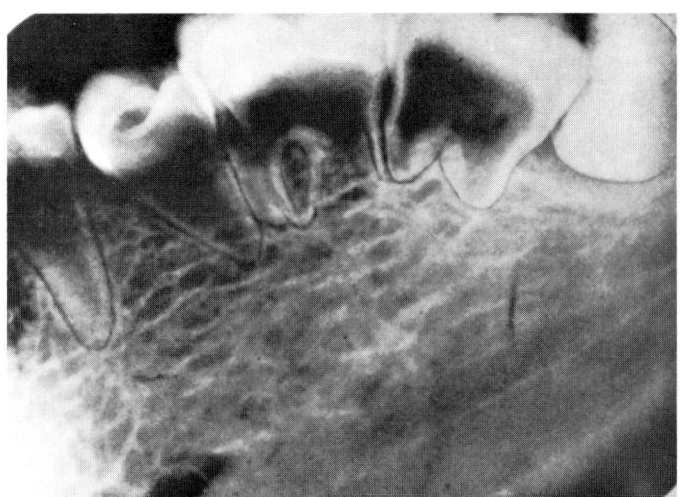

Figure 3-120 Shell teeth, a rare anomaly of dentin which has been described by Rushton. There is a thin layer of dentin surrounding the enormous pulp cavities. Roots are comparatively short. (From Rushton, M. A.: A new form of dentinal dysplasia: shell teeth. Oral Surg. Oral Med. Oral Path. 7:543-549, May, 1954.)

Anomalies of Eruption and Exfoliation

The age at which eruption and exfoliation of teeth occur varies widely. Many clinicians feel that there is a familial pattern of early or late eruption. A dramatic example of early eruption is the neonatal tooth, which is found occasionally in newborns. This has been reported to occur in 0.03 per cent of births (1 in 3,000) usually in the lower incisor area.[2]

Local or systemic factors can influence eruption or exfoliation of teeth. In the case of premature loss of primary teeth due to caries, the effect on eruption of the succedaneous tooth depends on the age at which the extraction takes place. If it occurs during the preschool period, eruption of the underlying tooth is usually somewhat retarded. If it occurs during the mixed dentition period and there is extensive bone pathology, eruption of the permanent tooth is accelerated. A frequent cause of retarded eruption of permanent teeth is the presence of embedded supernumerary teeth or ankylosed primary teeth.

Retarded eruption is associated also with such conditions as cleidocranial dysostosis, hypothyroidism, and hypopituitarism. Precocious exfoliation, on the other hand, may occur along with hypophosphatasia, acrodynia, and a form of reticular endotheliosis, such as Hand-Schüller-Christian disease.

Anomalies of Position of Teeth

In this classification there might properly be included all deviations from normal position—this would embrace all disharmonies of occlusion. For simplification, this section is limited to illustrations of deviations in tooth position due to ectopic eruption, ankylosis, and impaction. For illustrations of crossbite, rotation, and similar conditions see Chapter 11, Space Maintenance and Interceptive Orthodontics.

V. ANOMALIES OF ERUPTION AND EXFOLIATION

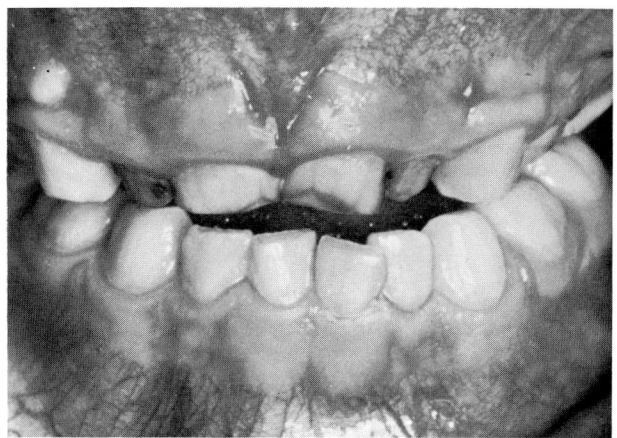

Figure 3-121 Delayed eruption of permanent teeth in an 8-year-old girl with cleidocranial dysostosis. In this hereditary condition the clavicles are absent, there are supernumerary teeth, and tooth eruption is delayed. (See also Figure 3-15.)

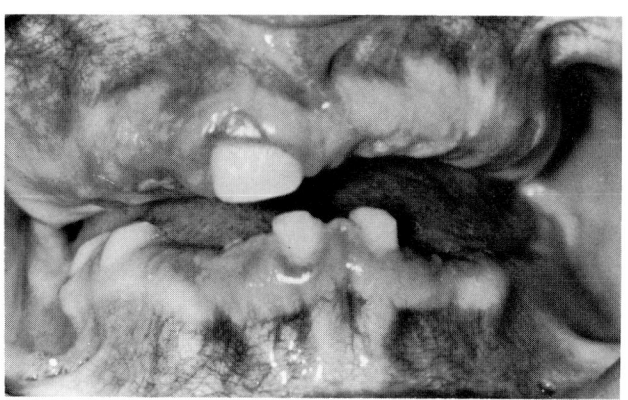

Figure 3-122 Intraoral view of 14-year-old girl with amelogenesis imperfecta (enamel hypoplasia type). Delayed eruption is sometimes associated with this anomaly.

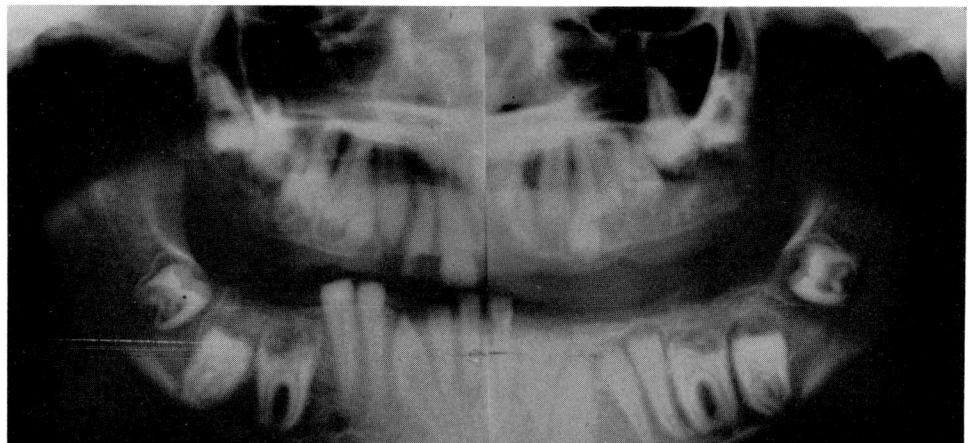

Figure 3-123 Radiographs of girl shown in Figure 3-122. Note multiple unerupted teeth.

V. ANOMALIES OF ERUPTION AND EXFOLIATION Continued

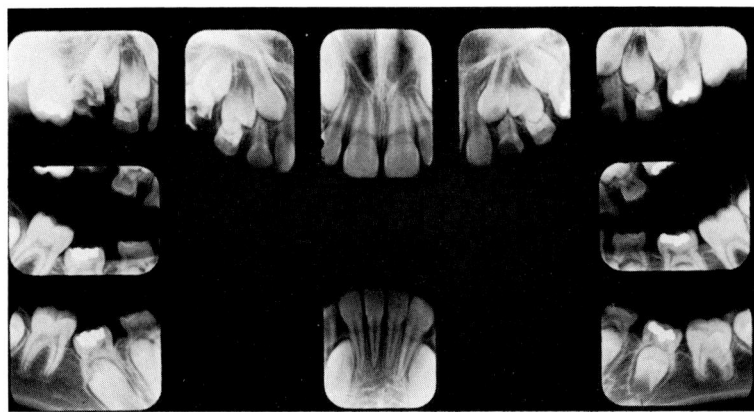

Figure 3-124 Radiographs of a 9-year-old girl with delayed eruption of all posterior permanent teeth. Some primary molars are ankylosed. There is no contact of teeth in the molar region, which might indicate lack of vertical bone growth.

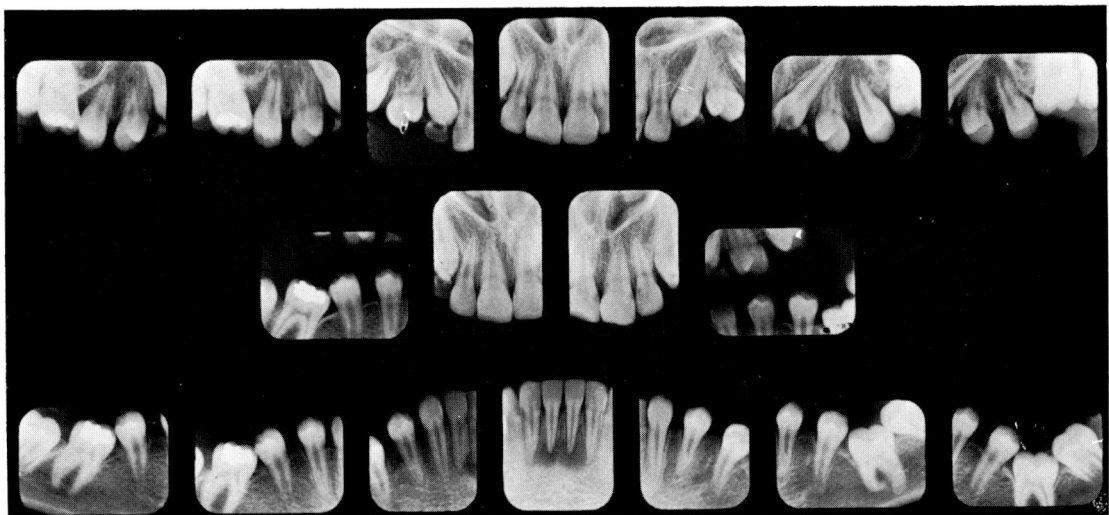

Figure 3-125 Same patient as seen in Figure 3-124, 2 years later. All primary teeth were extracted, but there is only limited eruption of posterior teeth. No other associated abnormalities were found.

ANOMALIES OF THE DENTITION

V. ANOMALIES OF ERUPTION AND EXFOLIATION *Continued*

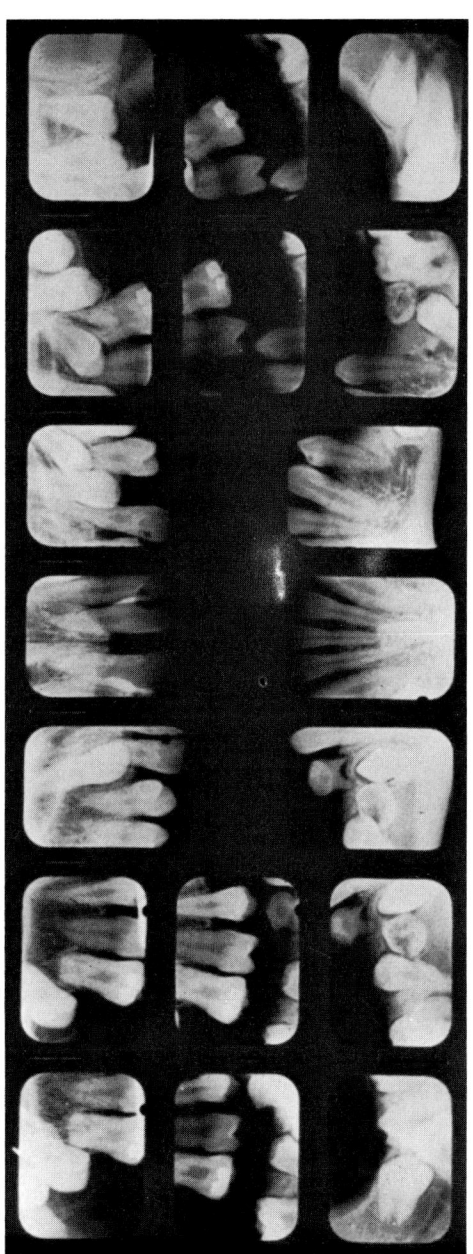

Figure 3-126 Delayed eruption in a 16-year-old boy with a history of hypothyroidism.

V. ANOMALIES OF ERUPTION AND EXFOLIATION Continued

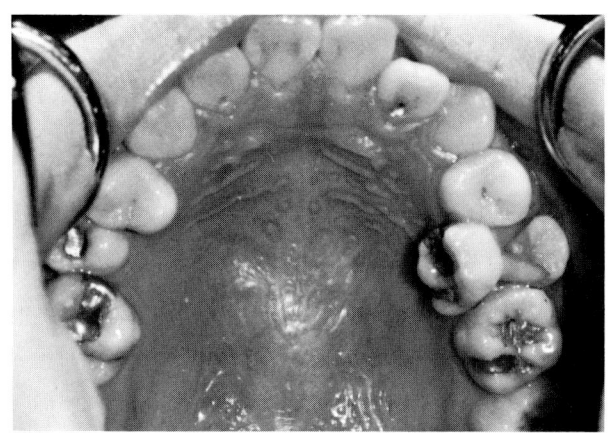

Figure 3-128 Delayed exfoliation of maxillary left primary second molar resulting from failure of resorption of lingual root.

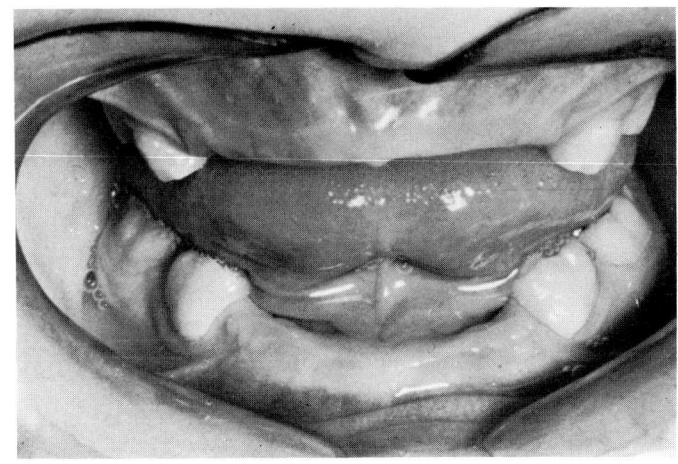

Figure 3-129 Precocious exfoliation of primary dentition in a 3-year-old boy with hypophosphatasia. This condition is transmitted as an autosomal recessive trait and is characterized by a deficiency of alkaline phosphatase. Because of the absence of cementum, the tooth is deprived of its normal periodontal attachment.

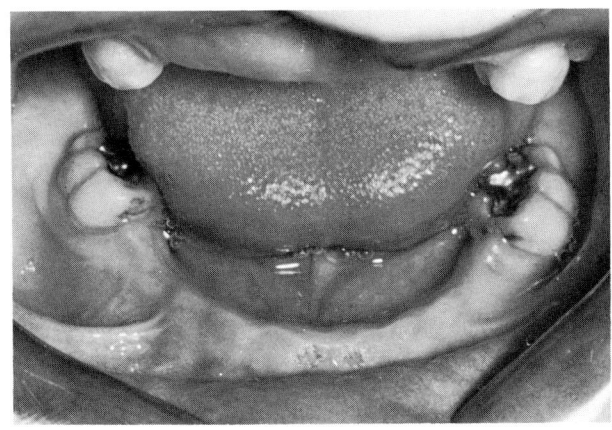

Figure 3-130 Same boy as shown in Figure 3-129, 1 year later. More teeth have loosened and been exfoliated. As this boy grew older, normal cementum developed around the permanent teeth and the periodontal attachment was normal.

VI. ANOMALIES OF POSITION

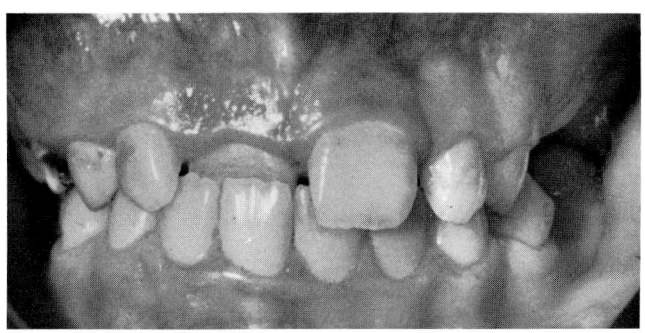

Figure 3-131 Anterior crossbite. Before treatment is started, radiographs should be obtained to ascertain the presence or absence of supernumeraries. There must be adequate room for the lingually locked tooth to move forward.

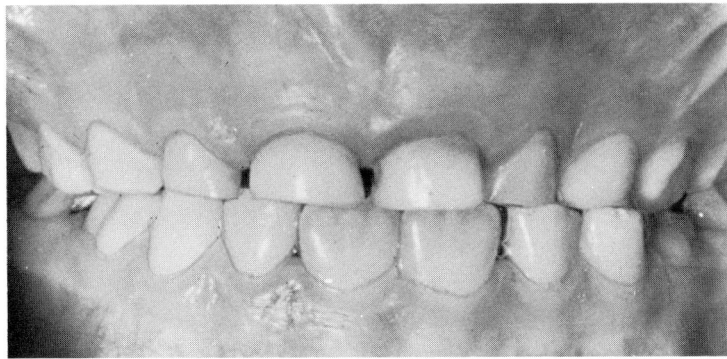

Figure 3-132 Posterior crossbite in the primary dentition. This condition can easily be overlooked. (See Chapter 11 concerning correction of anterior and posterior crossbites.) Note deviation of midline.

Figure 3-133 Labial eruption of maxillary permanent central incisor. Primary central incisors should be extracted. Some children exhibit over-retention of all primary teeth.

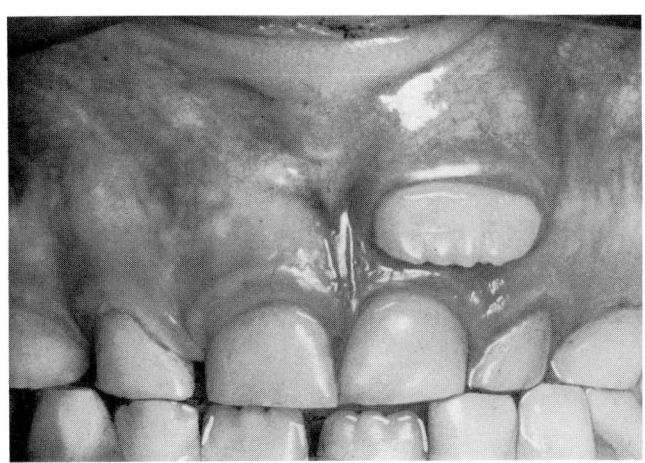

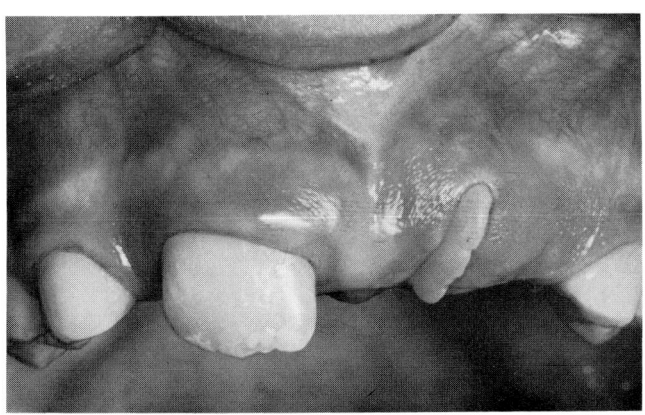

Figure 3-134 Permanent central incisor in abnormal position because of presence of a supernumerary tooth (mesiodens).

VI. ANOMALIES OF POSITION *Continued*

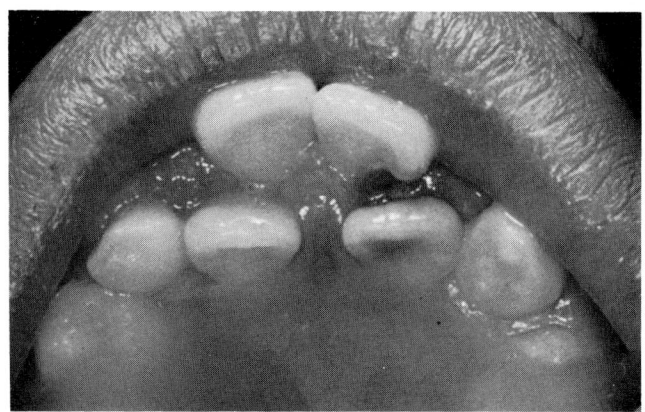

Figure 3-135 Extreme crowding in maxillary arch with lingual position of permanent lateral incisors. Orthodontic consultation should be sought.

Figure 3-136 Maxillary incisors crowded out of normal position due to presence of supernumerary tooth.

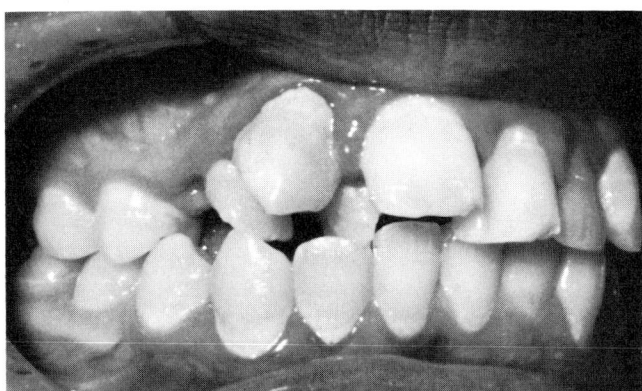

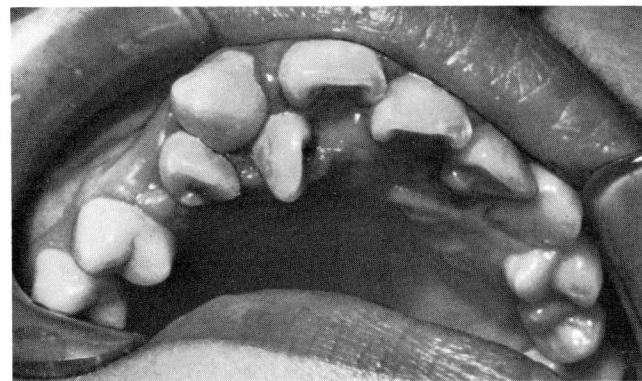

Figure 3-137 Occlusal view of patient shown in Figure 3-136. Extraction of the supernumerary tooth is indicated, followed by orthodontic treatment.

Figure 3-138 Ectopic eruption of mandibular permanent cuspids. Primary cuspids should be extracted and, if necessary, permanent cuspids repositioned.

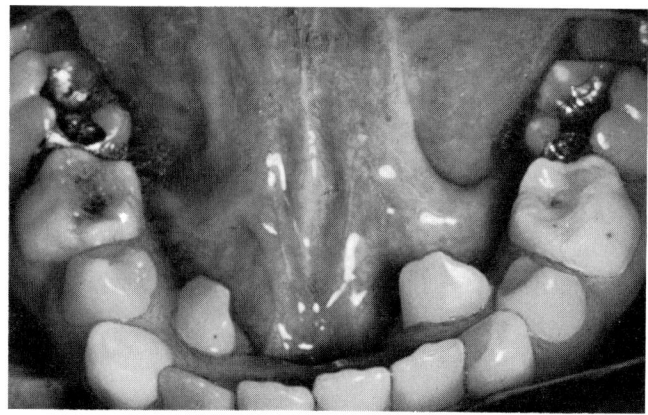

VI. ANOMALIES OF POSITION *Continued*

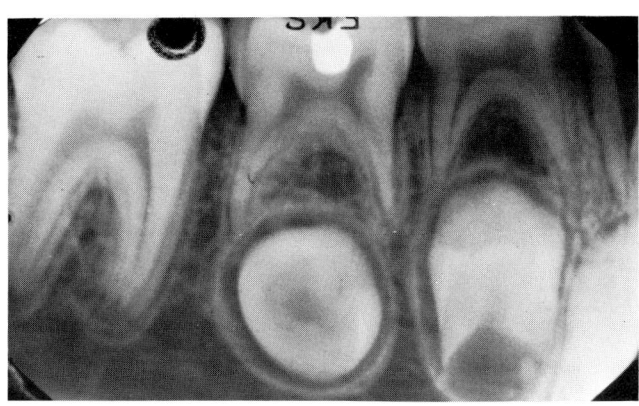

Figure 3-139 Rotated mandibular second bicuspid.

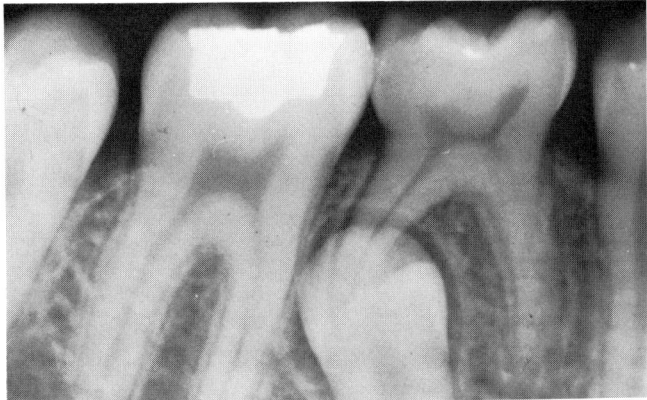

Figure 3-140 Over-retained second primary molar forces second bicuspid into distal position. The primary tooth should be extracted, the bone over the bicuspid removed, and the space maintained by a suitable appliance until the tooth erupts.

Figure 3-141 Ankylosed second primary molar has forced the second bicuspid to tip distally. The primary molar should be extracted and the space maintained until the permanent tooth erupts.

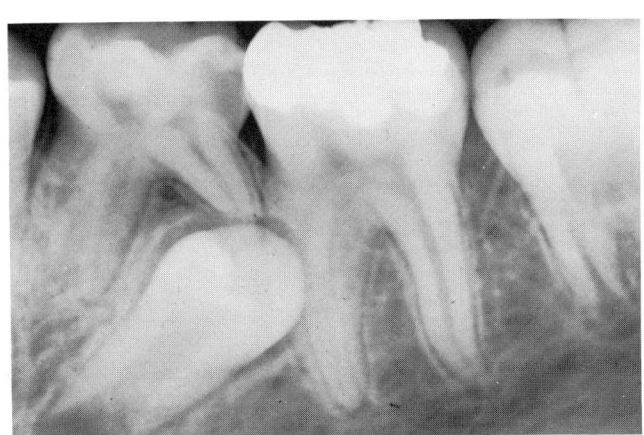

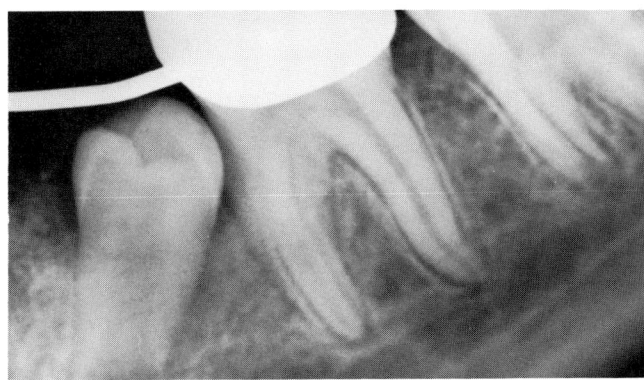

Figure 3-142 Same patient as in Figure 3-141, 3 months after extraction of the primary molar. The bicuspid is now upright and is erupting.

VI. ANOMALIES OF POSITION Continued

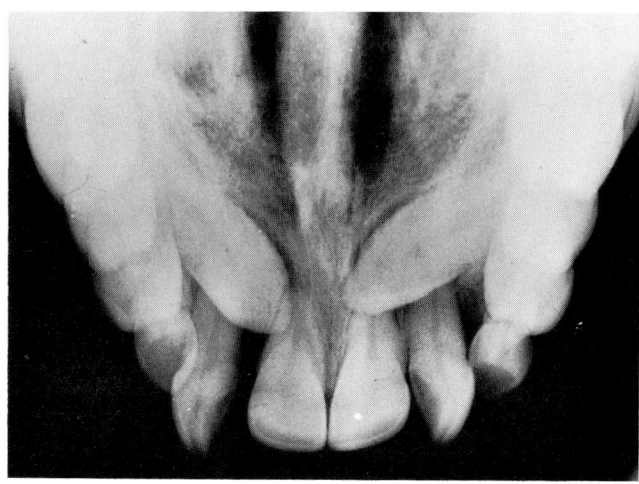

Figure 3-143 Permanent cuspids lying horizontally in the palate. Treatment of these cases should be done with the cooperation of the oral surgeon and the orthodontist.

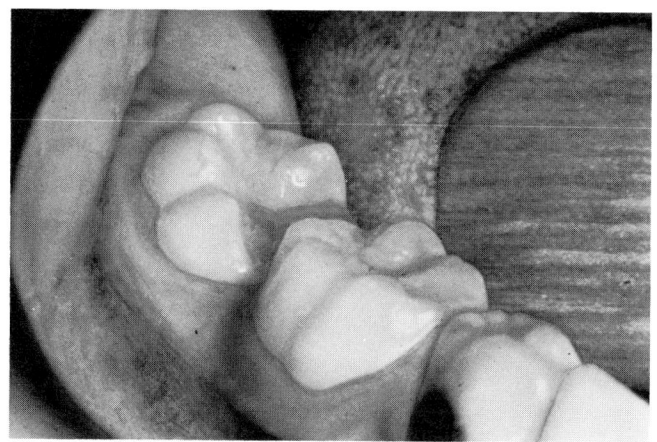

Figure 3-144 Ectopic eruption of mandibular first permanent molar. This is more commonly seen in the maxillary arch.

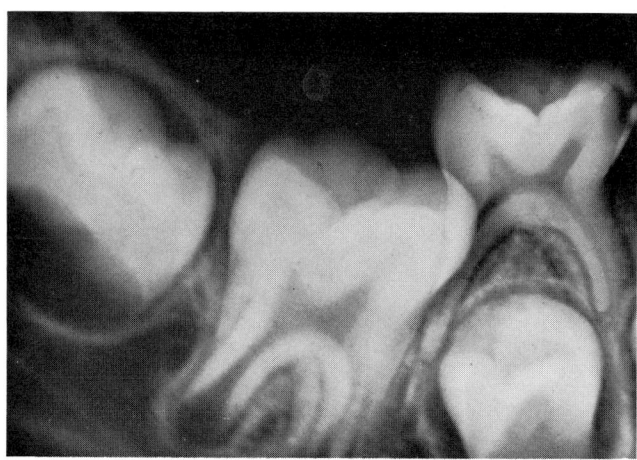

Figure 3-145 Radiograph of patient shown in Figure 3-144.

VI. ANOMALIES OF POSITION *Continued*

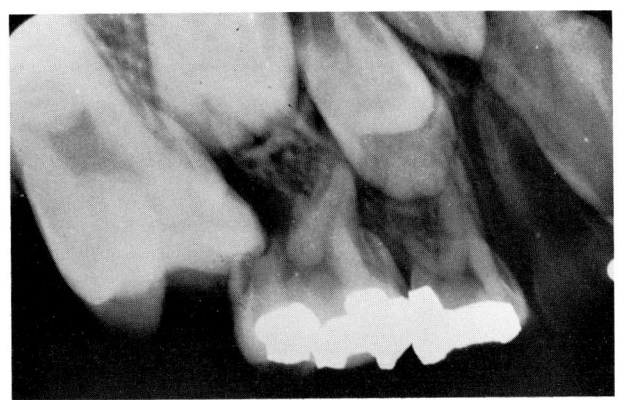

Figure 3-146 Ectopic eruption of maxillary first permanent molar. In a case as acute as this one, the primary second molar should be extracted and the patient should wear a corrective headgear to reposition the permanent molar.

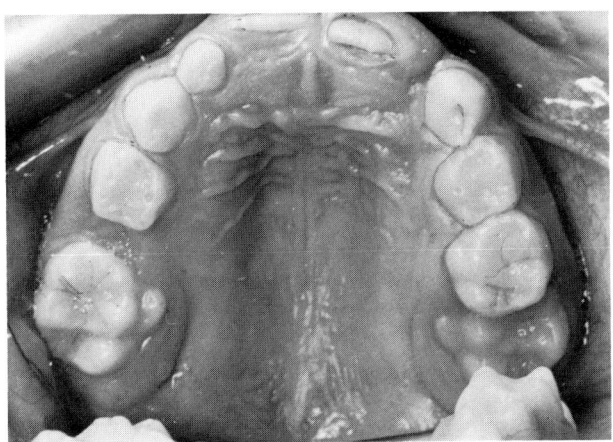

Figure 3-147 Maxillary occlusal view showing space loss created by an erupted ectopic first permanent molar that has not been treated. Note similar condition in opposite quadrant. Sometimes early intervention will prevent loss of second primary molar.

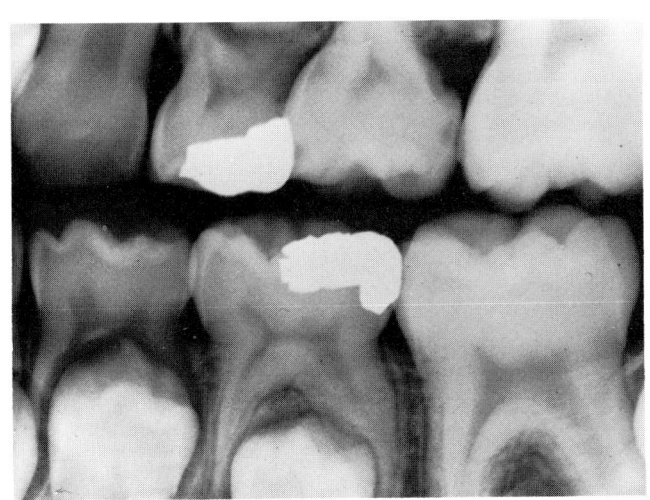

Figure 3-148 Bitewing radiograph illustrating a common situation: maxillary first permanent molar began to erupt ectopically, resorption took place, and the tooth assumed its proper position in the arch. Note the resorbed area on the distal root of the primary molar. Some ectopic eruptions are self correcting.

VI. ANOMALIES OF POSITION *Continued*

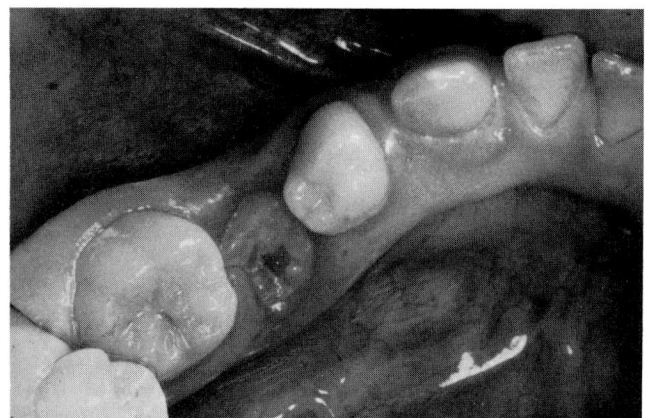

Figure 3-149 Ankylosis of a second primary molar. Growth of alveolar bone into lacunae on the root surface prevents normal vertical movement. The tooth should be extracted and the space maintained.

Figure 3-150 Ankylosis of mandibular primary molars. Loss of arch length can occur if ankylosed teeth fail to maintain proper position.

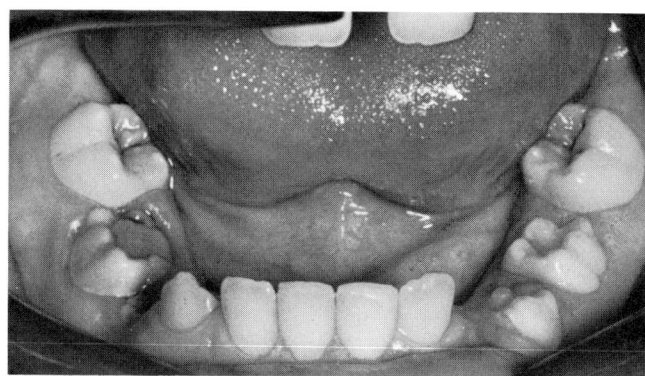

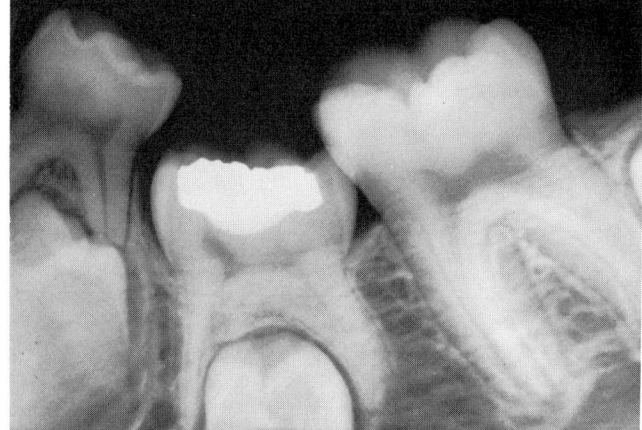

Figure 3-151 Radiograph of ankylosed primary second molar showing failure of tooth to maintain proper arch length. Extraction of the primary molar is indicated, followed by use of a suitable appliance to reposition the tipped first permanent molar.

Figure 3-152 Ankylosis of all maxillary and mandibular primary molars on the right side resulting in loss of masticatory function in this area.

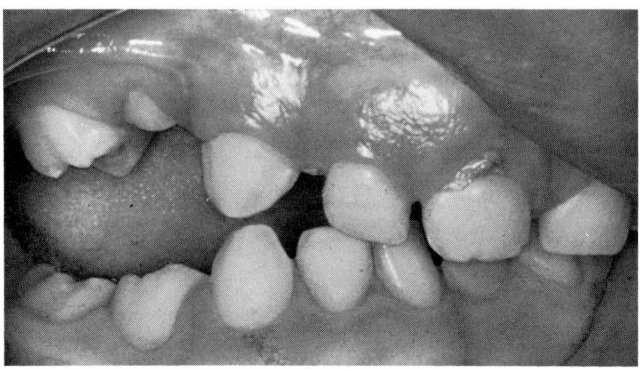

VI. ANOMALIES OF POSITION Continued

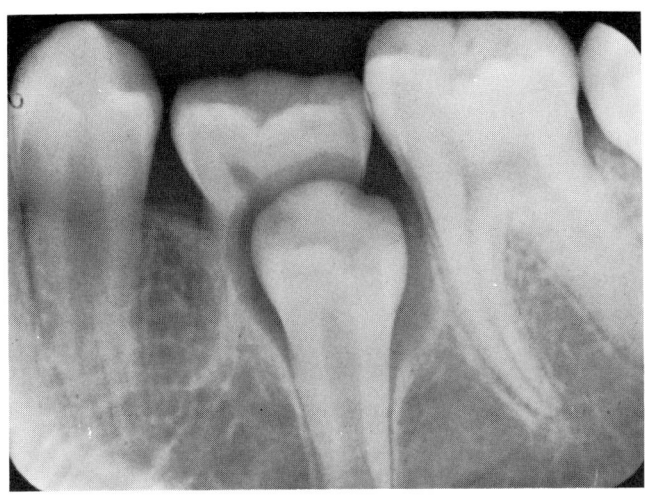

Figure 3-153 Ankylosis of mesial root of second primary molar interfering with eruption of second bicuspid.

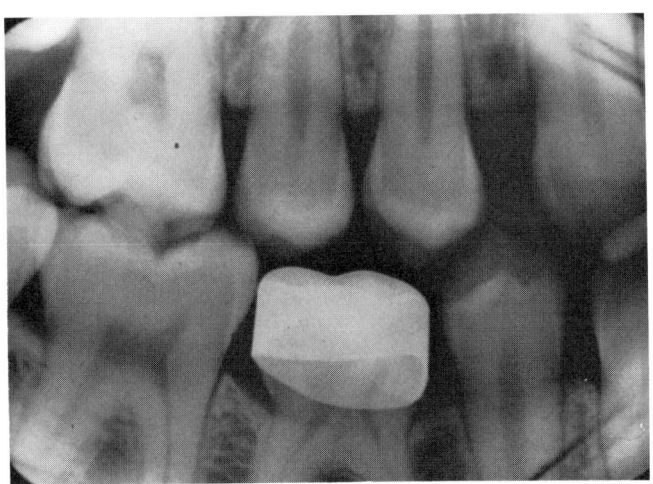

Figure 3-154 Use of a stainless steel crown to increase the height of an ankylosed molar and maintain arch length. This is advisable when the bicuspid is developmentally missing.

Figure 3-155 A cast gold crown can be constructed on an ankylosed primary molar, as shown here, to maintain arch length and occlusion. It is advisable to defer this type of restoration until vertical growth is attained, usually at 14 to 15 years of age.

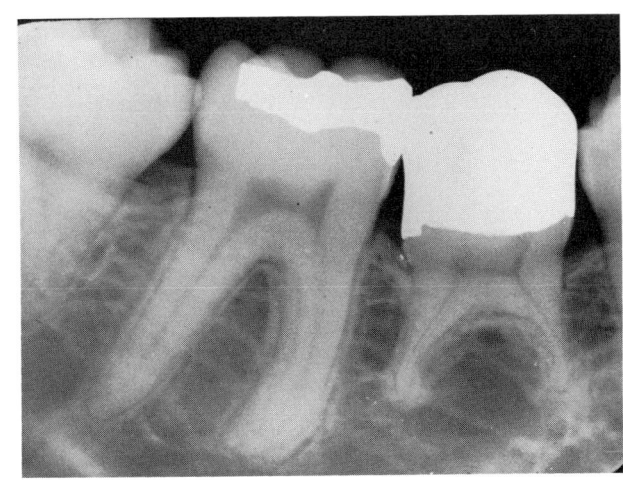

ANOMALIES OF THE DENTITION

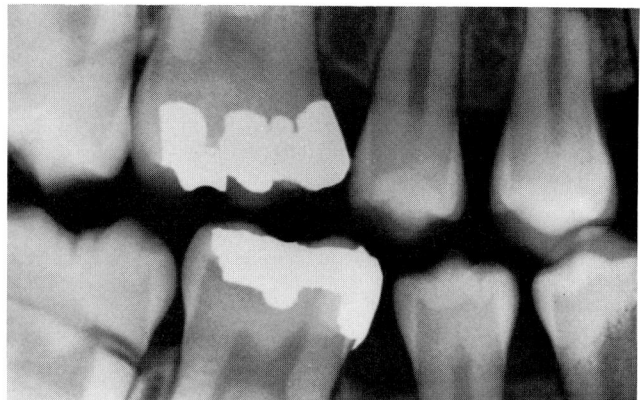

Figure 3-156 Permanent teeth seldom become ankylosed during the childhood years. This maxillary first permanent molar became ankylosed when the child was 12 years old, and was well below the line of occlusion by age 14, necessitating restorative treatment.

Figure 3-157 Same patient as seen in Figure 3-156, 2 years later. The extent of vertical bone growth that occurred during this period is indicated by the discrepancy in the line of occlusion and the occlusal relationship of the ankylosed tooth.

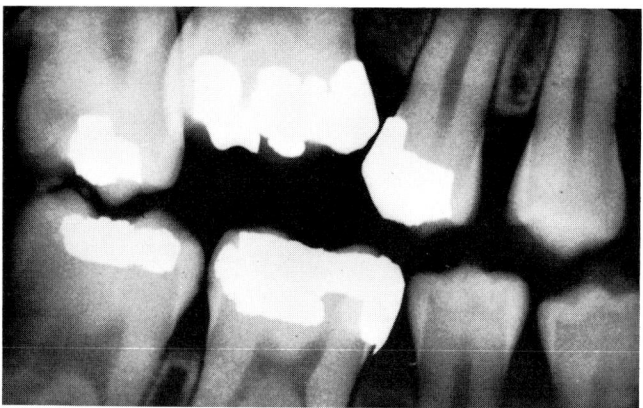

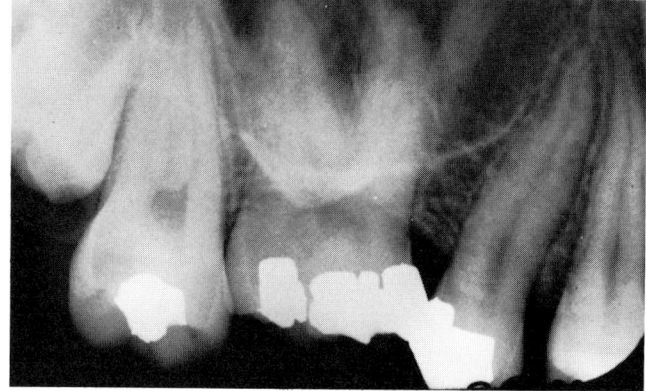

Figure 3-158 Periapical radiograph of ankylosed permanent molar shown in Figure 3-157. The exact areas of ankylosis cannot be detected.

Figure 3-159 Treatment of ankylosed permanent molar by construction of full cast gold crown, which has restored proper occlusion.

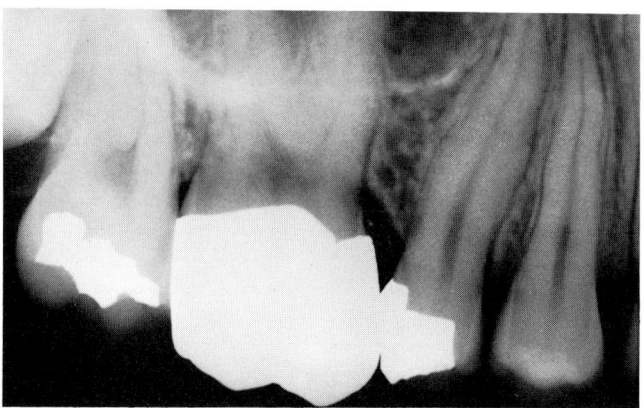

References

1. Blayney, J. R., and Hill, I. A.: Fluorine and dental caries. In Congenitally Missing Teeth. Special issue, J.A.D.A. *74*:298-299, Jan., 1967.
2. Bodenhoff, J.: Dentitio connatalis et neonatilis. Odont. Tidskrift. 67:645-695, 1959.
3. Brown, H. R., and Cunningham, U. M.: Some dental manifestations in mongolism. Oral Surgery *14*:664-676, 1961.
4. Castaldi, C. R., *et al.*: Incidence of congenital anomalies in permanent teeth of a group of Canadian children aged 6-9. J. Canad. Dent. Assoc. *32*:154-159, March, 1966.
5. Clayton, J. M.: Congenital dental anomalies occurring in 3,557 children. J. Dent. Child. *23*:206-208, 1956.
6. Grahnen, H.: Hypodontia in the permanent dentition. Odont. Revy. 7:Suppl. 3, 1956.
7. Grahnen, H., and Granath, L.: Numerical variations in the primary dentition and their correlation with the permanent dentition. Odont. Revy. *4*:348-357, 1961.
8. Menczer, L. F.: Anomalies of the primary dentition. J. Dent. Child. *22*:57, 1955.
9. Rushton, M.: A new form of dentinal dysplasia: shell teeth. Oral Surg. Oral Med. Oral Path. 7:543-549, May, 1954.
10. Witkop, C. J., Jr.: Genetics and dentistry. Eugenics Qtrly. 5:15-21, 1959.

RADIOGRAPHY

Chapter 4

Pedodontic diagnosis and treatment should be based upon a thorough clinical and radiographic examination. The radiographic technique should be practical in regard to useful information gained by the dentist, the safety and comfort of the patient, and the time required to perform such a survey.

If the child is cooperative at the first appointment, necessary radiographs can be obtained at this time. If the child is not cooperative, the procedure is best postponed until the second or even third appointment. Consultation and treatment are best withheld until good radiographs are available. Experience has indicated that if a child is cooperative in the filming of such a survey, then he is usually amenable to other dental treatment. The opposite is true also. Frequently the dentist bypasses the radiographic examination in his haste to begin operative treatment, or feels that his patient lacks the ability to tolerate such a survey. The dentist's error in neglecting this step in good diagnostic procedure often results not only in a poor diagnosis but also in future management problems.

The radiograph is a diagnostic tool which should be employed judiciously. First, every effort should be utilized to reduce the amount of radiation exposure to the minimum. Second, good radiographs may be particularly difficult to obtain in small children and it is necessary therefore to use a simple technique and have a specific reason for taking each view. The routine radiographic examination of a child below the age of 3 years generally does not necessitate the use of bitewing films, since the teeth in the posterior segment of the mouth usually are separated from each other.

It is desirable to make a complete dental radiographic survey of the child's primary and developing permanent dentition as soon as it is practicable. In a very young child, intraoral films, for which the cooperation of the patient is required in holding the film with a finger or a mechanical device, may be impractical. In such cases the lateral jaw or panoramic view may be the only one possible. By 4 or 5 years of age, the molars have generally come into contact with each other and thus bitewing films are necessary.

On the other hand, in mixed and permanent dentitions, clear apical views of all the teeth are desirable. Similarly, if all of the child's permanent teeth have erupted, periapical views are essential.

The following outline summarizes the radiographic views that are desirable in a routine radiographic examination of children of various ages.

SUMMARY OF SUGGESTED RADIOGRAPHIC VIEWS*

AGE	VIEW	NO. OF FILMS	TOTAL NO. OF FILMS
2-3 Years	Maxillary occlusal	1	
	Mandibular occlusal	1	
	Right lateral jaw	1	
	Left lateral jaw	1	4
	or		
	Panoramic	1	1
3-5 Years	Maxillary occlusal	1	
	Mandibular occlusal	1	
	Right lateral jaw	1	
	Left lateral jaw	1	
	Right bitewing	1	
	Left bitewing	1	6
	or		
	Panoramic	1	
	Right bitewing	1	
	Left bitewing	1	3
Mixed dentition	Maxillary central	1	
	Maxillary right cuspid	1	
	Maxillary left cuspid	1	
	Maxillary right primary molar	1	
	Maxillary left primary molar	1	
	Mandibular central	1	
	Mandibular right cuspid	1	
	Mandibular left cuspid	1	
	Mandibular right primary molar	1	
	Mandibular left primary molar	1	
	Right bitewing	1	
	Left bitewing	1	12
	or		
	Panoramic	1	
	Right bitewing	1	
	Left bitewing	1	3

*In practice the number of views necessary will vary depending on clinical findings.

Precautions for the patient's safety may be taken as follows: use shielded equipment that is in good working order, have patient wear a lead apron, and use film that produces the least possible exposure. The size of the film is determined only by the size of the child's mouth; the largest film possible is the most desirable one.*

Considerations† in taking dental radiographs are as follows:

1. The tip of the cone should always touch the face lightly.
2. The sagittal plane must be perpendicular to the floor.
3. The film must be placed tightly against the tissue.
4. For the incisor views, maxillary and mandibular, the crowns of the centrals should be perpendicular to the floor.
5. For posterior and canine views, the mean occlusal plane of the teeth to be exposed is placed parallel to the floor.
6. Gagging can be avoided by having patient breathe through nose.

*Some of the material in this chapter has been adapted from techniques suggested by Dr. Richard C. O'Brien in his *Dental Radiography*, W. B. Saunders Co., Philadelphia, 1966.
†Suggested by Dr. F. Lloyd Jacobson.

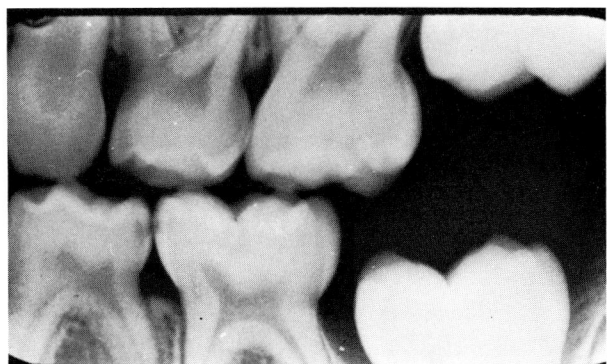

Figure 4-1 Bitewing radiograph (used primarily for caries evaluation).

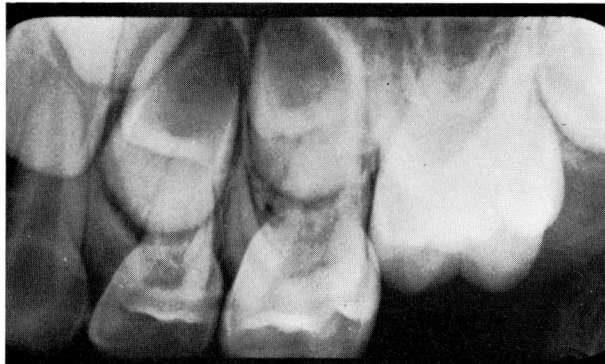

Figure 4-2 Periapical radiograph (used for evaluation of supporting structures and erupted and unerupted teeth).

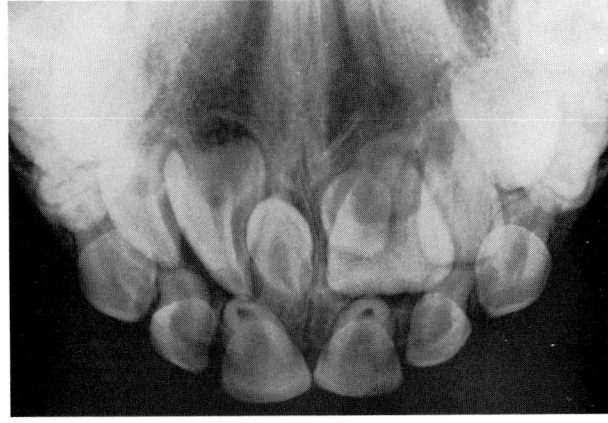

Figure 4-3 Occlusal radiograph (used for evaluation of supporting structures and erupted and unerupted teeth in the anterior dental arch, exposes a larger area than does the periapical view). A good exposure for young children whose maxillary or mandibular incisors have been subjected to trauma.

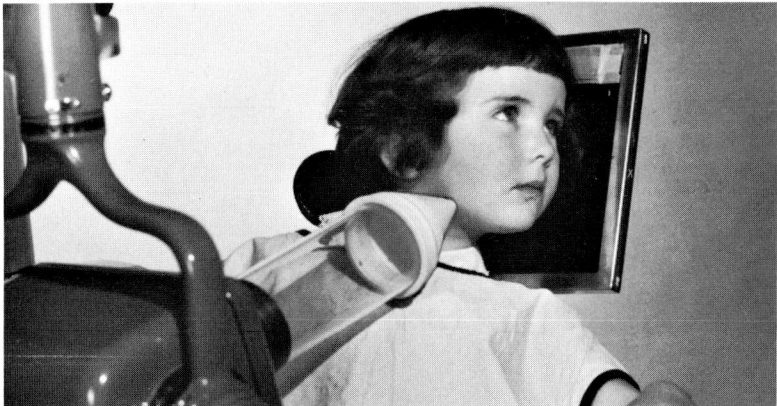

Figure 4-4 Position for taking a lateral jaw radiograph (used for evaluation of supporting structures and erupted and unerupted teeth in the posterior dental arch, exposes a larger area than does the periapical view). Frequently young children will tolerate this procedure better than a series of periapical views.

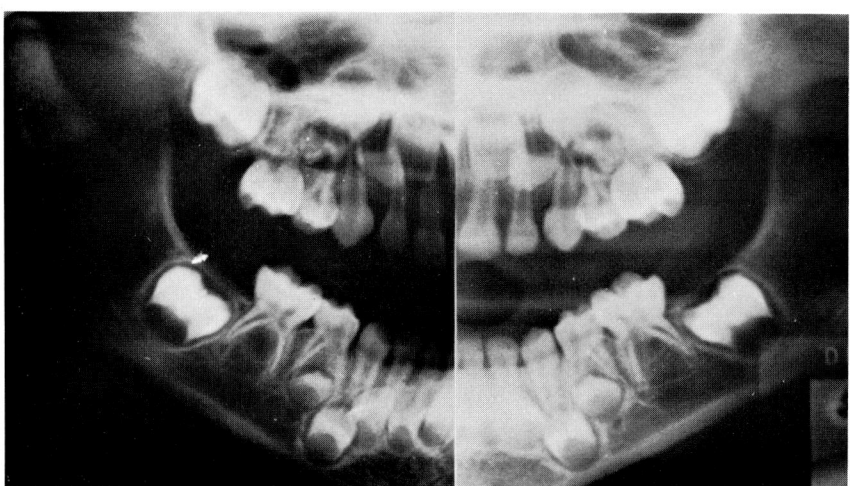

Figure 4-5 Panoramic radiograph (one exposure used for evaluation of supporting structures and erupted and unerupted teeth).

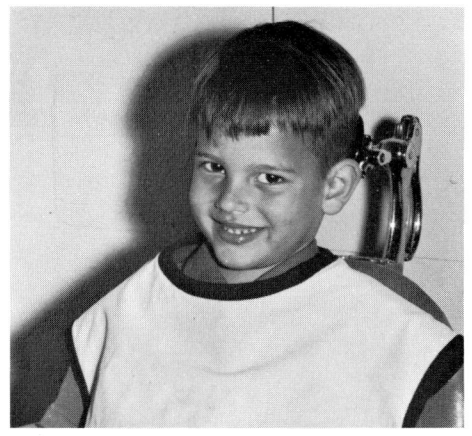

Figure 4-6 Lead apron worn by patient during radiographic examination.

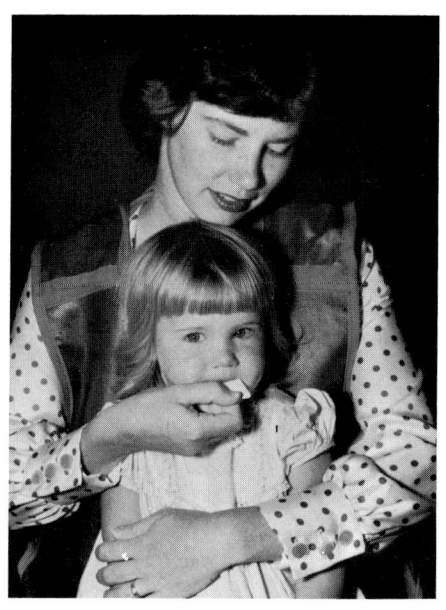

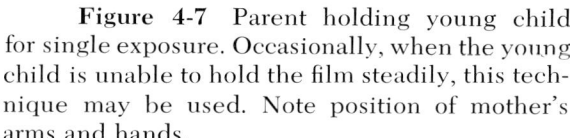

Figure 4-7 Parent holding young child for single exposure. Occasionally, when the young child is unable to hold the film steadily, this technique may be used. Note position of mother's arms and hands.

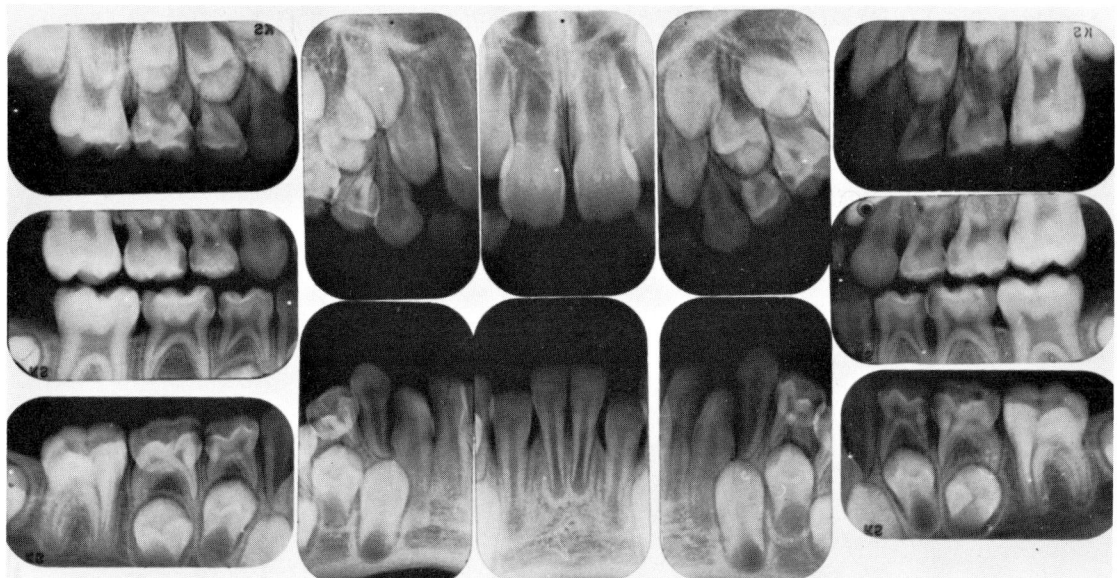

Figure 4-8 The suggested radiographic series for children under 12 years of age (10 periapical, and two bitewing exposures).

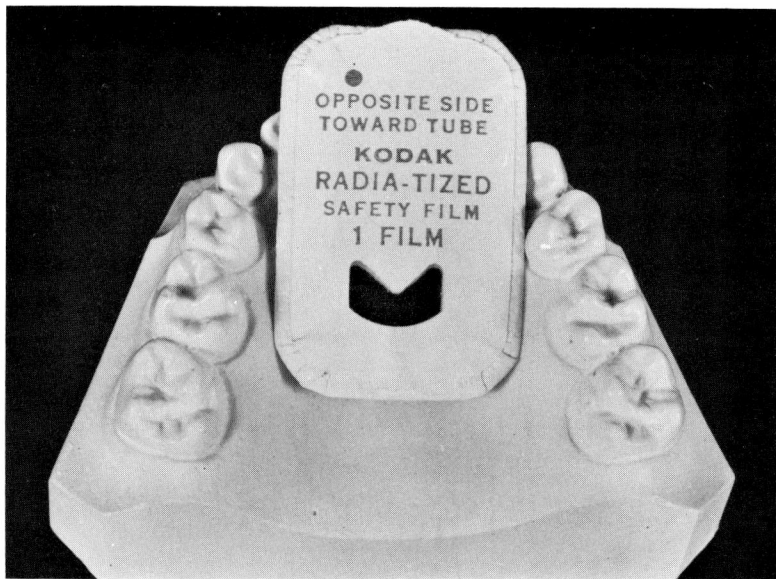

Figure 4-9 Placement of film for exposure of maxillary central and lateral incisors.

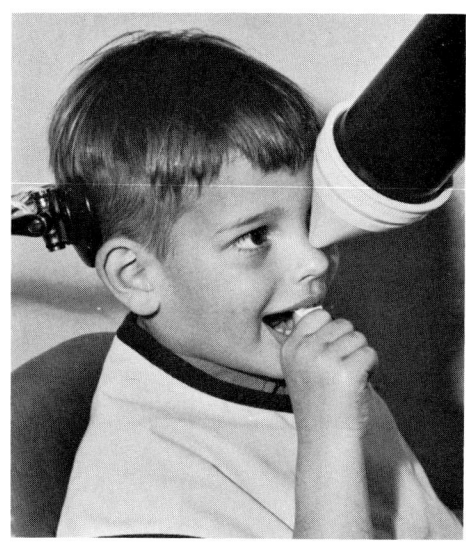

Figure 4-10 Angulation of cone in relation to patient and film for exposure of maxillary central and lateral incisors. The approximate vertical cone angulation is +45°.

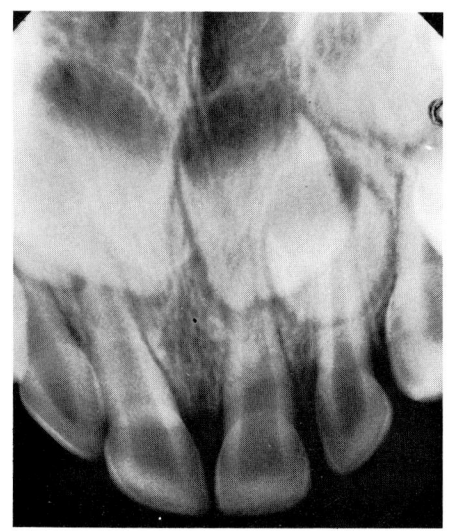

Figure 4-11 Resulting radiograph of maxillary central and lateral incisors.

RADIOGRAPHY

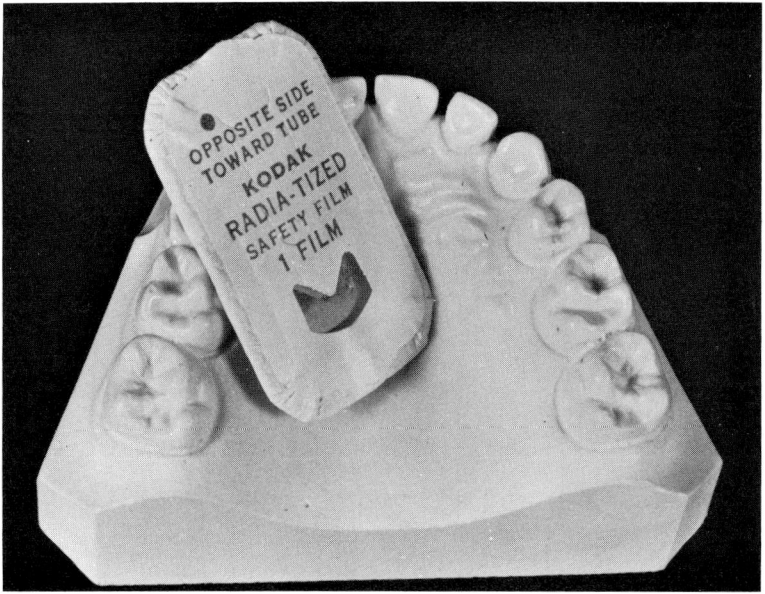

Figure 4-12 Placement of film for exposure of maxillary cuspid area.

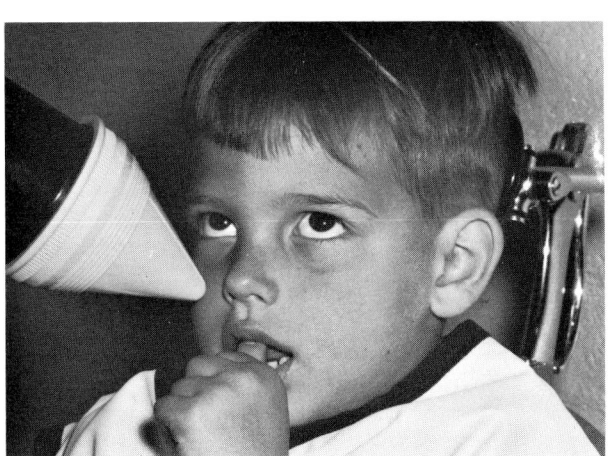

Figure 4-13 Angulation of cone in relation to patient and film for exposure of maxillary cuspid area. The approximate vertical cone angulation is +45°.

Figure 4-14 Resulting radiograph of maxillary cuspid area.

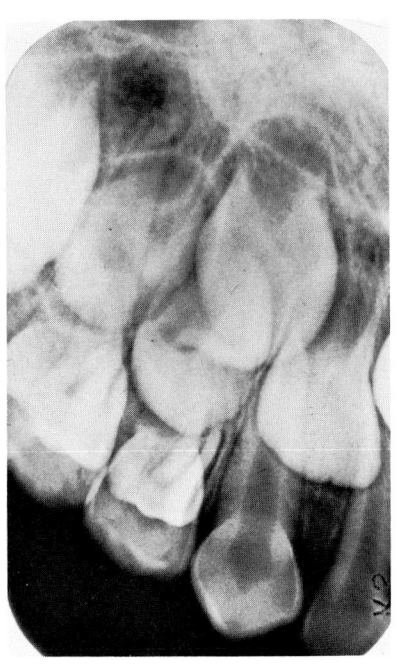

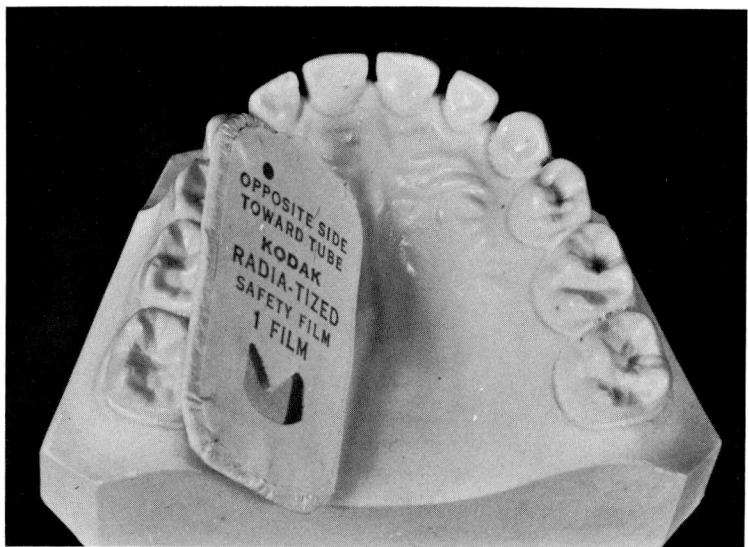

Figure 4-15 Placement of film for exposure of maxillary posterior area.

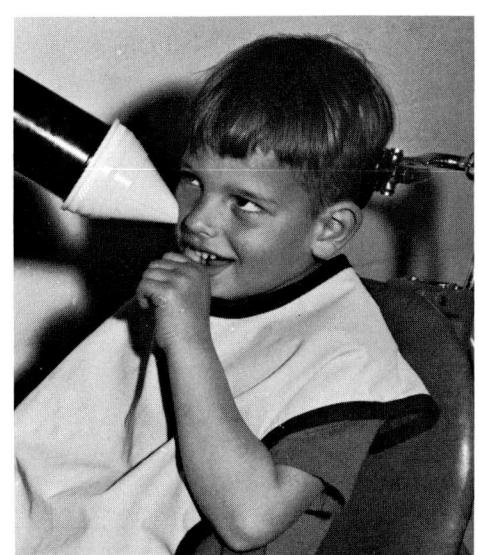

Figure 4-16 Angulation of cone in relation to patient and film for exposure of maxillary posterior area. The approximate vertical cone angulation is +35°.

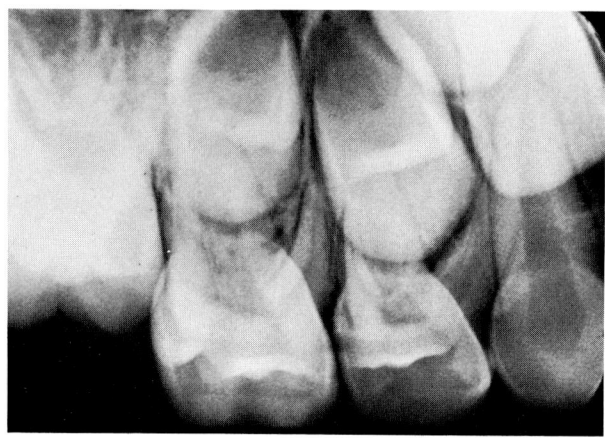

Figure 4-17 Resulting radiograph of maxillary posterior area.

RADIOGRAPHY

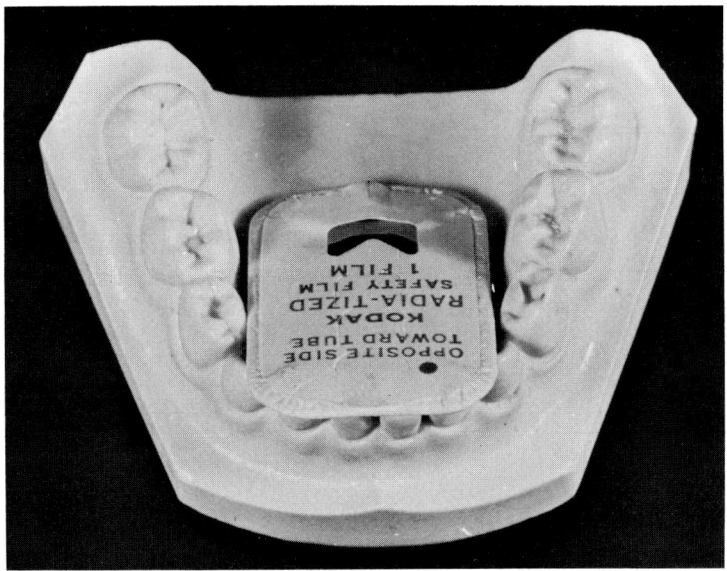

Figure 4-18 Placement of film for exposure of mandibular central and lateral incisors.

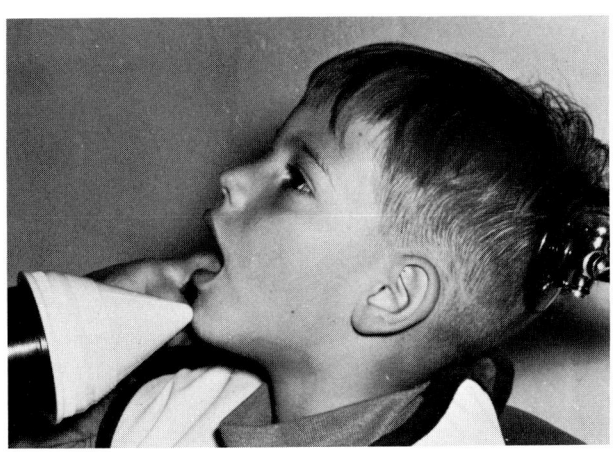

Figure 4-19 Angulation of cone in relation to patient and film for exposure of mandibular central and lateral incisors. The approximate vertical cone angulation is −20°.

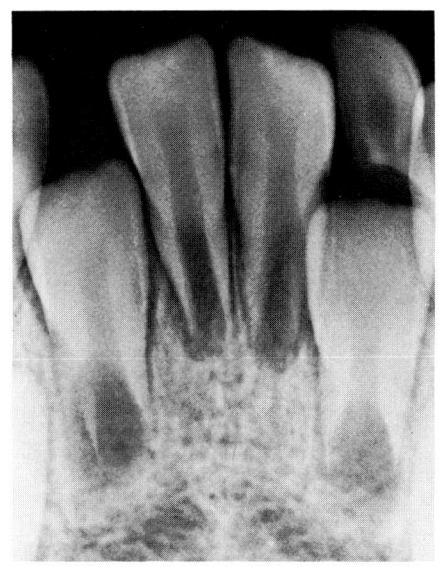

Figure 4-20 Resulting radiograph of mandibular central and lateral incisors.

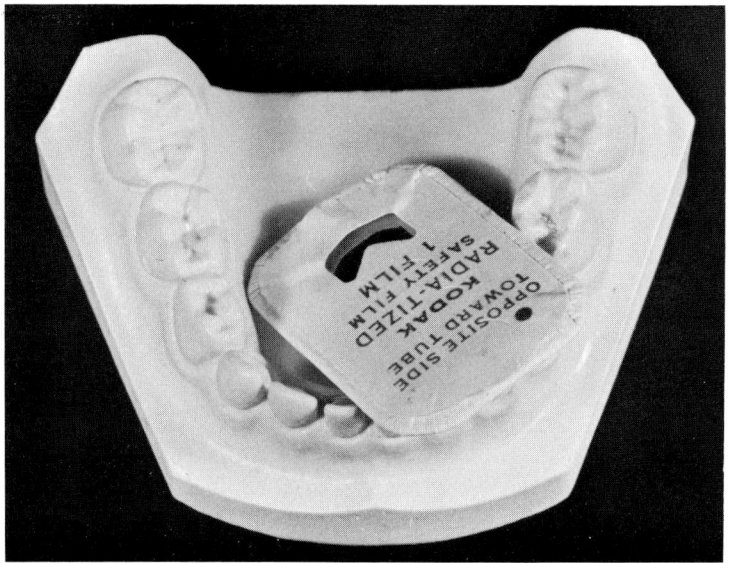

Figure 4-21 Placement of film for exposure of mandibular cuspid area.

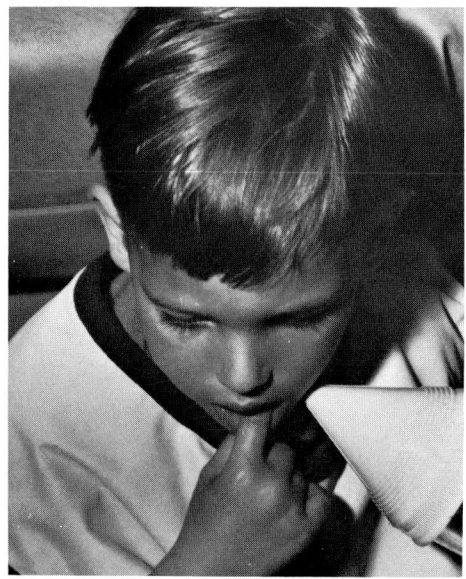

Figure 4-22 Angulation of cone in relation to patient and film for exposure of mandibular cuspid area. The approximate vertical cone angulation is −25°.

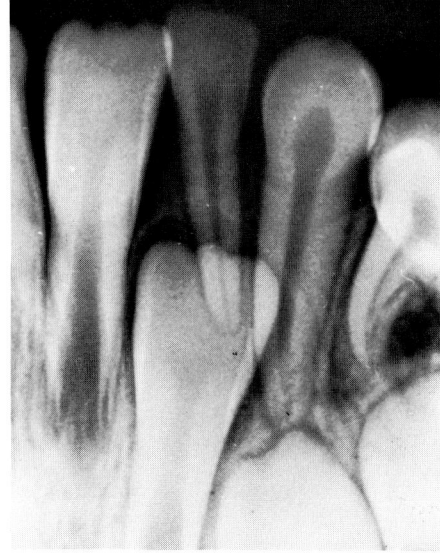

Figure 4-23 Resulting radiograph of mandibular cuspid area.

RADIOGRAPHY

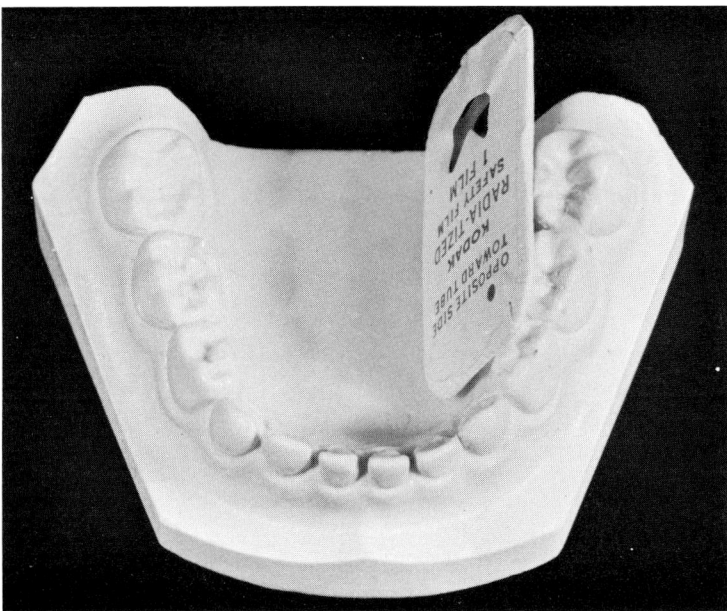

Figure 4-24   Placement of film for exposure of mandibular posterior area.

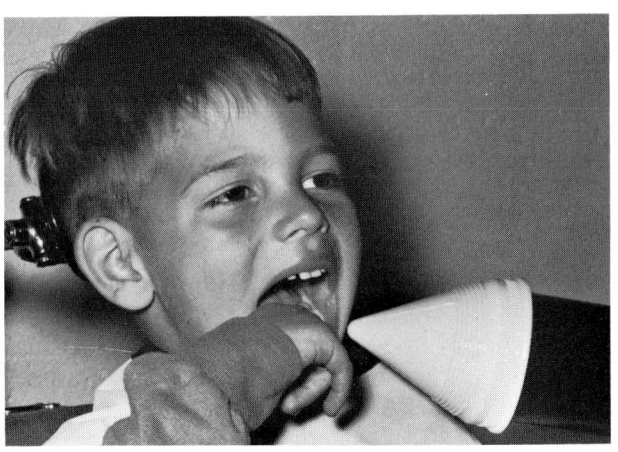

Figure 4-25   Angulation of cone in relation to patient and film for exposure of mandibular posterior area. The approximate vertical cone angulation is −15°.

Figure 4-26   Resulting radiograph of mandibular posterior area.

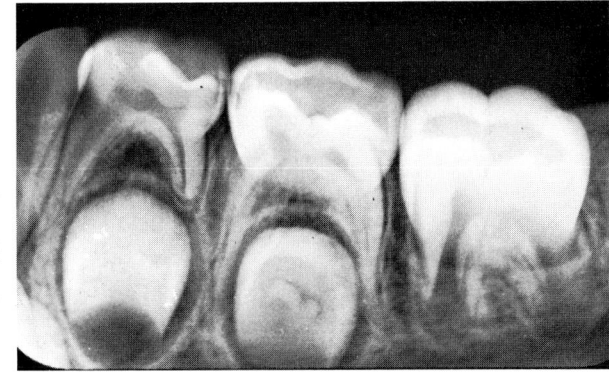

124 RADIOGRAPHY

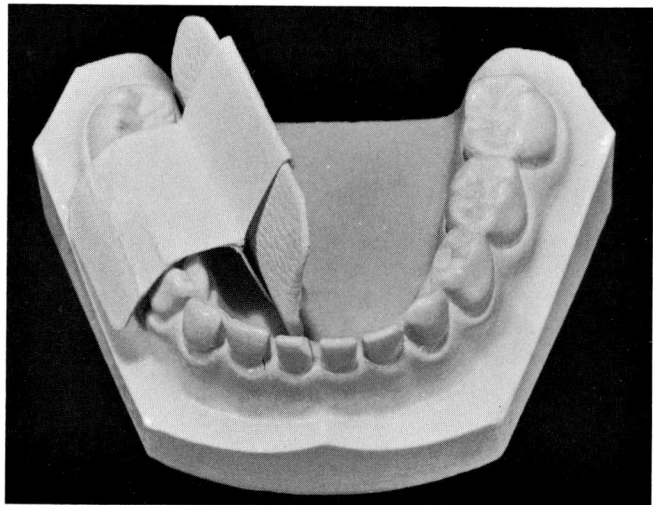

Figure 4-27 Placement of film for posterior bitewing exposure.

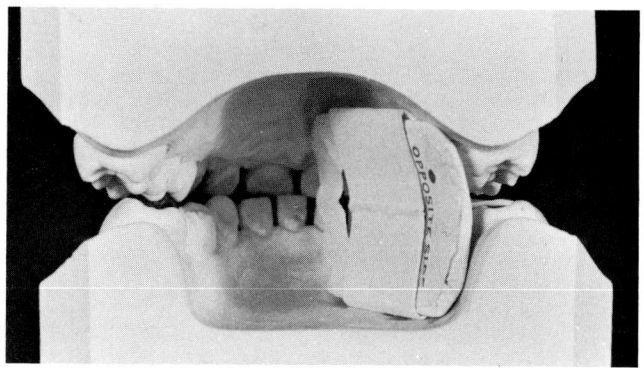

Figure 4-28 Placement of film for posterior bitewing exposure with teeth in occlusion.

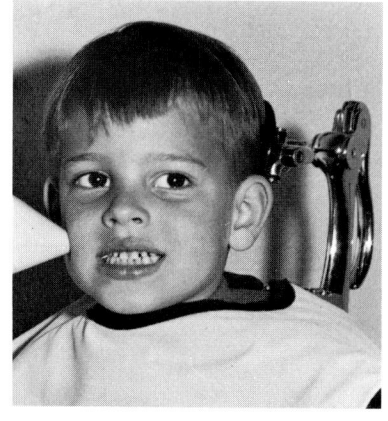

Figure 4-29 Angulation of cone in relation to patient and film for posterior bitewing exposure. The approximate vertical cone angulation is +10°.

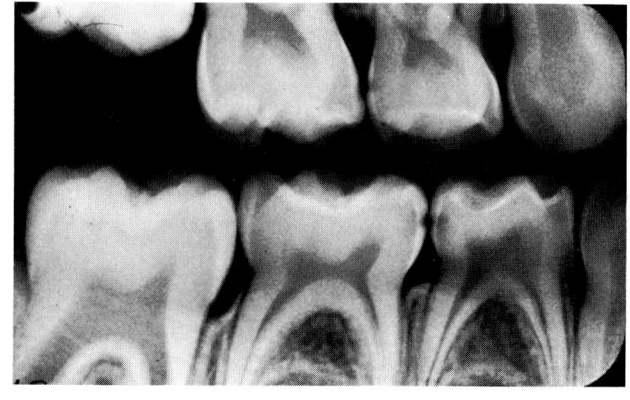

Figure 4-30 Resulting radiograph of posterior bitewing exposure.

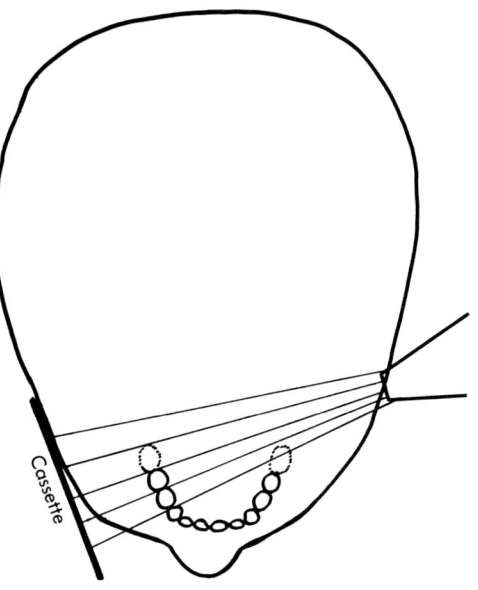

Figure 4-31 Diagrammatic sketch of patient illustrating placement of film and horizontal cone angulation for a lateral jaw exposure. (From O'Brien, R. C.: *Dental Radiography*, 1966, p. 104.)

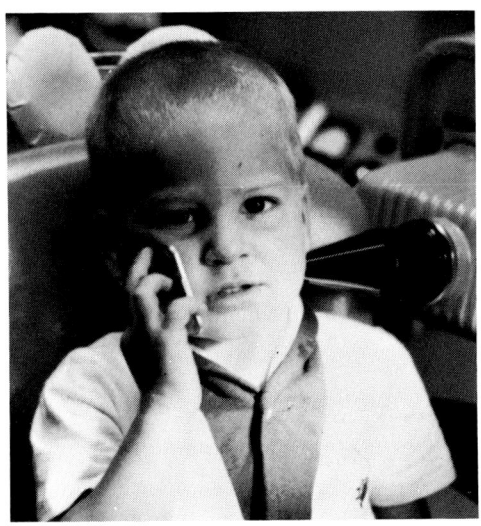

Figure 4-32 Correct position of the patient, film, and cone tip for a lateral jaw exposure. (From O'Brien, R. C.: *Dental Radiography*, 1966, p. 104.)

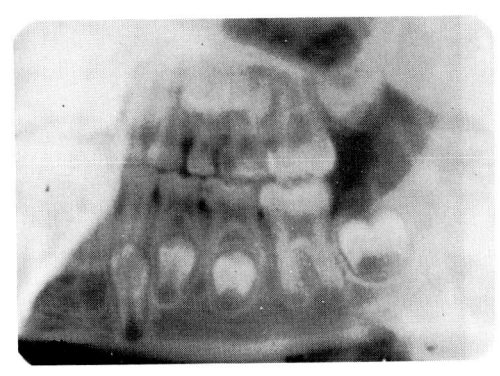

Figure 4-33 Resulting radiograph of a lateral jaw exposure. (From O'Brien, R. C.: *Dental Radiography*, 1966, p. 104.)

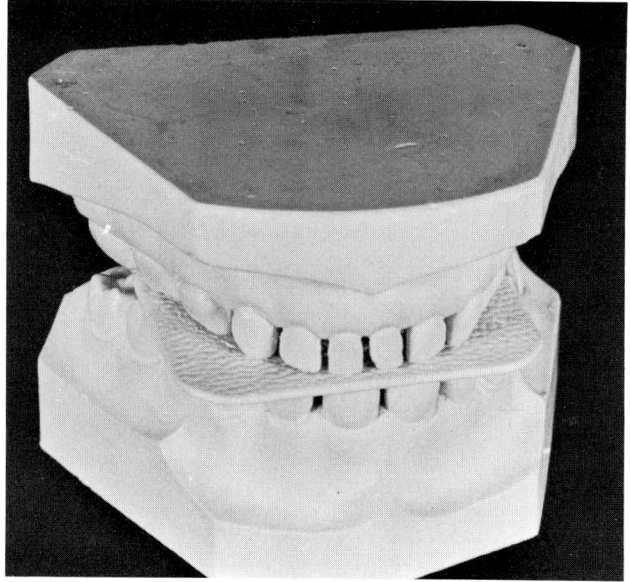

Figure 4-34 Placement of film for maxillary occlusal exposure.

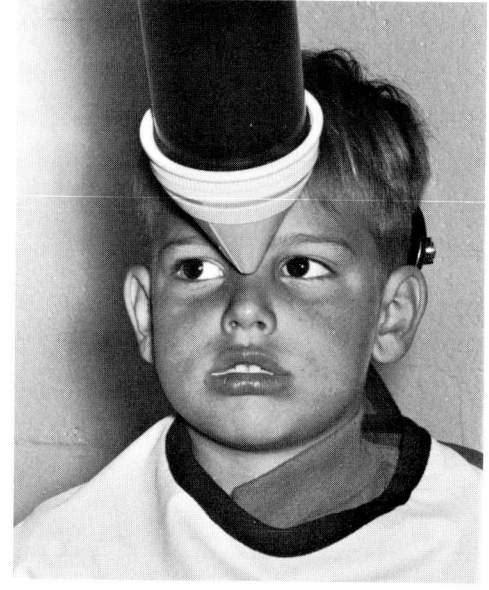

Figure 4-35 Angulation of cone in relation to patient and film for maxillary occlusal exposure. The approximate vertical cone angulation is +65°.

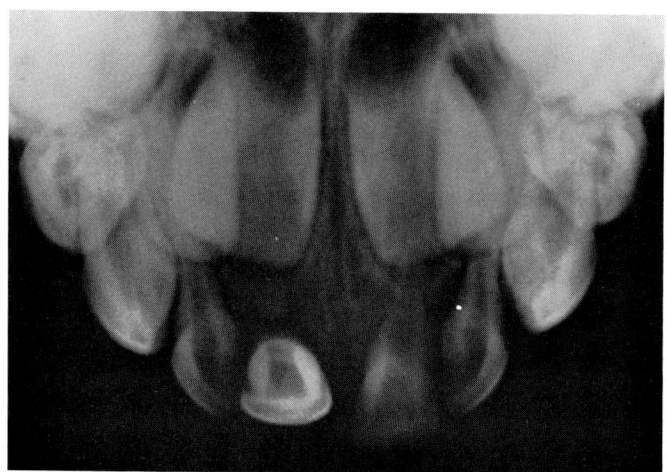

Figure 4-36 Resulting radiograph of maxillary occlusal exposure.

RADIOGRAPHY 127

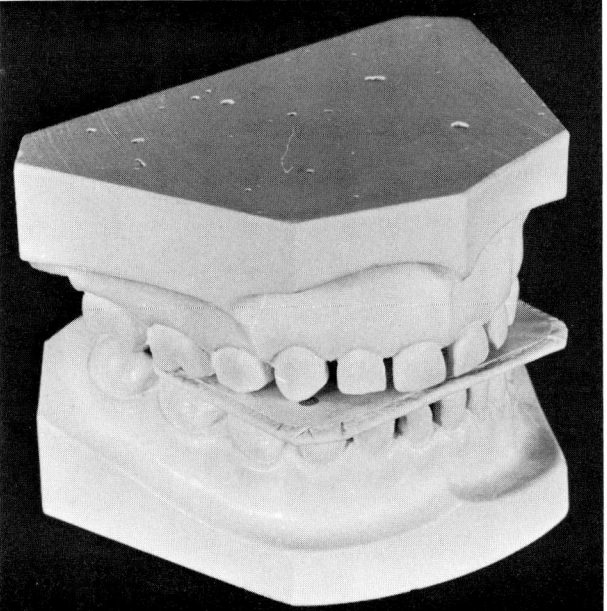

Figure 4-37 Placement of film for mandibular occlusal exposure.

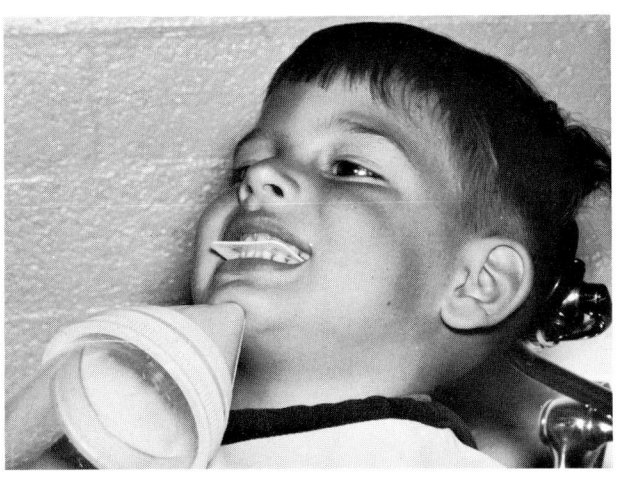

Figure 4-38 Angulation of cone in relation to patient and film for mandibular occlusal exposure. The vertical cone angulation for this exposure is dependent on how far back the patient's head is tipped. The film and cone should be in approximately this relation.

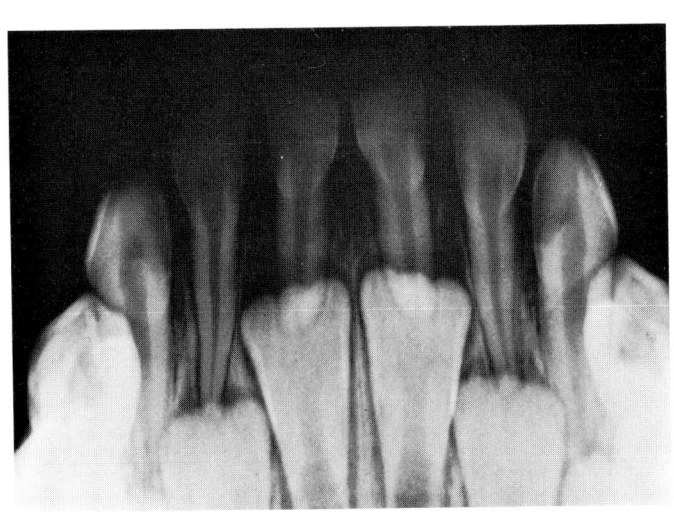

Figure 4-39 Resulting radiograph of mandibular occlusal exposure.

128 RADIOGRAPHY

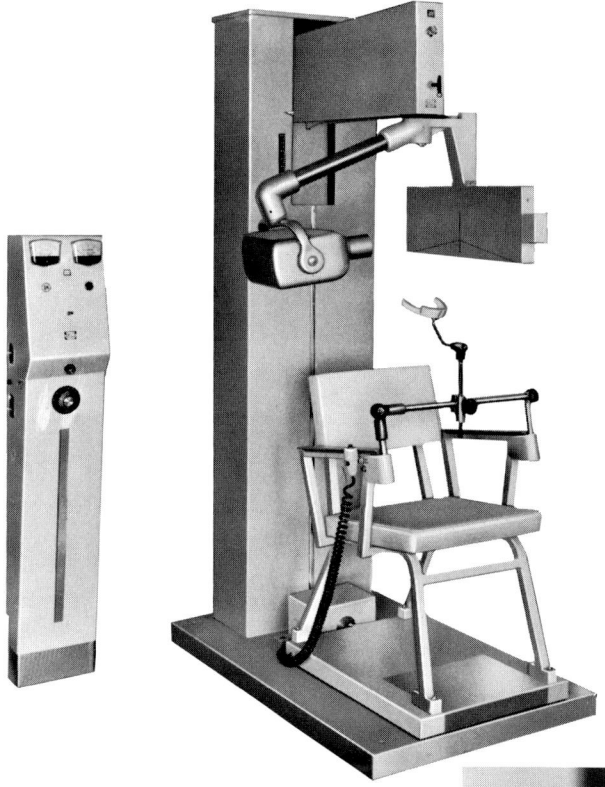

Figure 4-40 Panoramic x-ray unit.

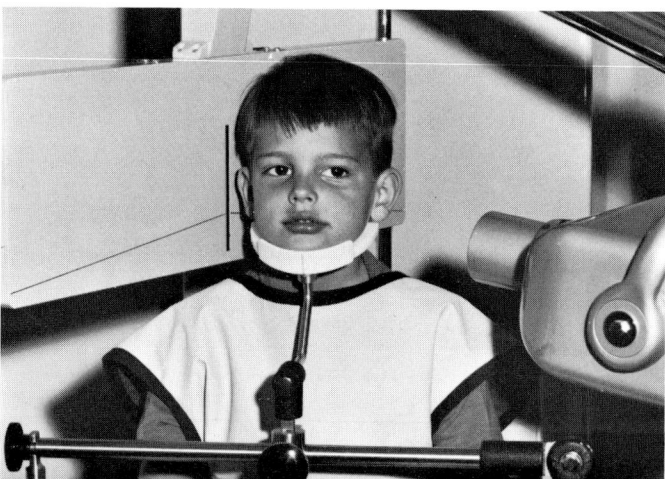

Figure 4-41 Child seated in panoramic x-ray unit prior to exposure.

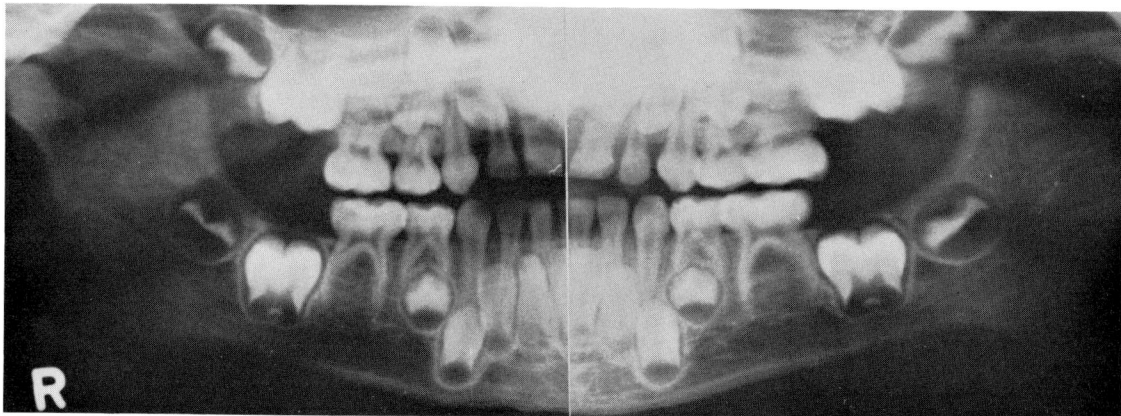

Figure 4-42 Resulting panoramic radiographic exposure.

RADIOGRAPHY 129

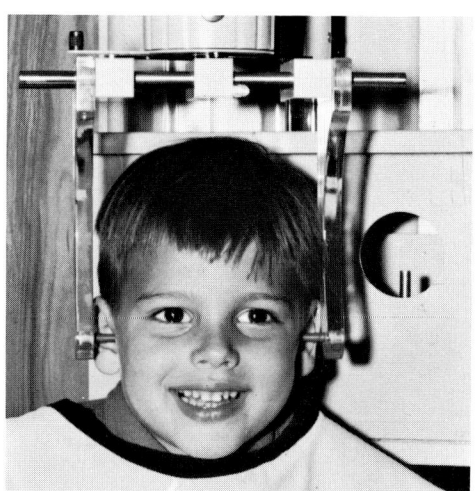

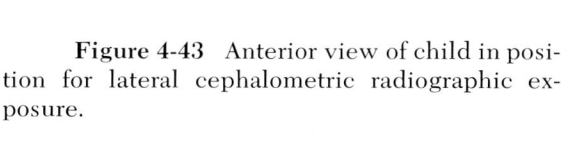
Figure 4-43 Anterior view of child in position for lateral cephalometric radiographic exposure.

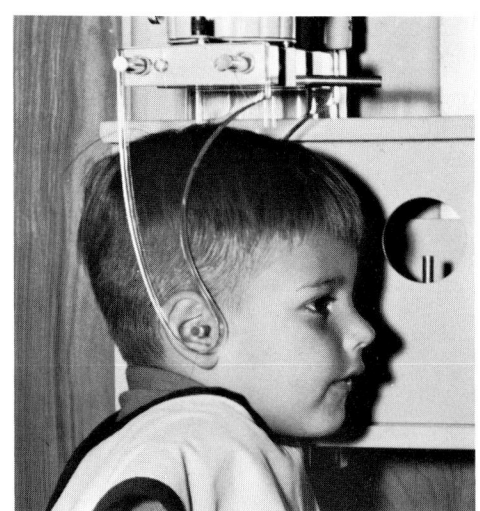

Figure 4-44 Lateral view of child in position for lateral cephalometric radiographic exposure.

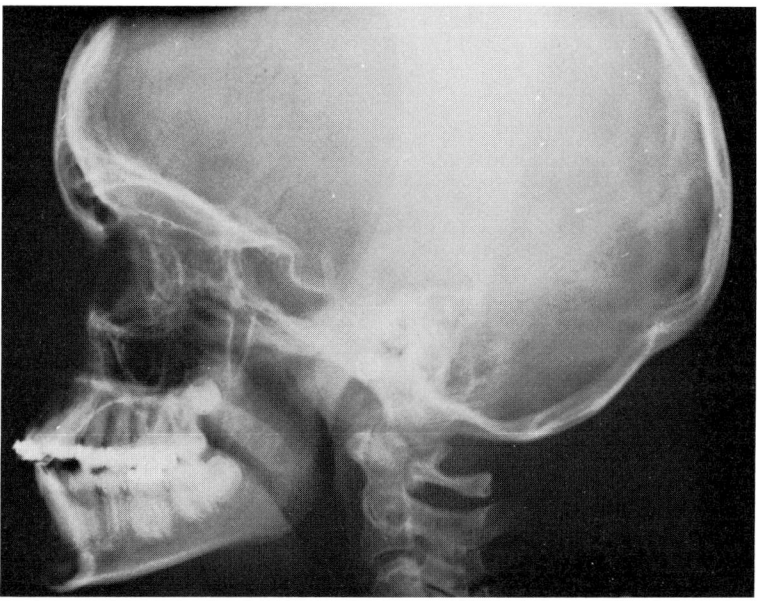

Figure 4-45 Lateral cephalometric radiograph (used primarily for growth evaluation).

CARIES PREVENTION

Chapter 5

Caries control is an essential part of the practice of preventive dentistry in children. It is especially important that the dentist keep abreast of scientific advances in this area if he is to offer the best service to his patients. Recent research has reinforced certain observations about the role of sugars, particularly sucrose, in the production of carious lesions. The utmost effort should therefore be made to educate parents and children on the need for children to curtail their consumption of foods with high sugar content, particularly cookies, candies, jams, jellies, and other adhesive carbohydrates. Frequency of eating can be a decisive factor in rampant caries as can the habit of eating before bedtime.

The importance of the dental plaque in the caries process has likewise received renewed attention. Oral hygiene procedures correctly taught and practiced after mealtimes can help to reduce plaque accumulation on accessible surfaces.

The use of fluorides probably represents the most promising approach to caries control when incorporated in a program that also includes sugar restriction and emphasis on oral hygiene. Community water fluoridation provides the most effective means for fluoride ingestion during the formative years. If it is not available, the dentist should prescribe a daily dietary supplement of fluoride. It is recommended that every child, whether or not he is ingesting fluoride, should have twice yearly topical treatments. Saturation of the outer enamel layer does not occur with a fluoride concentration of one part per million, and the topical treatments provide the necessary supplementation. Stannous or acidulated fluoride may be used depending on the preference of the dentist.

No preventive program will be effective unless the child is seen by the dentist on a regular and periodic basis. Recall visits permit early radiographic detection of caries, application of topical fluorides, and reinforcement of home care procedures. If the dentist first sees the child when he is between 2 and 3 years of age, and continues to see him on a semiannual basis, significant benefits will be realized. The following material illustrates the need for utilizing more than one approach to the problem of caries prevention.

Effect of Oral Hygiene on Caries Inhibition by Topical Fluoride*

	Poor Oral Hygiene (Mean DMFS)	Good Oral Hygiene (Mean DMFS)
Control, no fluoride	4.83	3.51
Fluoride treated teeth	2.70	1.41
Reduction	44%	60%

*Wellock, W. D., Maitland, A., and Brudevold, F.: Caries increments, tooth discoloration, and state of oral hygiene in children given single annual applications of acid phosphate-fluoride and stannous fluoride. Arch. Oral Biol. 10:453-460, 1965.

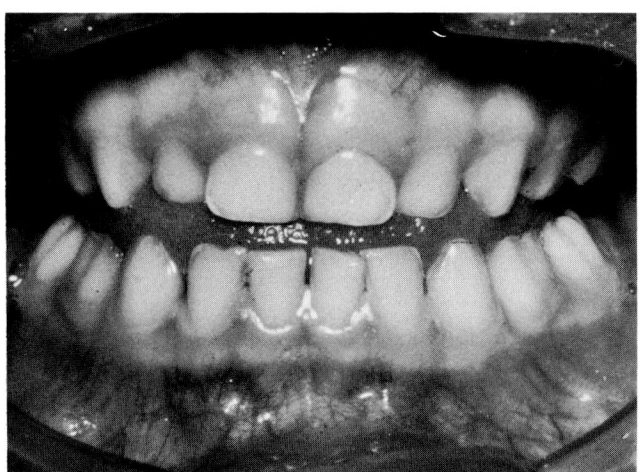

Figure 5-1 A caries-free mouth in the primary dentition. This is the goal of an adequate program of prevention started in the first years of life.

CARIES PREVENTION 133

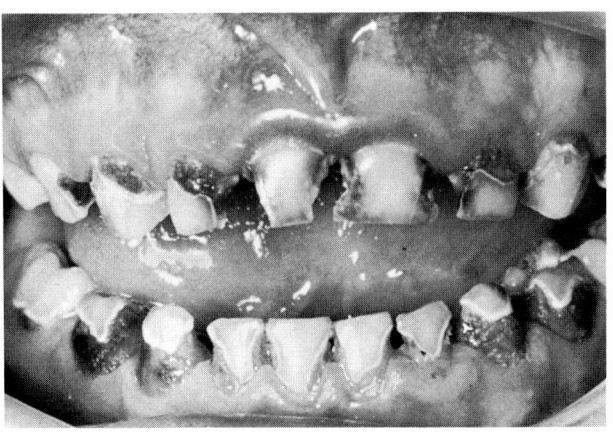

Figure 5-2 Rampant caries in the primary dentition. This condition has resulted from a combination of factors, including a high sugar diet, lack of oral hygiene, and lack of professional care and supervision.

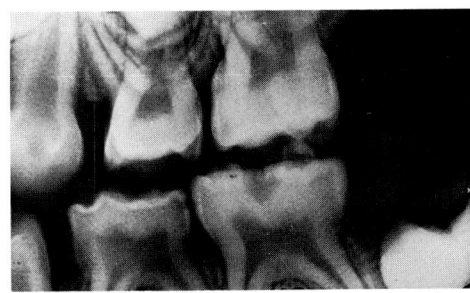

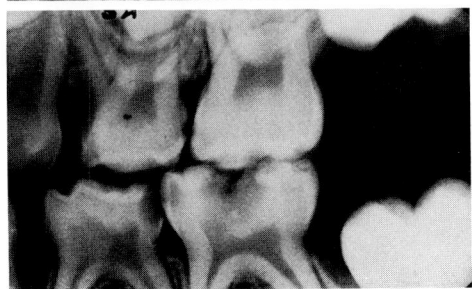

Figure 5-3 Radiographs showing 1 year's progress of carious lesions in a preschool child. Periodic recalls are essential if the child is to be kept free of serious dental problems.

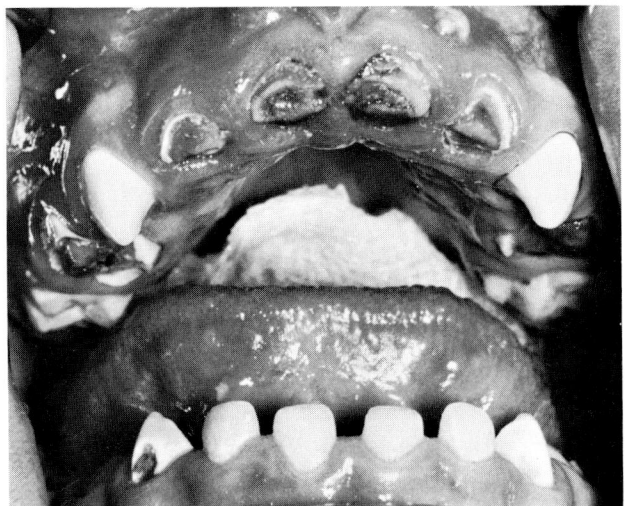

Figure 5-4 Anterior primary teeth involved with extensive carious lesions, sometimes called "baby bottle syndrome." Very young children may experience caries in these areas from prolonged sucking on a bottle containing sweetened juice. Parents should be counseled on the need to restrict consumption of sweets.

Figure 5-5 Gingival caries in the primary molars. Adequate brushing after meals will materially aid in preventing caries in such accessible areas.

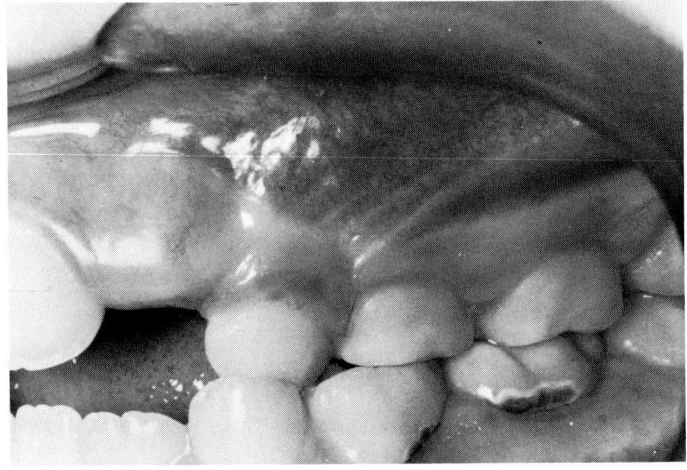

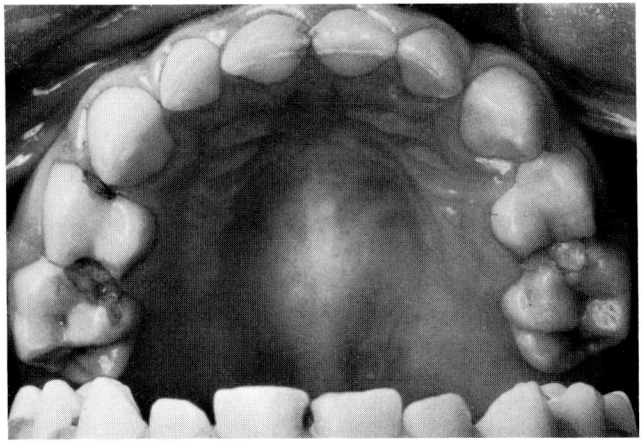

Figure 5-6 Interproximal carious lesions in the maxillary primary molars. These lesions should have been detected in the early stages of the disease and restorations placed to prevent further tooth destruction.

CARIES PREVENTION 135

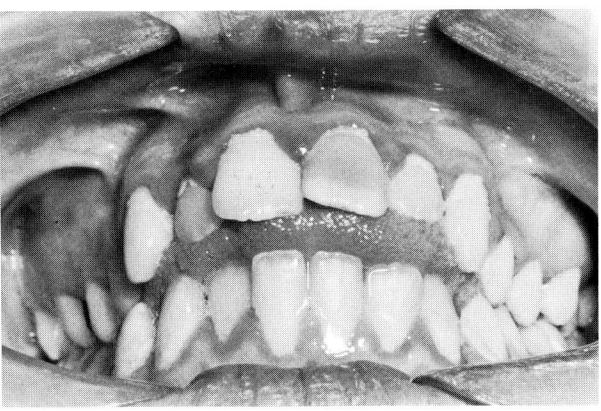

Figure 5-7 Anterior view of a teenager with poor oral hygiene practices. Note debris around gingival of maxillary incisors permitting the formation of a bacterial plaque.

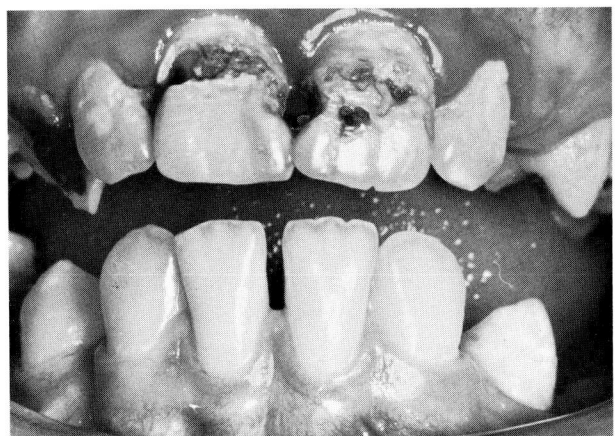

Figure 5-8 Anterior view of a teenager who neglected oral hygiene and consumed large quantities of highly cariogenic foods. Carious lesions are evident in areas easily accessible to the toothbrush.

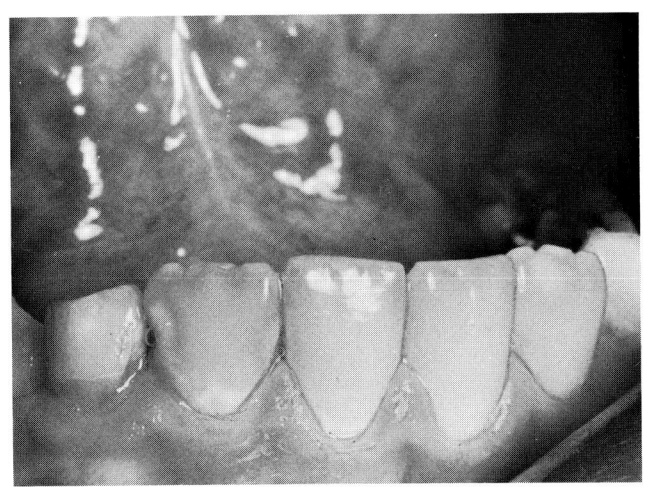

Figure 5-9 Interproximal caries in lower permanent incisors in a 9-year-old boy. These teeth are the least susceptible to caries. In such a case the child should be placed on a stringent program of oral hygiene, sugar restriction, and fluoride therapy.

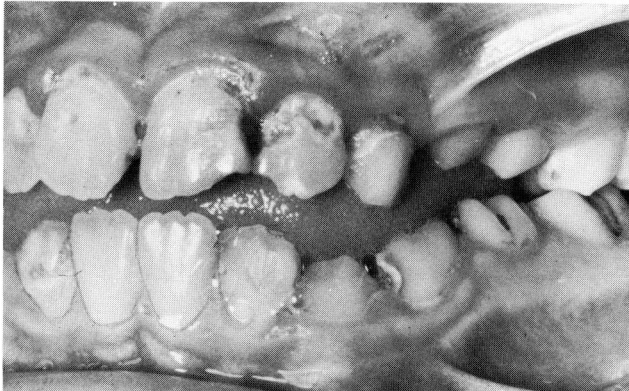

Figure 5-10 An open bite prevented this child from getting the benefit of masticatory scouring action on the left side. Increased susceptibility to caries resulted. Careful brushing of these areas is necessary.

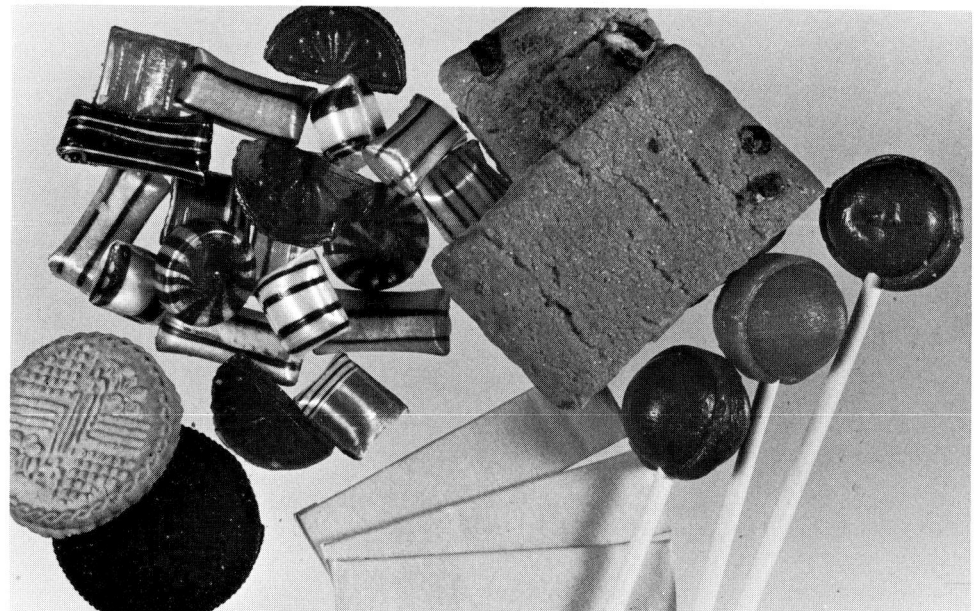

Figure 5-11 Sticky sweet foods must be restricted to help prevent caries.

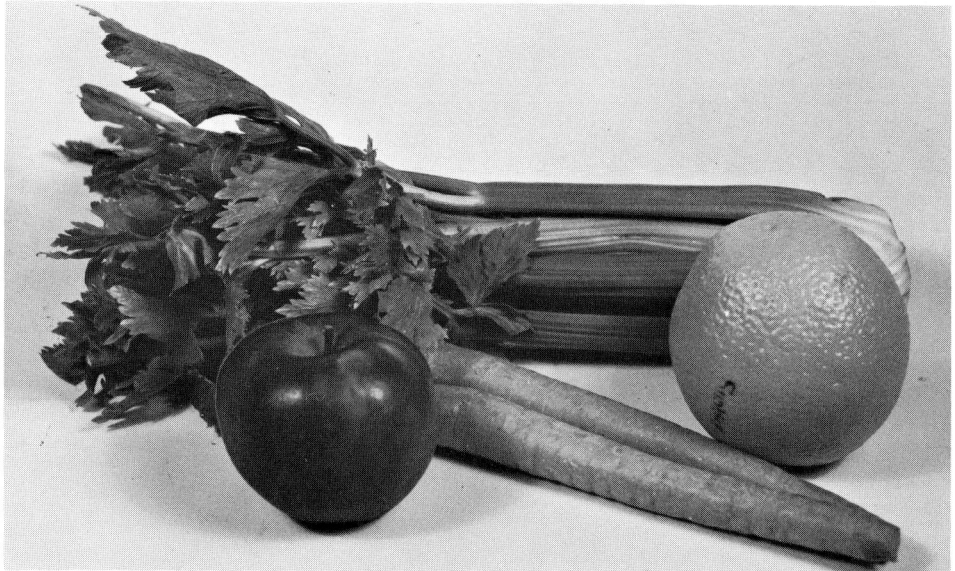

Figure 5-12 Raw vegetables and fresh fruits are acceptable substitutes for sweets and have considerable cleansing action as well.

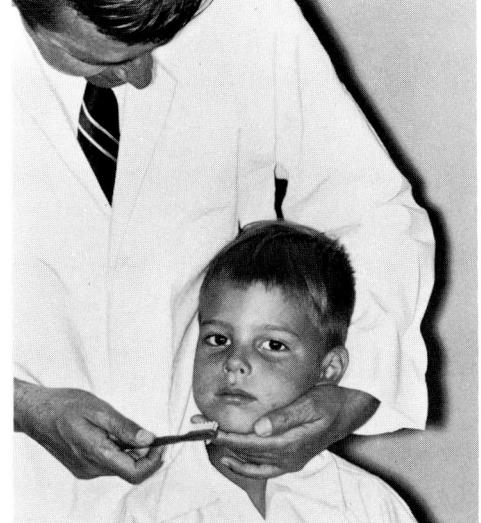

Figure 5-13 Correct position of parent and child in preparation for brushing the child's teeth. The head is cradled between the body and arm, and the fingers of the left hand retract the lips.

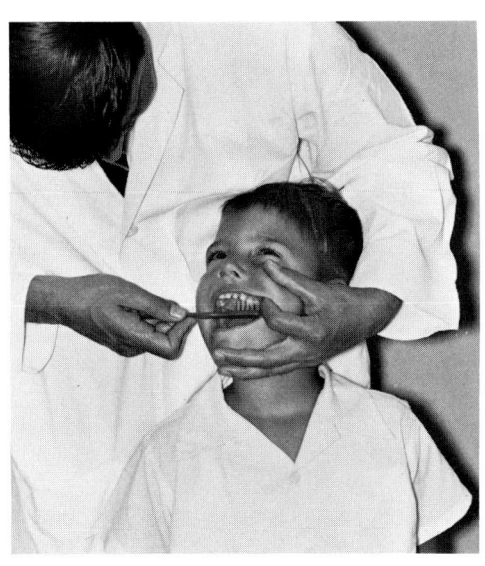

Figure 5-14 Correct position of parent and child in preparation for brushing the child's upper teeth.

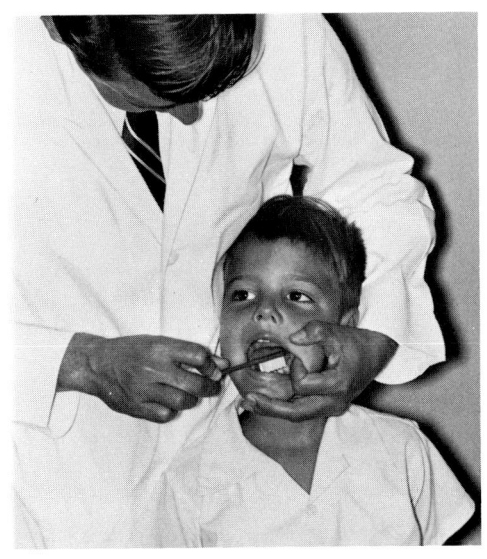

Figure 5-15 Correct position of parent and child in preparation for brushing the child's lower teeth.

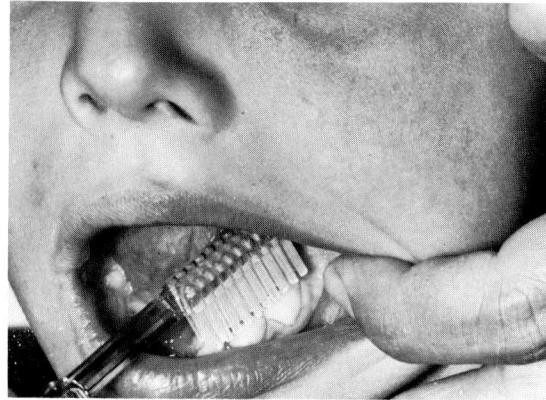

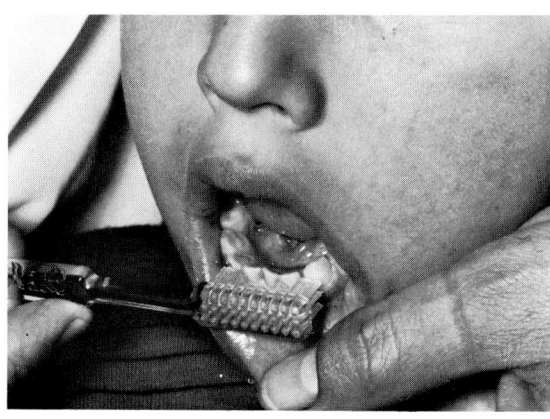

Figure 5-16 Brushing the occlusal surfaces of the lower molars.

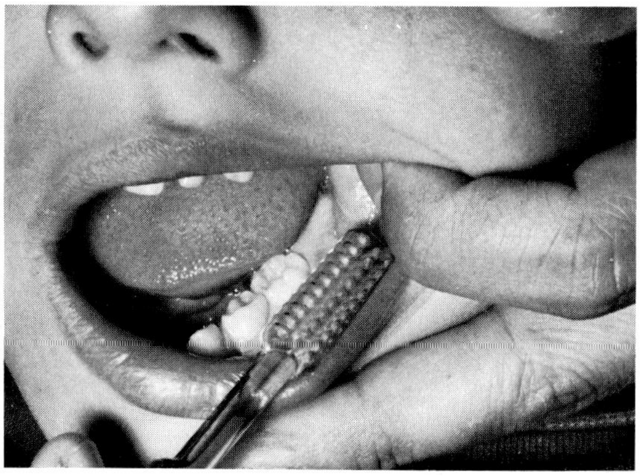

Figure 5-17 Brushing the buccal surfaces of the lower molars. Note lip retraction.

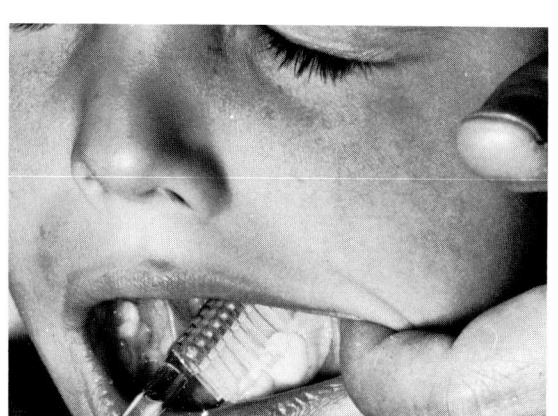

Figure 5-18 Brushing the lingual surfaces of the lower molars.

Figure 5-19 Brushing the labial surfaces of the lower incisors. Note how the lip is retracted.

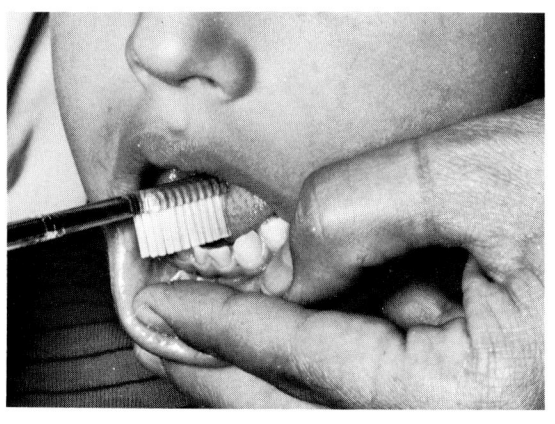

Figure 5-20 Brushing the lingual surfaces of the lower incisors.

Figure 5-21 Brushing the occlusal surfaces of the upper molars.

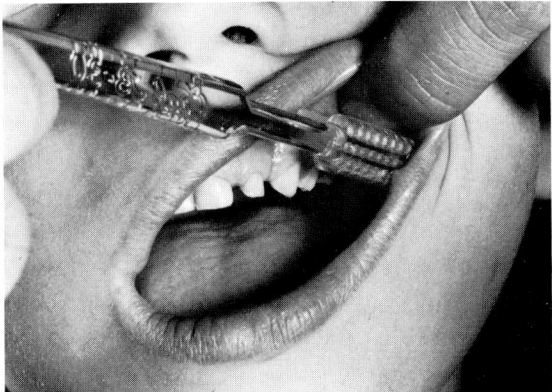

Figure 5-23 Brushing the lingual surfaces of the upper molars.

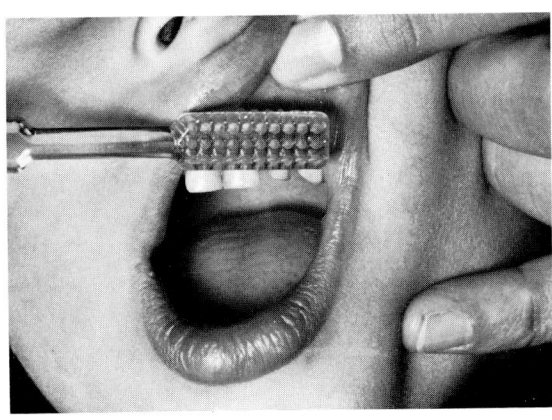

Figure 5-25 Brushing the lingual surfaces of the upper incisors.

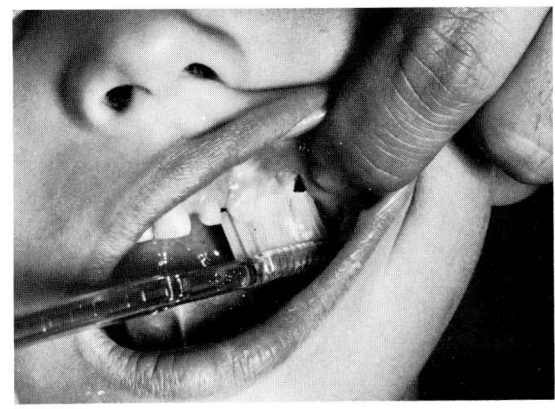

Figure 5-22 Brushing the buccal surfaces of the upper molars. Note lip retraction.

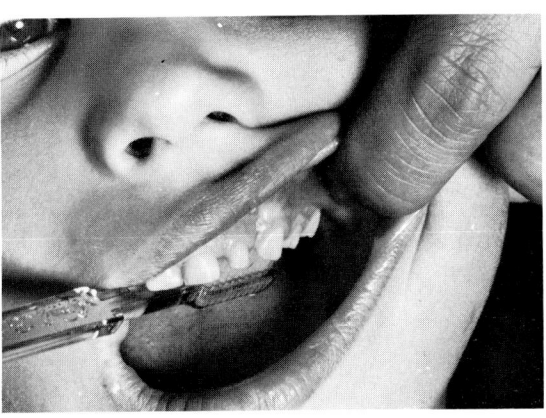

Figure 5-24 Brushing the labial surfaces of the upper incisors. Note how the lip is retracted.

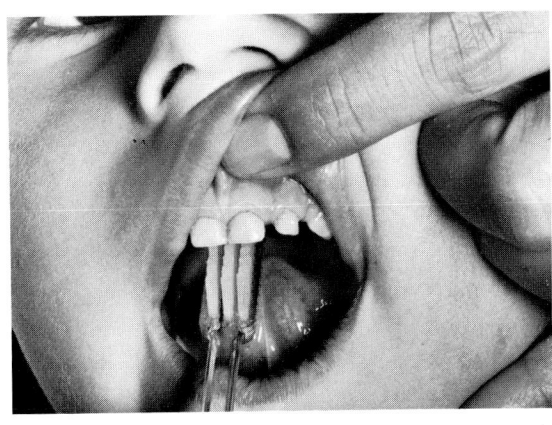

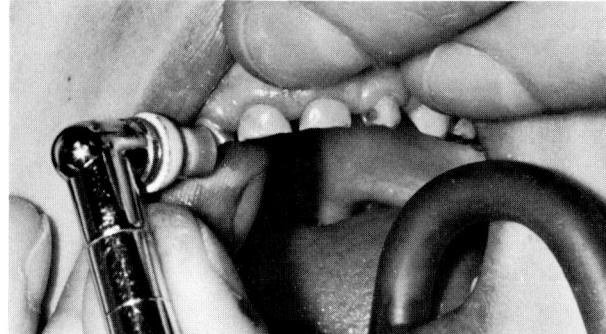

Figure 5-26 Teeth polished with a prophylaxis cup and paste.

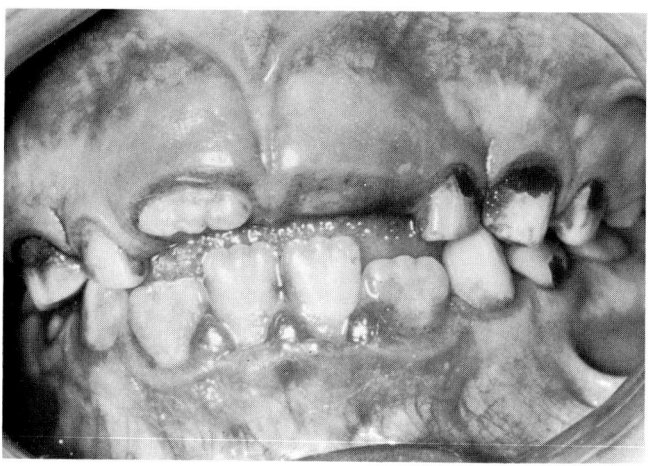

Figure 5-27 Disclosing solution applied to the teeth before prophylaxis. This is a convenient aid for indicating areas of plaque formation which must be removed during prophylaxis.

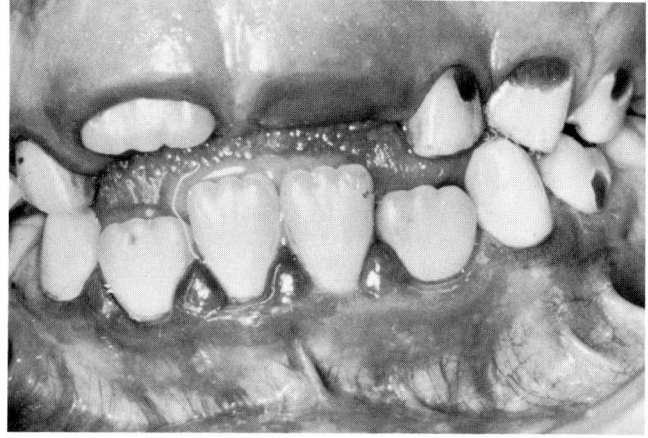

Figure 5-28 Patient seen in Figure 5-27 following prophylaxis and reapplication of disclosing solution. The solution should be applied after the prophylaxis in order to expose any uncleaned areas. It is also recommended that children use disclosing tablets periodically at home. This is a good aid in determining whether all areas have been cleaned thoroughly.

Figure 5-29 Dental floss (preferably unwaxed) with paste is used to polish the interproximal contact areas.

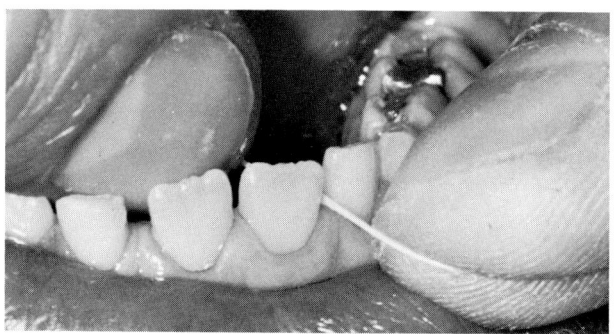

Figure 5-30 Condit Jr. cotton roll holder used to keep teeth dry while topical fluoride is applied. A cotton roll may be used to obstruct the flow of saliva from Stenson's duct (parotid gland) and a saliva ejector to remove excess saliva. Topical fluoride treatment is given every 6 to 12 months. Acidulated sodium fluoride and sodium fluoride solutions must be stored in polyethylene containers. Stannous fluoride solutions must be prepared fresh immediately prior to treatment.

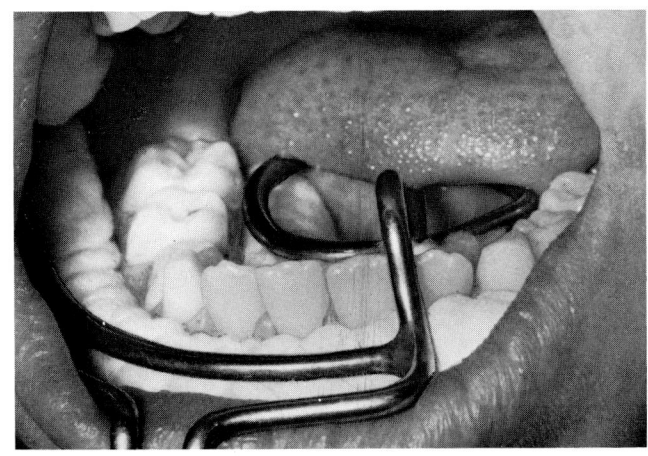

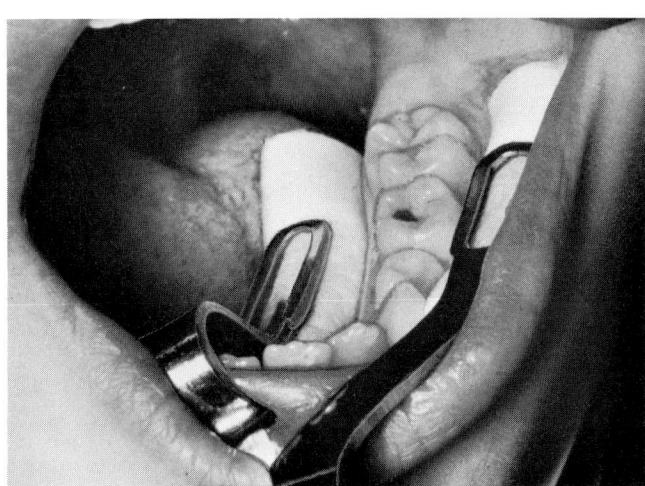

Figure 5-31 Garmer cotton roll holder used to keep teeth dry while topical fluoride is applied.

Figure 5-32 Application of fluoride solution; cotton ball is held by cotton pliers.

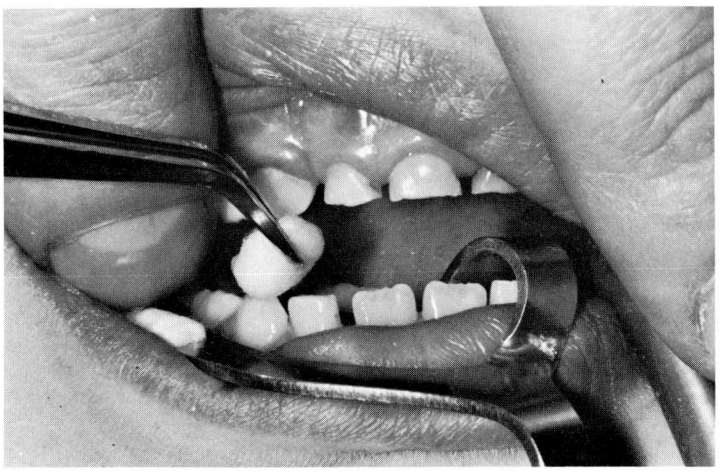

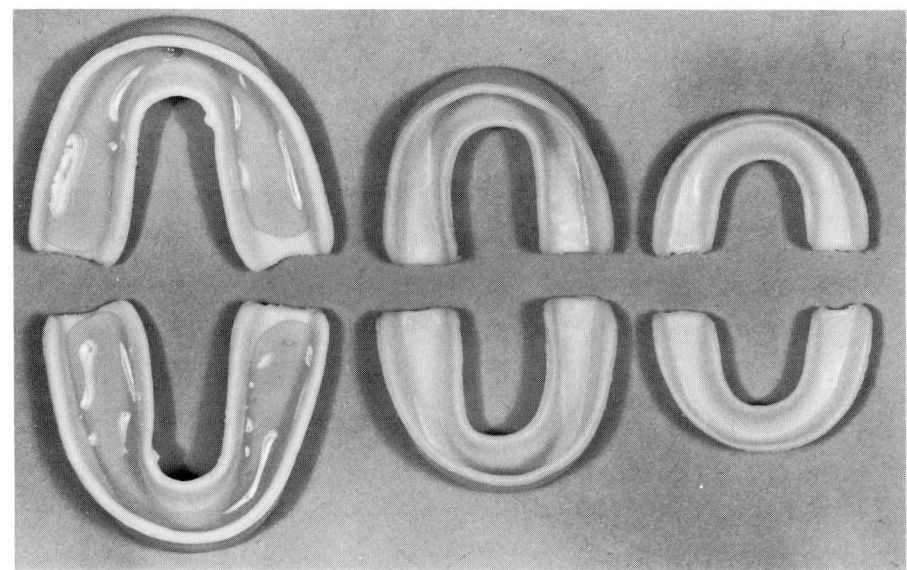

Figure 5-33 Adaptable trays may be used for the application of topical fluoride. The size which most closely fits the patient's dental arch should be used.

Geographical areas that do not have fluoride in the water require that the dentist prescribe fluoride supplements for home use. Table 5-1 suggests the proper amount of fluoride for different age levels in areas where less than optimal fluoride exists in the water supply.

Table 5-1 Administration of Fluoride Supplements*

Proper daily allowance of fluoride ion for a child 3 years or over. Reduce these amounts by one-half for children 2 to 3 years old. For children under 2 years of age, use prepared bottled water, 1 ppm fluoride concentration, in formula and food preparation.

Fluoride in H_2O	Adjusted Allowance	
ppm	Sodium Fluoride mg. per day	Provides Fluoride ion mg. per day
0.0	2.2	1.0
0.2	1.8	0.8
0.4	1.3	0.6
0.6	0.9	0.4

*From *Accepted Dental Remedies*, 32nd ed., American Dental Association, Chicago, 1967, p. 162.

Chapter 6 — ANESTHESIA

Local Anesthesia

Skillful administration of a local anesthetic affords the practitioner an excellent opportunity to give the child the optimum advantage of modern dentistry. When a child has a painful injection experience or if no anesthetic at all is used during operative procedures, patient management problems are more likely to occur. After a pleasant injection experience, the child will become confident in the dental environment and accept local anesthesia as part of routine dental treatment. A smooth injection technique is the cornerstone to painless dentistry and successful patient management.

Fundamental requirements of good local anesthetic technique should include the following:

1. A good case history to assure that the child can physically withstand a local anesthetic procedure.

2. A knowledge of the type of anesthetic necessary to perform the specific operation.

3. The type of injection needed to fulfill the goal of anesthesia.

4. Sterile and sharp needles.

5. A technique which will minimize the child's fear and condition him to be amenable to future treatment.

The anesthetic of choice is the one which is the least toxic, most profound, and of shortest duration for the particular procedure at hand. Undesirable side effects, such as lip biting, may occur if the anesthetic is of long duration.

For most injections on pedodontic patients, short needles are desirable. The 1¼ inch stainless steel disposable needle of a fine gauge (27) can be successfully used to obtain suitable anesthesia for most treatment involving the primary and mixed dentitions. The slight added cost of disposable needles over the standard needles is minimal compared with the advantages gained, such as freedom from cross-infection and sharpness of the point which decreases the initial unpleasant sensation.

The use of a topical anesthetic is desirable both in cleansing the site of the injection and in producing partial anesthesia in the area of the injection.

The child's acceptance of local anesthetics can best be obtained if the operator makes his motions gracefully and with a sense of confidence. Though the dentist should forewarn the child immediately prior to the injection, he should not allow him much time to speculate about the procedure nor should he be allowed to actually see the instruments used. It has been found most helpful to have the patient's eyes open so that the operator may, by the use of facial expression as well as words, offer reassurance and instill confidence in spite of the fact that some discomfort may be experienced.

There is always a possibility that a dental emergency might arise from the use of a local anesthetic. Consequently, it is important to have oxygen resuscitation equipment close at hand. All personnel in the dental office should be taught the use of the equipment and know where it is kept.

General Anesthesia

The use of general anesthesia in the treatment of certain pedodontic patients has gained wide acceptance. Patients upon whom this method is used should be rigidly selected and the method and place of administration carefully determined. It is possible that complications may arise from the use of a general anesthetic. Therefore, it should be employed on those children who are either severely physically handicapped or mentally unable to cooperate under a local anesthetic. Occasionally the extent of necessary treatment combined with the distance of residence to the professional office makes general anesthesia the method of choice. In some cases involving very young children, it is the only method by which treatment can be accomplished satisfactorily. General anesthesia for pedodontic patients should be carried out only in a location where complete emergency and recovery facilities and trained professional personnel are available. In most instances, the ideal facilities are found in a hospital. The desirable team of professional personnel includes a pediatrician, anesthesiologist, registered nurse, and dentist. When these individuals work in close harmony in a well-equipped hospital, the ideal environment is established for rendering full-mouth restorative care of children under general anesthesia.

TABLE 6-1. NERVES AND AREAS INNERVATED*

Inferior alveolar n.	Mandibular teeth to midline. Frequently the central incisor and its investing labial soft tissues are innervated by fibers of the opposite inferior alveolar nerve.
Lingual n.	Lingual investing soft tissues to midline and anterior two-thirds of tongue.
Long buccal n.	Mucosa of the cheek and the buccal investing soft tissues of the posterior teeth and a portion of the labial investing soft tissues of the canine.
Posterior superior alveolar n. (zygomatic)	Maxillary permanent and primary molars and their buccal investing soft tissues.
Middle superior alveolar n.	Mesiobuccal root of the first permanent molar, primary molars, premolars, the buccal investing soft tissues of these teeth as well as a part of the labial investing soft tissues of the canine. This nerve is frequently missing, and, in such instances, the posterior superior alveolar nerve is the nerve supply for these structures.
Anterior superior alveolar n.	Incisors and canine and their labial investing soft tissues.
Anterior palatine n.	Palatal investing soft tissues of the primary and permanent molars and premolars and a portion of the palatal investing soft tissues of the canine.
Nasopalatine n.	Palatal investing soft tissues of the incisors and a portion of the palatal investing soft tissues of the canine. Contributes to the innervation of the central and lateral incisors.

*From Mink, J. R., and Spedding, R. H.: An injection procedure for the child dental patient. Dental Clin. North Amer. July, 1966, p. 315.

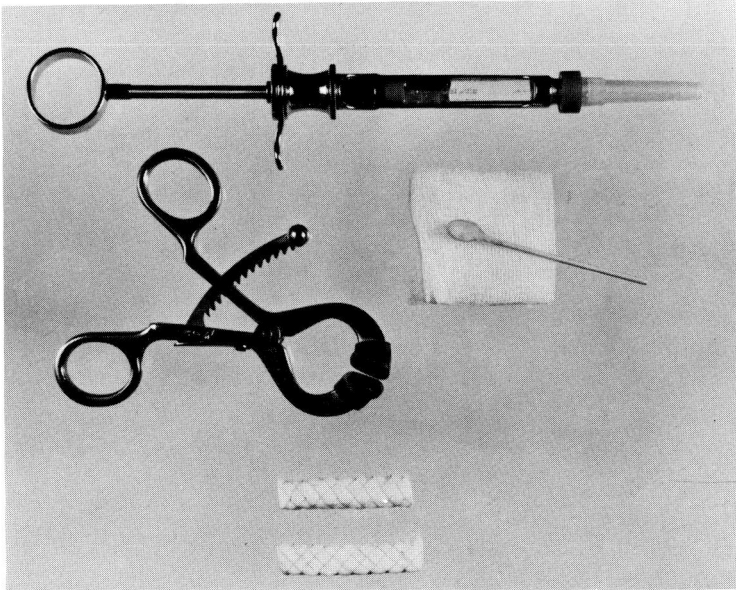

Figure 6-1 Suggested equipment for local anesthesia. Note aspirating syringe, disposable 27 gauge needle, topical anesthetic, 2 × 2 gauze sponge, mouth prop, and cotton rolls. The aspirating syringe enables the operator to reposition the needle if blood is aspirated in the anesthetic carpule, avoiding intravascular injection of anesthetic fluid.

146 ANESTHESIA

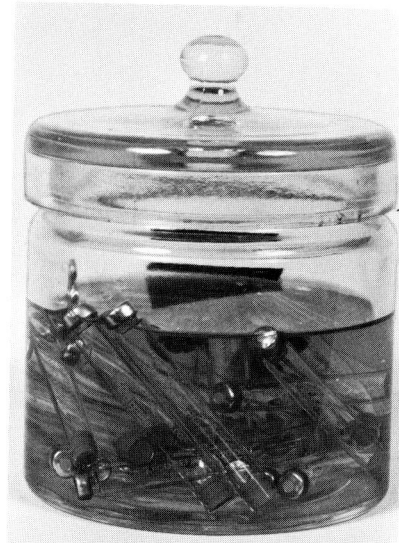

Figure 6-2 Storage of anesthetic carpules in a germicidal solution.

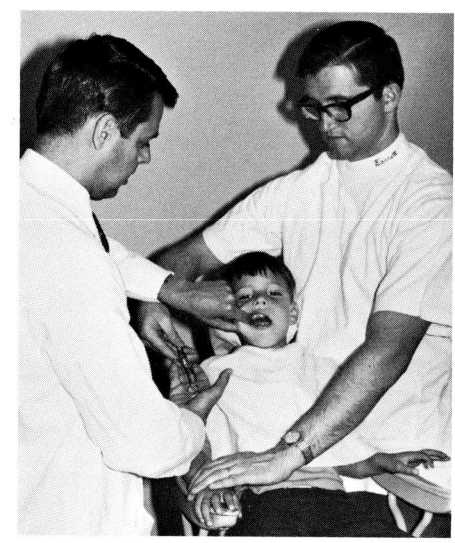

Figure 6-3 Assistant passing syringe from right side of patient for injections in the maxillary and mandibular right quadrants. Note the hands of the assistant gently resting over the hands of the patient ready to prevent any sudden movements during the injection procedure.

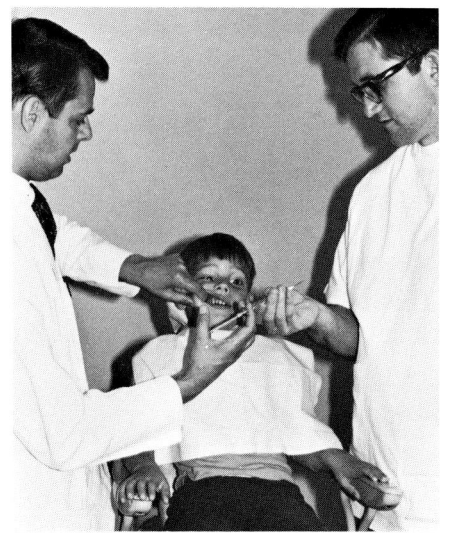

Figure 6-4 Passing the syringe in front of the child before injecting is very likely to cause management problems and should be emphatically discouraged.

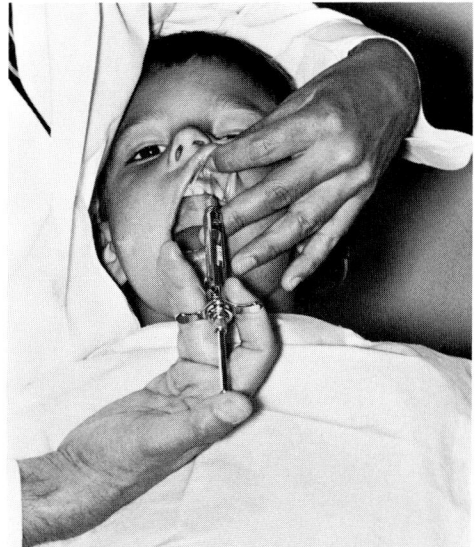

Figure 6-5 Position of operator's arms for injecting the maxillary anterior area. Fingers are used for stabilization.

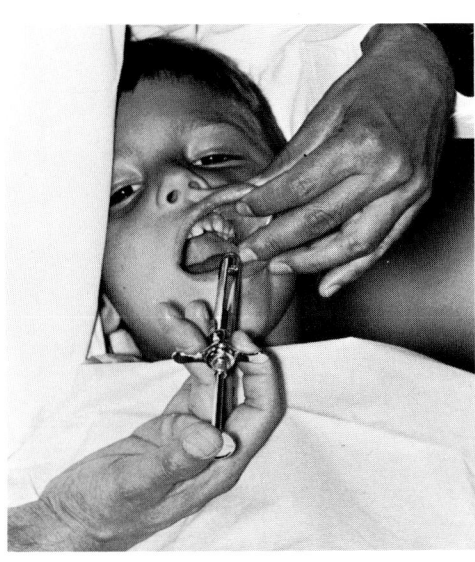

Figure 6-6 Position of operator for injecting maxillary posterior area. Arms are used to stabilize operator and patient. Note finger and forearm position of the dentist.

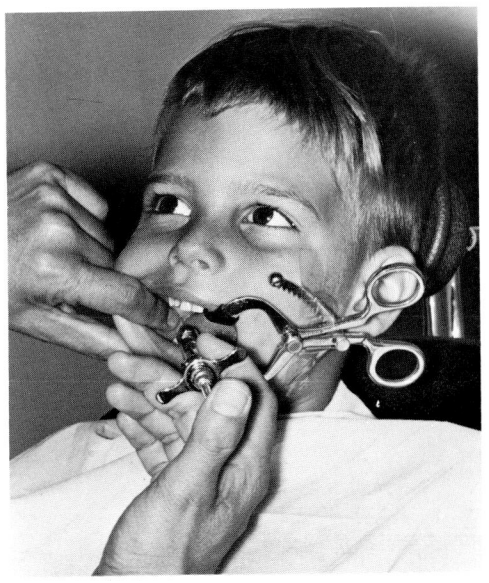

Figure 6-7 For the handicapped child who has difficulty in keeping his mouth open, the Molt mouth prop may be used during the inferior alveolar block injection.

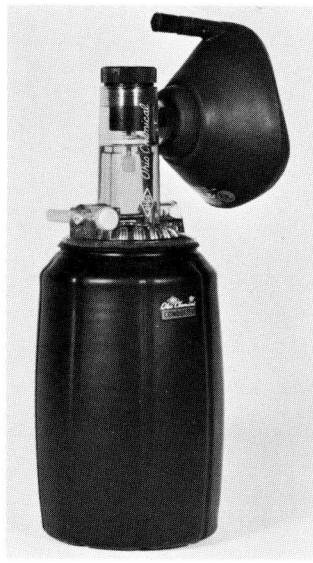

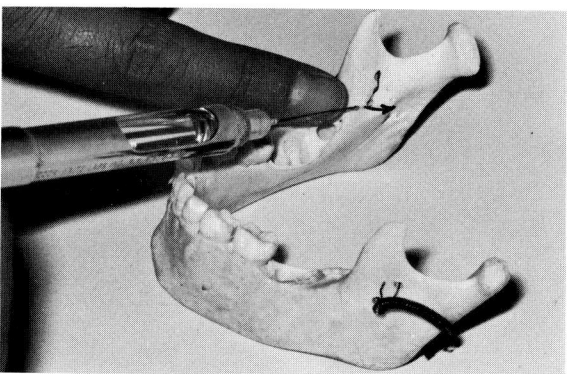

Figure 6-8 Resuscitation equipment should always be close at hand whenever a local anesthetic is used. Oxygen should be available for connection to this type of apparatus.

Figure 6-9 Procedure for the inferior alveolar injection. The index finger or thumb is moved up and down along the anterior border of the ramus until the greatest concavity is palpated (the coronoid notch). The finger is then moved lingually onto the internal oblique ridge. The needle is inserted from the opposite side of the mouth and should bisect the fingernail as the tissue is penetrated. A very small amount of anesthetic is injected upon entering the tissue and continued until the needle gently touches bone (the lingual nerve is usually anesthetized at this time). When bone is touched the needle should be withdrawn slightly, the syringe aspirated, and anesthetic injected slowly provided no blood is aspirated. All injections should be made slowly, taking at least 1 minute. When this is done the injection is almost painless and produces a more profound state of anesthesia. Arrow designates area of mandibular foramen.

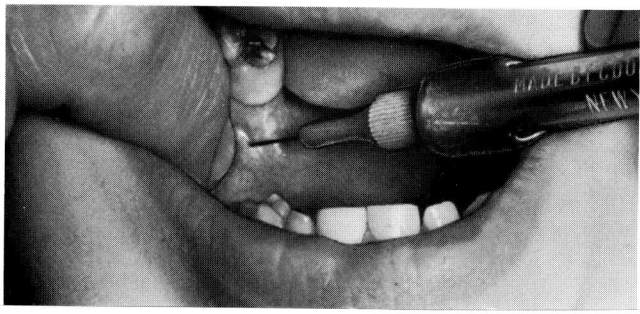

Figure 6-10 Inferior alveolar injection in 4-year-old child.

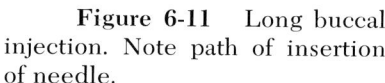

Figure 6-11 Long buccal injection. Note path of insertion of needle.

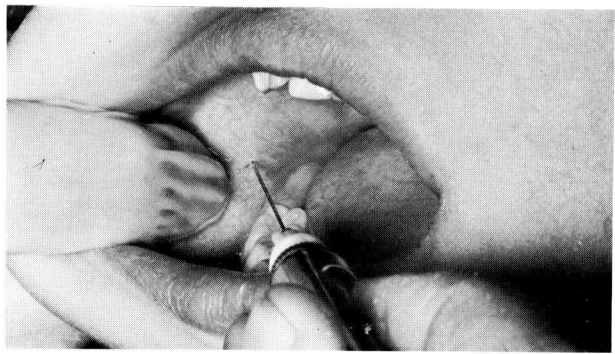

ANESTHESIA 149

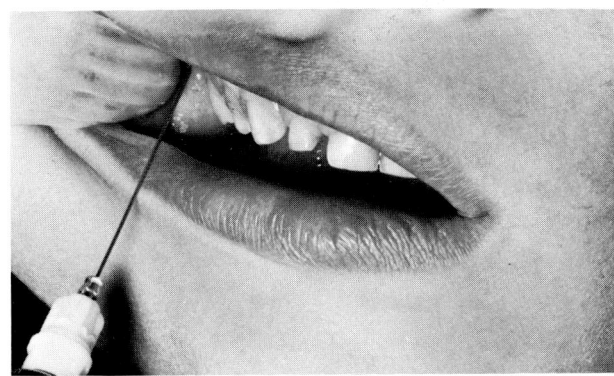

Figure 6-12 Posterior superior alveolar injection. A long needle is used in Figures 6-12 and 6-13 only for demonstration purposes, as previously stated. A short needle is usually adequate for injections on children.

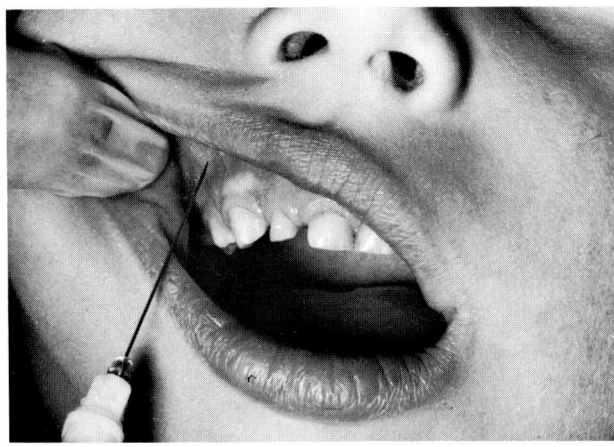

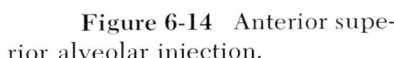

Figure 6-13 Middle superior alveolar injection.

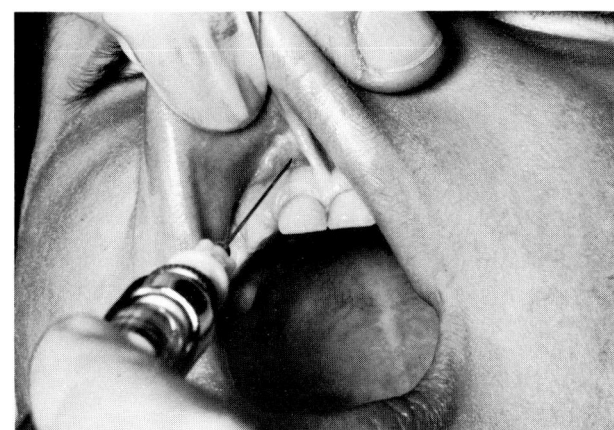

Figure 6-14 Anterior superior alveolar injection.

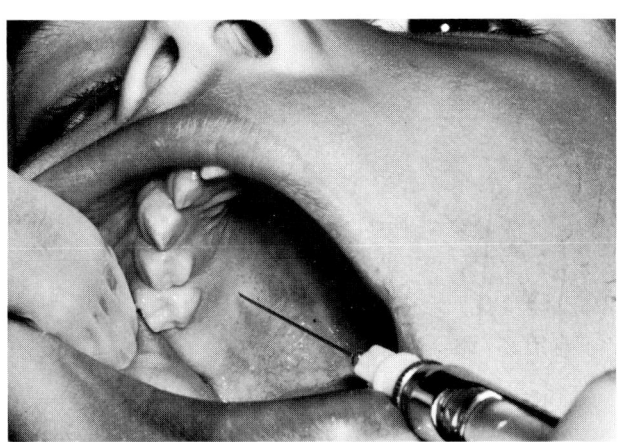

Figure 6-15 Palatal injection. This may be a painful injection. Both topical and pressure anesthesia from the cotton applicator held in place during the injection will reduce the sensation of pain considerably.

150 ANESTHESIA

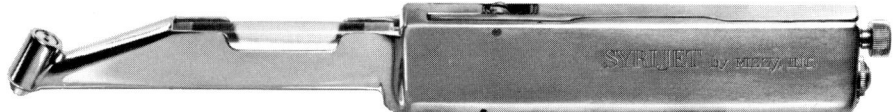

Figure 6-16 Pressure injection device (Mizzy Syrijet) for forcing anesthetic solution into superficial tissues. Useful in obtaining painless topical anesthesia prior to needle injection.

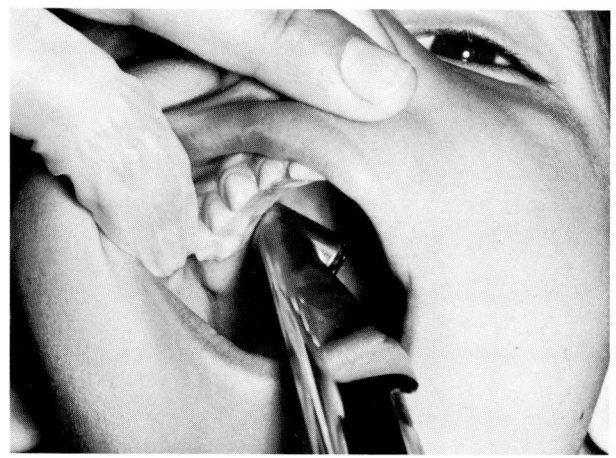

Figure 6-17 Same instrument as seen in Figure 6-16, being used on lingual of maxillary right first primary molar.

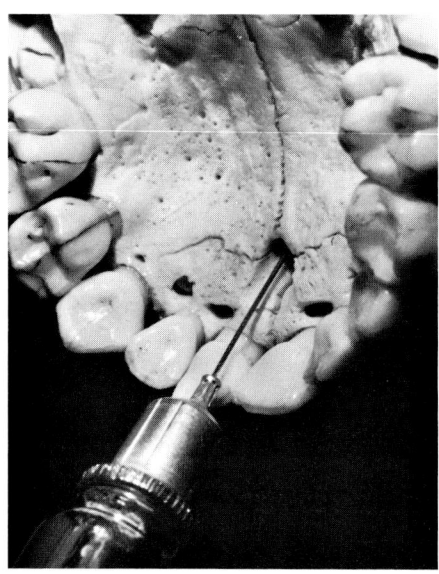

Figure 6-18 Anatomy of nasopalatine injection. Note how the needle parallels the long axis of the anterior teeth in order to enter the foramen.

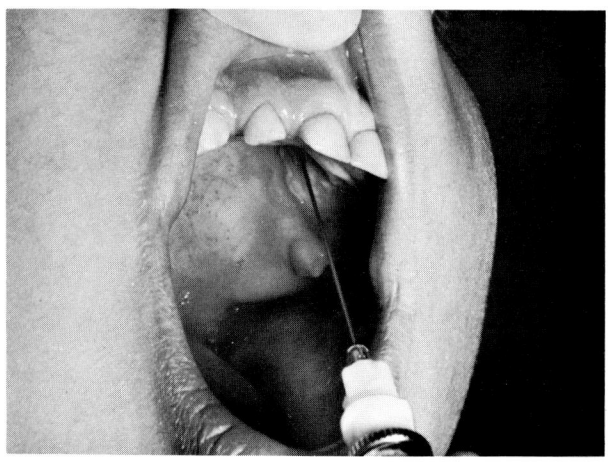

Figure 6-19 Nasopalatine injection. This can also be a painful injection and the same technique as described in Figure 6-15 or 6-17 may be used.

ANESTHESIA 151

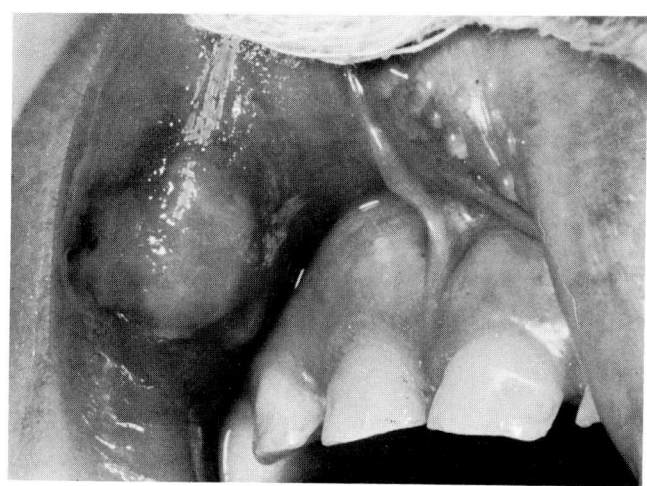

Figure 6-20 Trauma resulting from biting the upper lip after infiltration with local anesthetic was made over the maxillary right primary cuspid. If the area is still anesthetized when the child is dismissed, the parent and patient should be told of the trauma which will ensue if the child bites on the lip as the anesthetic wears off.

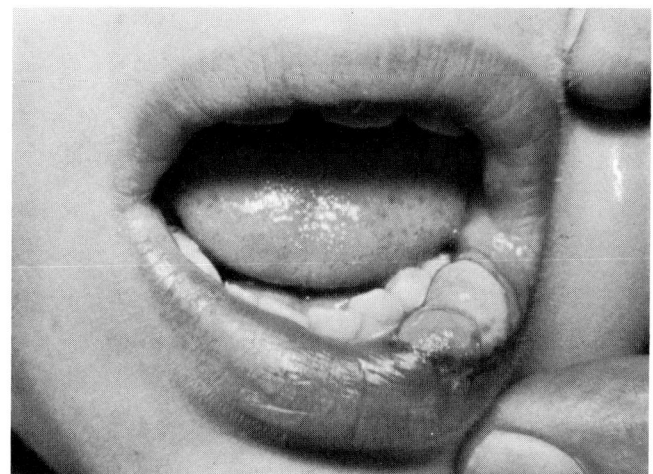

Figure 6-21 Trauma resulting from biting the lower lip. An inferior alveolar block injection was given prior to treatment, and after dismissal the child chewed on the lip as the anesthetic was wearing off. It usually takes from 5 to 7 days for these traumatized areas to heal.

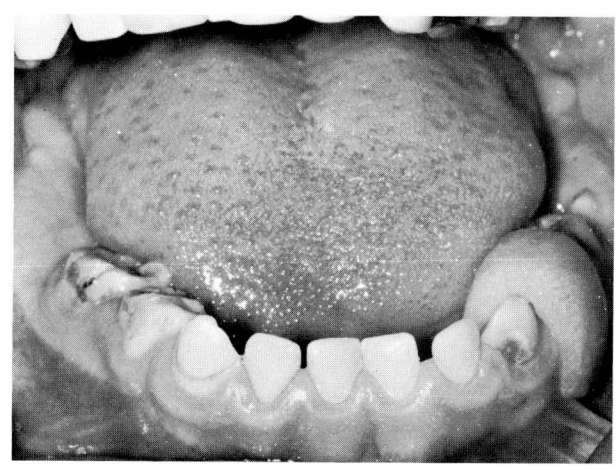

Figure 6-22 Plastic strip (Squibb Oradhesive) placed over freshly restored tooth on patient's left side to prevent cheek or lip biting for duration of anesthesia.

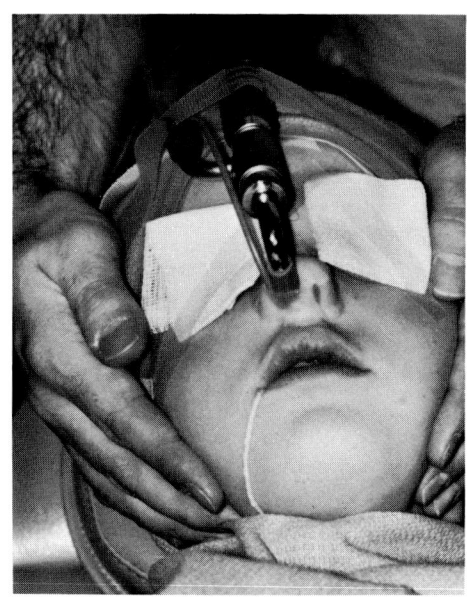

Figure 6-23 Nasotracheal intubation. This is the intubation method of choice for full-mouth dental treatment under general anesthesia.

Figure 6-24 Orotracheal intubation. On a rare occasion the anesthesiologist will not be able to pass a nasal tube, but instead will have to intubate through the oral cavity. Note how the operating area in the oral cavity is restricted for the dentist when this method of intubation is used.

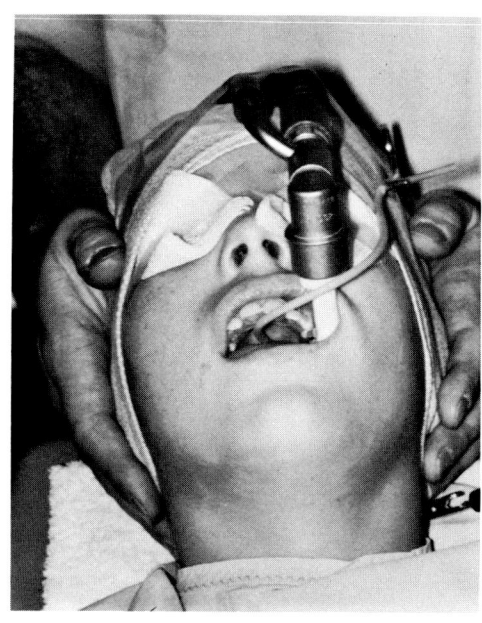

RUBBER DAM

Chapter 7

The use of the rubber dam provides many advantages in treating children, most important of which is the high degree of patient control during operative procedures. Involuntary movements of the mandible and associated muscles combine to make other techniques less satisfactory than the rubber dam. If it is not used with some children, the area of operation becomes contaminated with saliva despite all efforts of the dentist to keep it dry. In addition to moisture control, use of the rubber dam results in the following:

1. A greater degree of protection for the patient against swallowing or aspirating foreign bodies that may come in contact with the posterior areas of the mouth. This is especially important during general anesthesia.

2. Better restriction of the tongue, cheeks, and lingual muscles from involuntary movements as in cases of cerebral palsy.

3. Decreased operating time because of better patient control and operator visibility.

4. Improvement in parent education since the dentist can more clearly illustrate to the parent his specific treatment.

The use of the rubber dam has been found to be reasonably well received by children. They are able to swallow and to make themselves understood with the dam in place. The speed and accuracy in completion of the operation with the use of the rubber dam easily offset any inconvenience to the patient at the beginning of treatment. The psychological effect upon the dentist is to make procedures seem easier to accomplish.

The following technique has been found to be the most expedient and practical for the dam's placement and maintenance:

1. Use 5 × 5 inch dam of heavy black rubber.
2. Largest hole is used for rubber dam clamp.

3. Holes are punched close together—2 mm. between outsides of holes.

4. Include only those teeth that must be involved in the treatment. The second primary molar is usually the best tooth to clamp because of its configuration.

5. Desirable clamps for most pedodontic cases include Ivory (carbon steel) numbers 14, 8A, and 00.

6. Place clamp on dam and dam on frame before inserting into the mouth. The dam is secured on the frame by exerting tension in the vertical direction to permit maximum flexibility in the horizontal direction.

7. Use floss to depress the dam around the gingivae of the teeth and to ligate where needed.

8. Use wooden wedges if needed to depress interproximal areas. The wedges may be left in position throughout the cavity preparation phase of the operation.

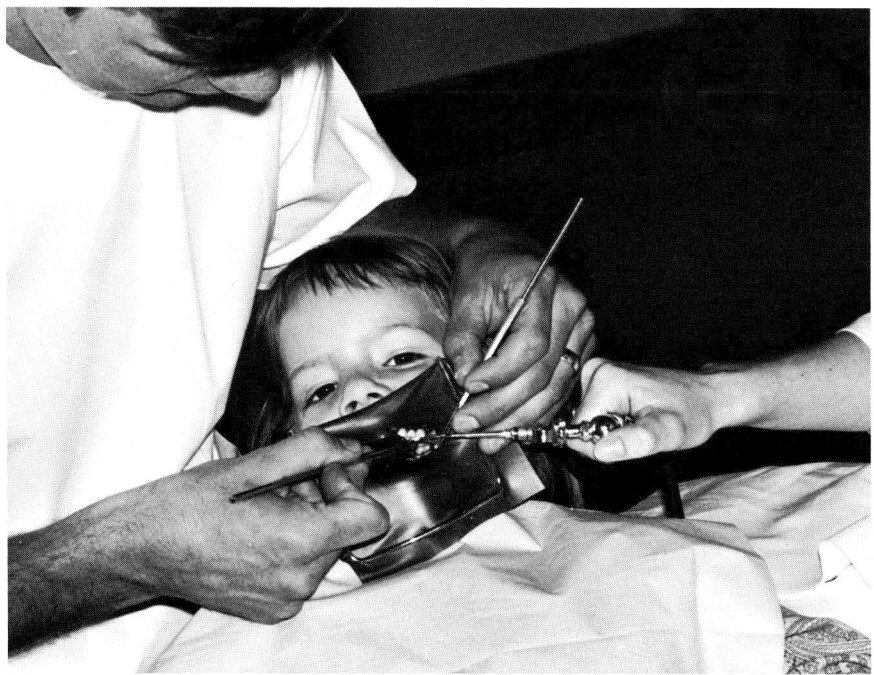

Figure 7-1 Rubber dam in place and patient ready for restorative procedures in the maxillary left quadrant. Note how the rubber dam isolates the teeth and provides a clean dry field of operation.

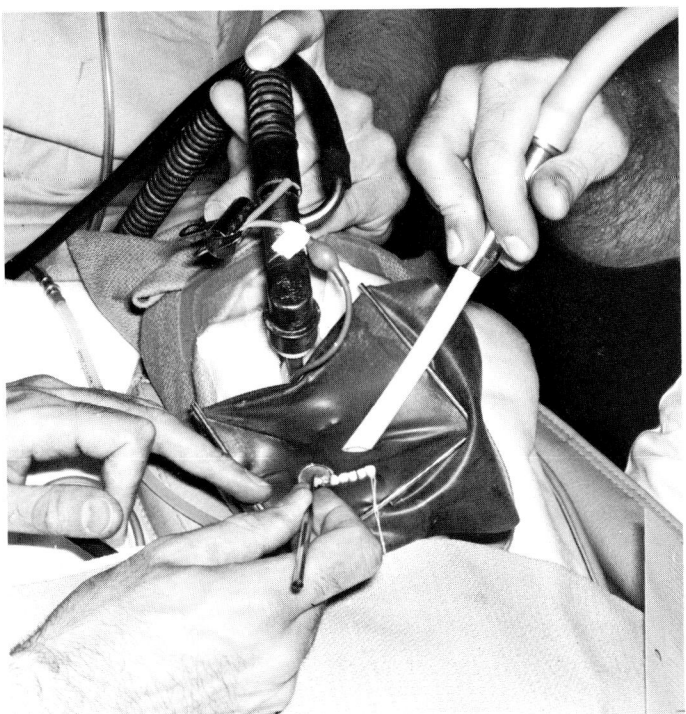

Figure 7-2 Rubber dam in place for routine operative procedures under general anesthesia. Throat pack should be placed prior to seating rubber dam.

156 RUBBER DAM

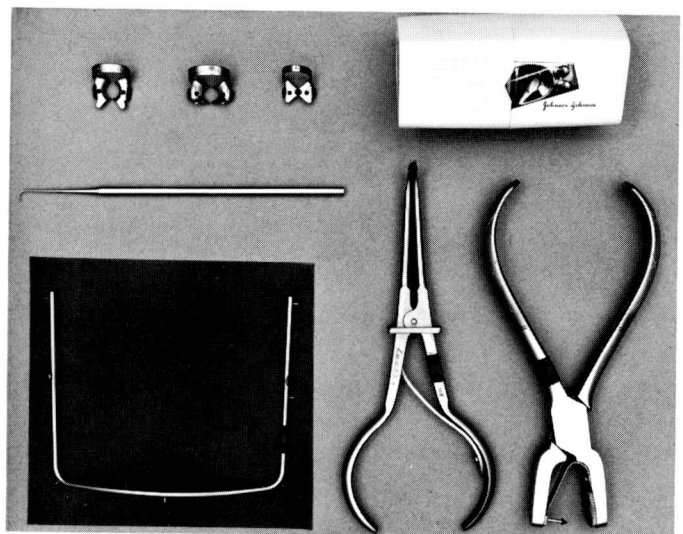

Figure 7-3 Tray setup for placement of rubber dam.

Figure 7-4 Ivory clamp No. 14 (carbon steel) used to clamp second primary molar and first permanent molar (erupted).

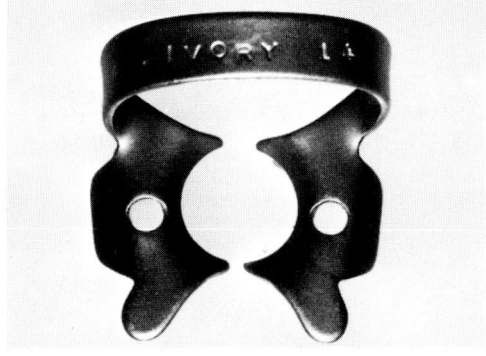

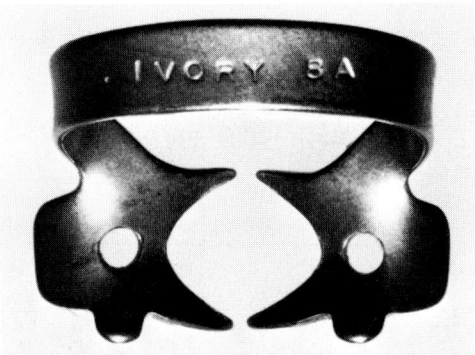

Figure 7-5 Ivory clamp, No. 8A (carbon steel), used to clamp partially erupted first and second permanent molars.

Figure 7-6 Ivory clamp No. 00 (carbon steel) used to clamp primary cuspids and first primary molars.

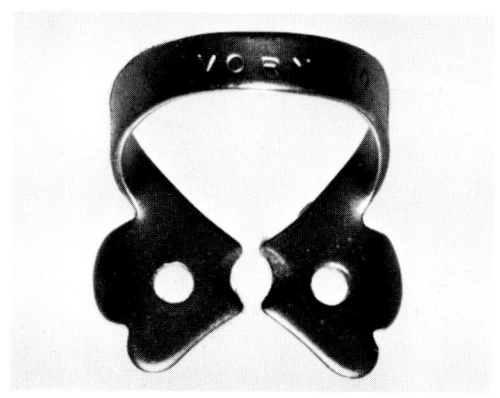

Figure 7-7 Holes punched in a 5 × 5 inch rubber dam for routine operative work in the mandibular arch (right side). This same punched rubber dam may be used on the left side of the mandibular arch by turning it over. Observe the following:
1. The largest hole of the punch is used for the tooth to be clamped.
2. Holes are punched 2 mm. apart (outside measurements).
3. Holes are punched at a 45 degree angle.

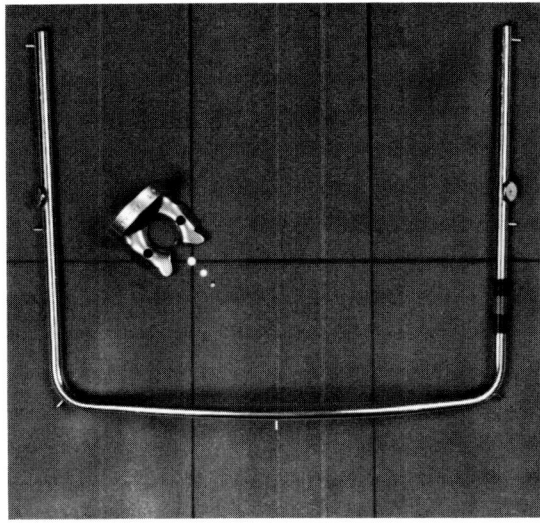

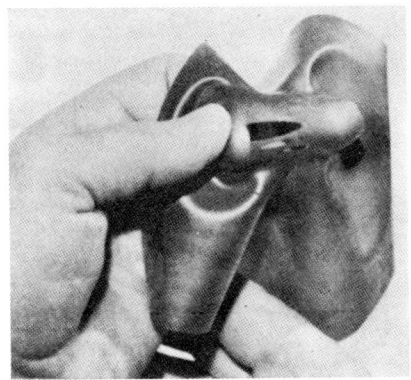

Figure 7-8 Dam stretched for insertion of clamp. Note how the thumb and index finger are used to hold the dam while the middle finger stretches it. (From Jinks, G. M.: Rubber dam technique in pedodontics. Dent. Clin. North America, 327-340, July, 1966.)

Figure 7-9 Wings of clamp inserted in rubber dam. Note its appearance in Figure 7-8. (From Jinks, G. M.: Rubber dam technique in pedodontics. Dent. Clin. North America, 327-340, July, 1966.)

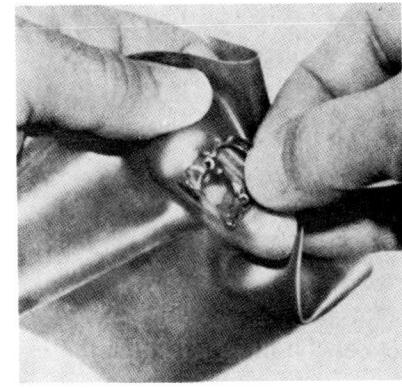

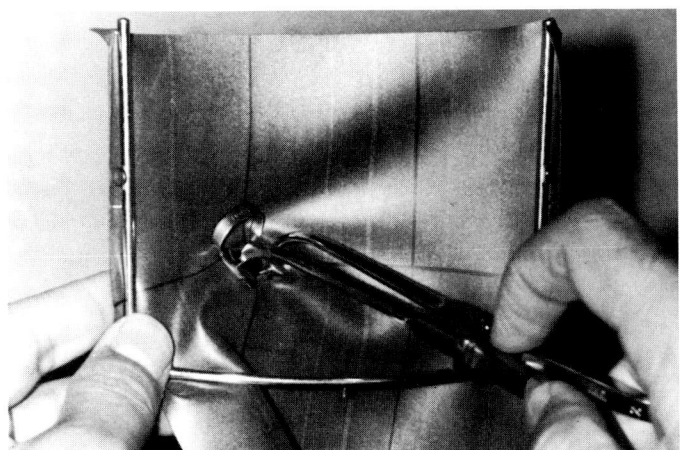

Figure 7-10 Rubber dam and clamp ready to be carried to the mouth attached to the Young's frame. Note that the frame is held to the dam by a slight tension in the vertical direction so as to permit maximum flexibility in the horizontal direction for easier placement in the mouth.

158 RUBBER DAM

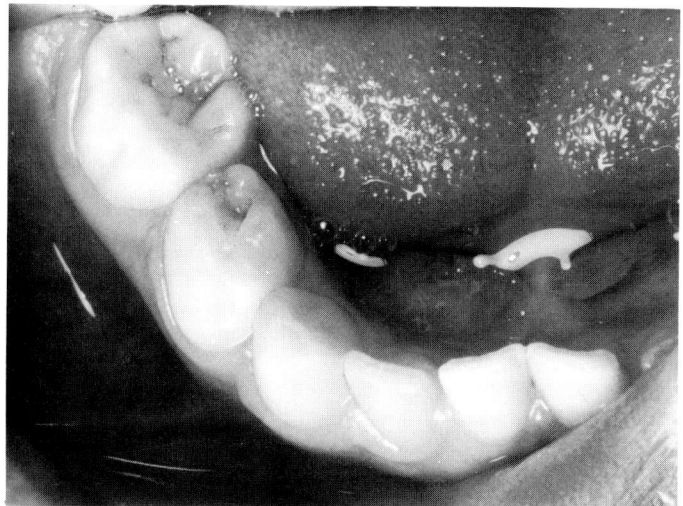

Figure 7-11 Right mandibular quadrant in a preschool child. Rubber dam will be placed on the second primary molar, first primary molar, and primary cuspid to facilitate operative procedures.

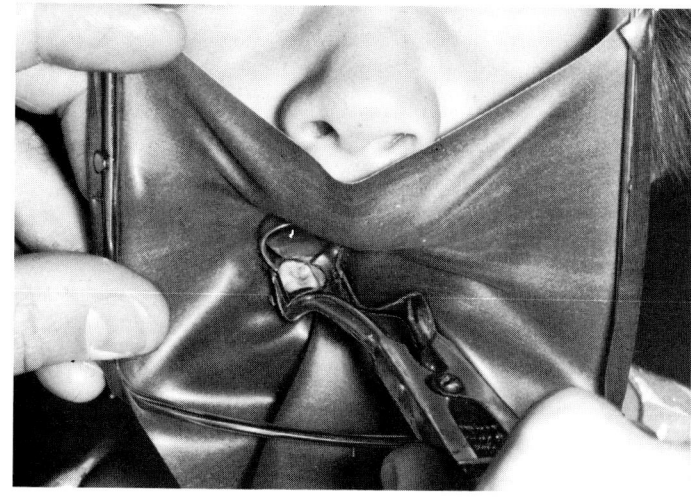

Figure 7-12 Rubber dam, clamp and Young's frame carried to the mouth. The clamp is always on the outside with the wings engaged only in the dam. This prevents accidental aspiration of the clamp in the event that it slips off the tooth during placement.

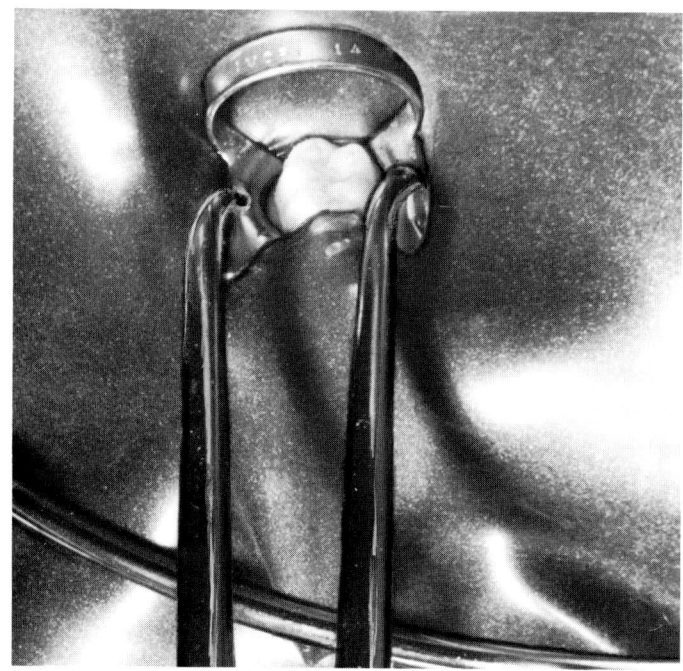

Figure 7-13 Clamp is seated on tooth with firm pressure. Minimal tissue damage is assured by carefully sliding clamp down the tooth.

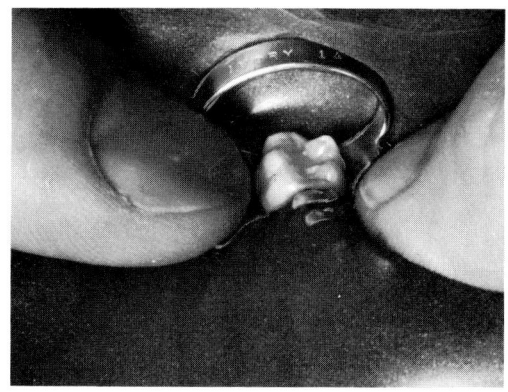

Figure 7-14 Upon releasing clamp, the operator must use thumbs or forefingers to further seat clamp firmly on the tooth. Such action will prevent the clamp from snapping off.

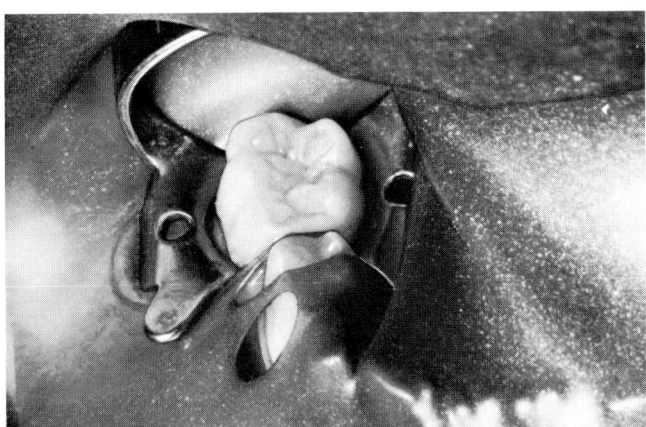

Figure 7-15 Clamp and dam in position prior to adjustment of rubber around teeth. Note the rubber has not been snapped under the clamp yet.

Figure 7-16 Rubber dam is snapped under the clamp and stretched around the remaining teeth by use of the fingers and dental floss. The edges of the dam around the teeth are then tucked into the gingival crevice with an explorer. Warm air blown around the teeth as the dam is tucked facilitates this procedure.

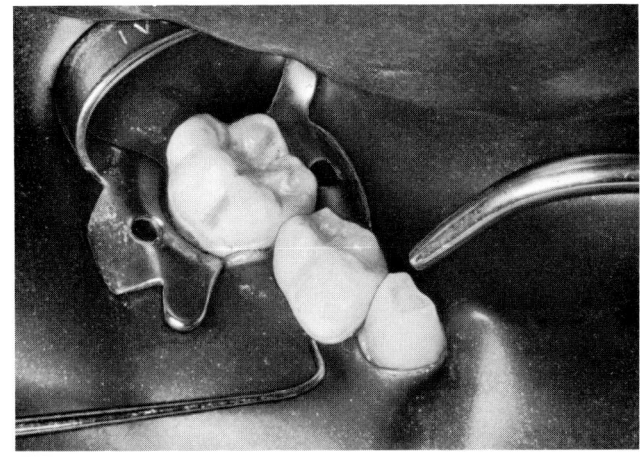

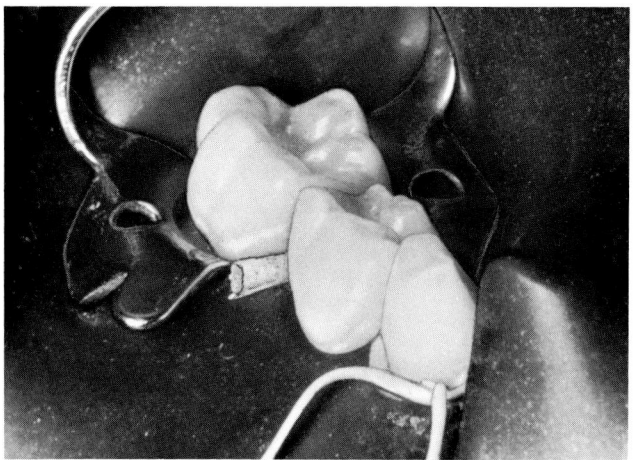

Figure 7-17 An interproximal wedge and simple ligature (dental floss) may be used to retract the dam and prevent it from slipping off the teeth. The gingival constriction of primary teeth makes ligature application very effective. When preparing Class II cavities, preparation may be carried into the wedge itself.

Figure 7-18 Rubber dam in position assuring a clean, dry field. The mouth is held open and accessory actions of tongue and lips are controlled. The Young's frame does not restrain the child unduly and he is able to move his head without disturbing the placement of the dam. If it is desirable to cover the nose with the rubber dam, the series of holes is punched in the same direction, but ½ to 1 inch lower on the dam.

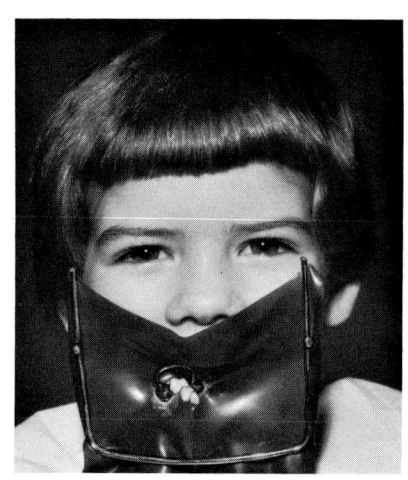

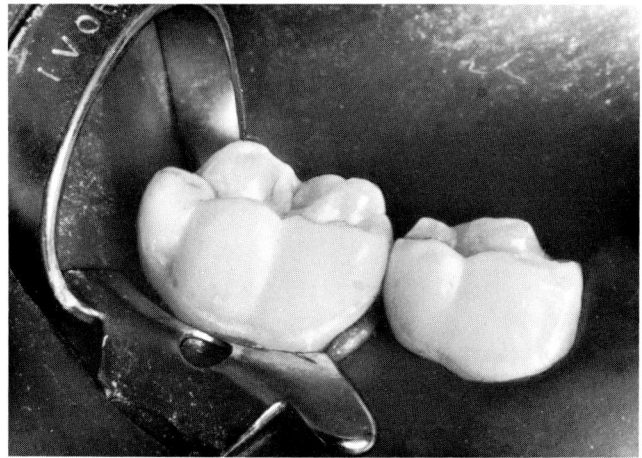

Figure 7-19 Buccal view of rubber dam when only two teeth are included. In many cases it is desirable to include in the dam only those teeth which are to be treated, plus the tooth to be clamped.

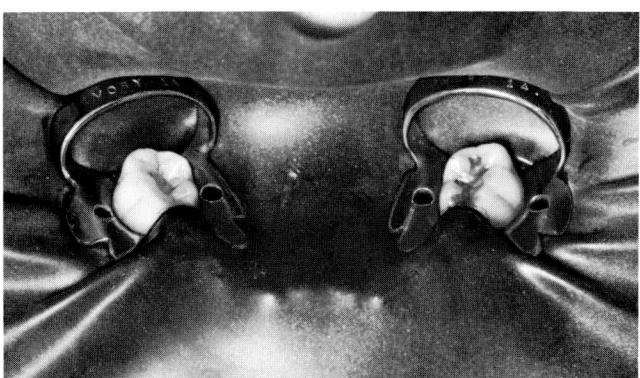

Figure 7-20 Bilateral clamping of mandibular first permanent molars to accomplish occlusal restorations in a single appointment. This procedure is particularly effective when a patient is treated under general anesthesia.

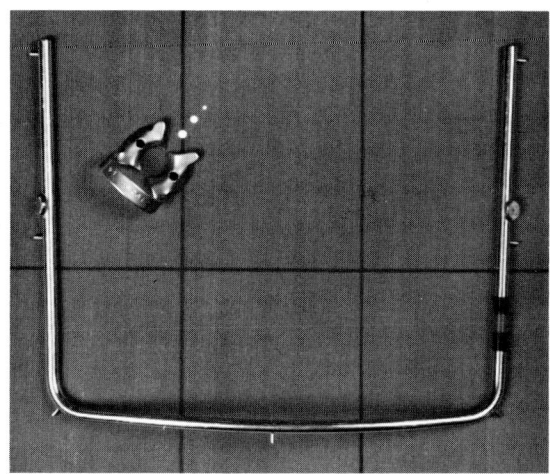

Figure 7-21 Holes punched in a 5 × 5 inch rubber dam for routine operative work in the maxillary arch (right side). This same punched rubber dam may be used on the left side of the maxillary arch by turning it over (see Figure 7-1). Note close proximity of holes to one another and 45 degree inclination toward center of dam.

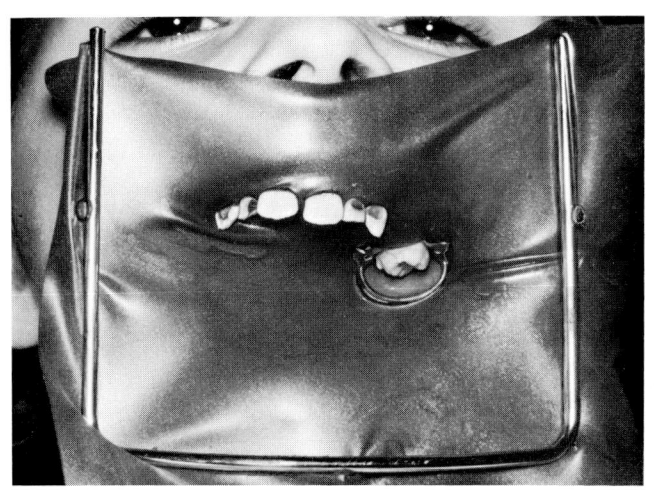

Figure 7-22 Position of rubber dam for treatment of anterior teeth. Stability of dam is best achieved by clamping a molar tooth. Wedges and ligatures are frequently used.

Chapter 8

OPERATIVE DENTISTRY

Historically, restorative procedures for the child patient have constituted the major consideration for the practicing dentist. The rapidity of onset of caries in the primary dentition has presented a challenge to the conscientious operator who sought to provide durable well-finished restorations. Over the years better understanding of child behavior plus the use of local anesthetics have enabled the motivated practitioner to accomplish operative procedures for the child that are equal to those in the adult. In addition, there has been the impact of the advent of new materials. The development of the full coverage steel crown, for example, has been a major breakthrough in economically solving the problem of restoring the badly broken down tooth in the primary and mixed dentition. It can be predicted, however, that with the wider use of fluorides and other caries control agents now being tested, operative procedures in the child patient will gradually become less necessary and a shift will be seen in the direction of greater emphasis on other problems of the early years such as preventive orthodontics, habit control, and treatment of the handicapped.

The technical approach to cavity preparation in the primary dentition originated as a modified version of the conventional cavity design for amalgam in permanent teeth. The primary tooth being smaller and the pulp chamber relatively large, it was necessary not only to scale down the usual cavity preparation, but to change it in certain respects. A shallower pulpal floor was indicated, and since the contact areas of the primary molars are flat, the extension of the interproximal cavity had to be wider to attain a self-cleansing area. No bevel on the gingival was needed since the enamel rods on primary teeth incline occlusally in the gingival third. In addition, various authors recommended specific modifications which they felt would improve the interproximal cavity design in particular. Brauer[1] has suggested the need to make the occlusal or "neck" portion one half the width of the buccolingual occlusal area. Sweet[5] proposed a wide occlusal step, rounding of all angles to reduce stress, deepening of the central portion of the pulpal floor, and creation of buccal and lingual lateral walls that are parallel to the external surfaces. Lampshire,[2] on the basis of limited impact and photoelastic studies, suggested that rounded line angles throughout the cavity preparation are indicated to reduce stresses. He also recommended a wide isthmus in the interproximal preparation, a rounded pulpal wall, and buccal and lingual retention grooves in the proximal box.

Recent studies by Terkla and Mahler,[6] by Nadal, Phillips, and Swartz,[4] and by MacRae, Zacherl, and Castaldi[3] indicate that marginal defects are the greatest failure occurring in Class II amalgam restorations in both primary and permanent teeth. They emphasize the need to eliminate traumatic cuspal occlusion and the desirability of a conservative occlusal outline to minimize marginal defects. Modifications such as grooving, rounding of floors, and gingival reverse bevels have not been demonstrated to improve resistance to bulk proximal fracture as tested in vivo.[6] It has been repeatedly demonstrated that amalgam can be successfully adapted to sharp angles (45 degrees or more) and since these angles permit less removal of sound tooth structure than the rounded version, they present a conservative design. The interproximal cavity preparation in the primary molar will involve an isthmus one-third the intercuspal dimensions of the tooth, and for practical purposes, a converging outline on the proximal buccal and lingual walls. Special care will be required in the correction of opposing cusp interferences prior to commencing cavity preparations. It is felt that such a cavity design will minimize accidental pulp exposure and reduce the incidence of marginal breakdown of amalgam. However, it should be pointed out that other factors such as lack of removal of caries, improper amalgam manipulation, and faulty condensation can result in failure regardless of the operator's philosophy of cavity preparation.

Carving and polishing of amalgam restorations in primary teeth should be carried out with the same care as in permanent teeth. Usually it is not desirable to carve deep central and secondary grooves when restoring primary molars. It is necessary to check the occlusion a second time with articulating paper after final carving and removal of the rubber dam. The same precaution should be followed at the polishing appointment and at subsequent recall appointments to avoid undesirable cuspal trauma. Final polishing of all amalgam restorations is necessary, since it reduces corrosion and marginal deterioration and results in more comfort for the patient.

OPERATIVE DENTISTRY 165

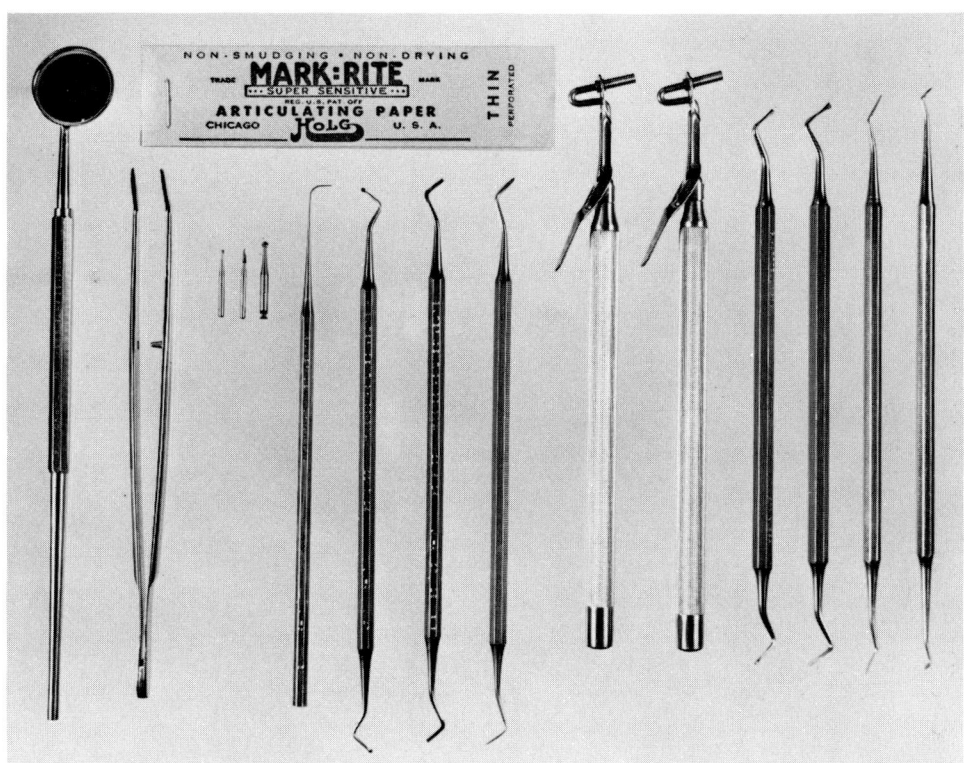

Figure 8-1 Tray setup for routine operative procedures includes mirror, cotton forceps, inverted cone bur, fissure bur, round bur, explorer, double-ended spoon excavator, enamel hatchets, amalgam carriers, amalgam condensers, and amalgam carvers.

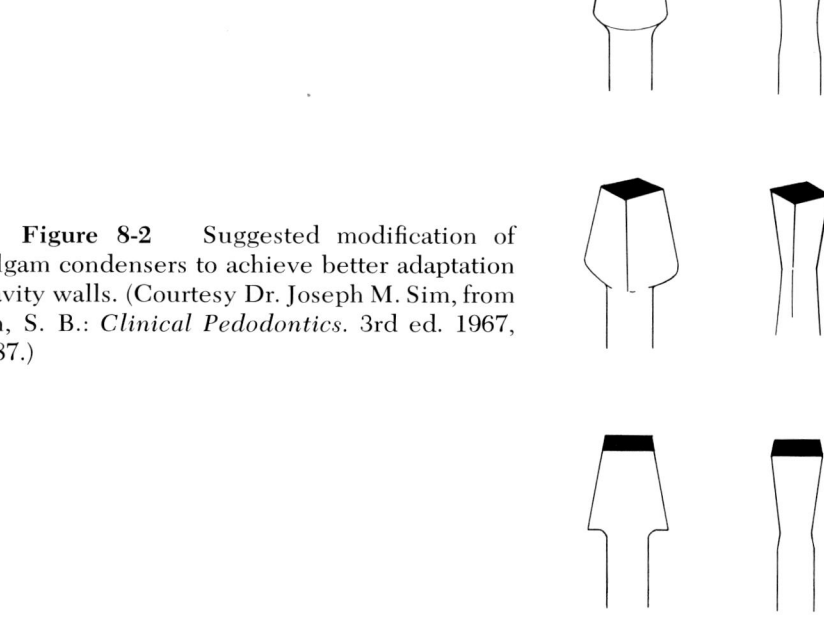

Figure 8-2 Suggested modification of amalgam condensers to achieve better adaptation to cavity walls. (Courtesy Dr. Joseph M. Sim, from Finn, S. B.: *Clinical Pedodontics*. 3rd ed. 1967, p. 187.)

Conventional   Altered

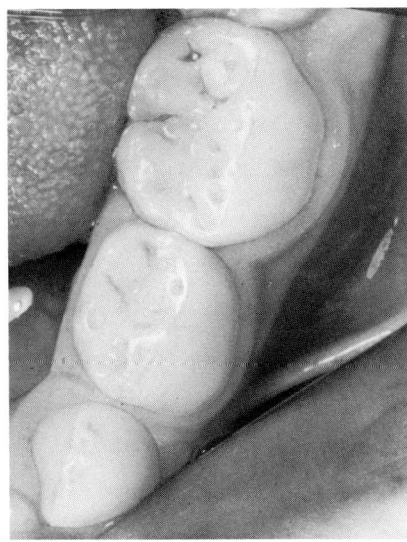

Figure 8-3 Anatomy of the primary mandibular molars. Note typical flat contacts. Numerous supplementary fissures are characteristic of the occlusal of the mandibular second primary molar.

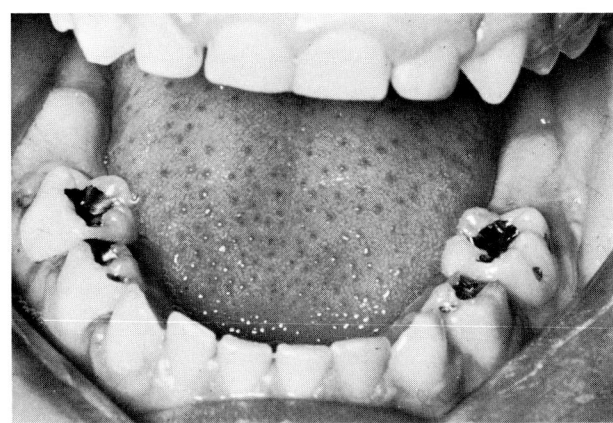

Figure 8-4 Occlusal amalgam restorations on mandibular second primary molars. All fissures must be included in the cavity preparation.

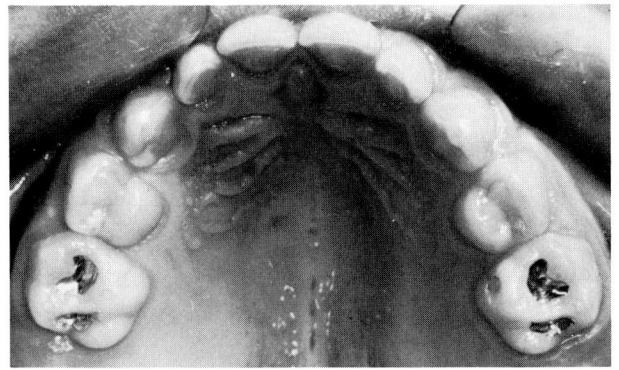

Figure 8-5 Occlusal amalgam restorations on maxillary second primary molars. Outline form is minimal because of absence of supplementary grooves.

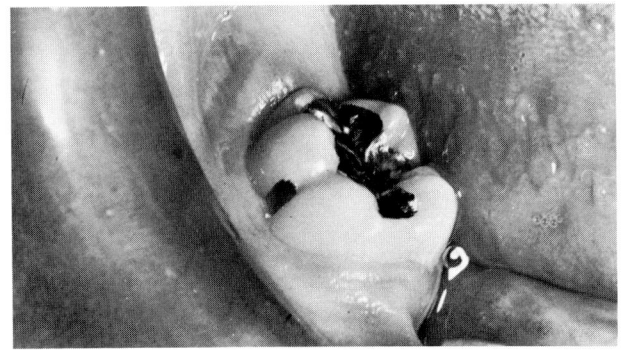

Figure 8-6 Occlusal amalgam restoration on mandibular first permanent molar. Note anatomical carving of the amalgam. This is important in the young permanent teeth to maintain proper cuspal interdigitation.

Figure 8-7 Plaster model of mandibular first primary molar illustrating disto-occlusal cavity preparation with conservative isthmus, flat floor, and sharp angles.

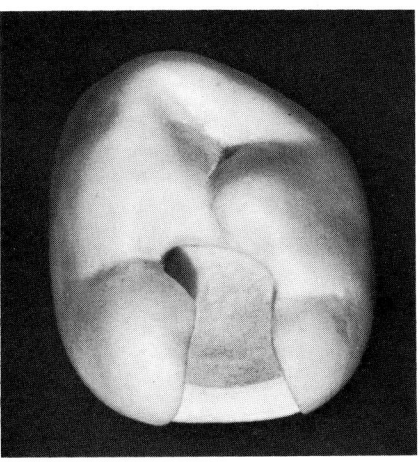

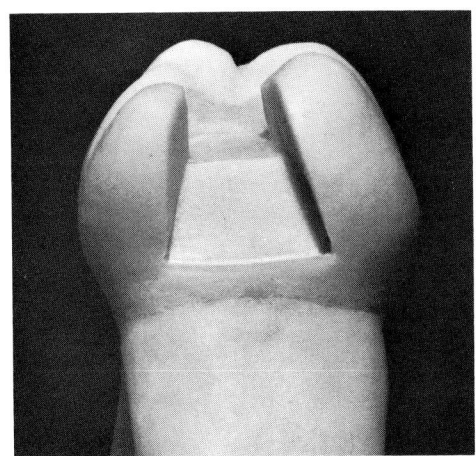

Figure 8-8 Proximal view of model shown in Figure 8-7, illustrating converging proximal walls and sharp buccogingival and linguogingival line angles. Sharp angles are more conservative of tooth structure and are also retentive.

Figure 8-9 A sharp-angled cavity preparation restored with amalgam and cut in cross-section to show good adaptation to cavity walls. Use of good condensing force and properly shaped trapezoidal condensers is necessary to secure adaptation of the amalgam.

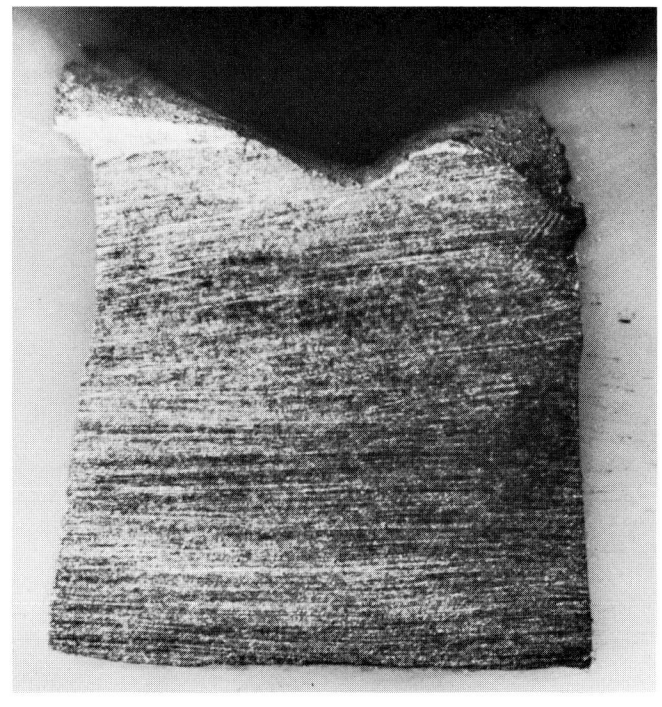

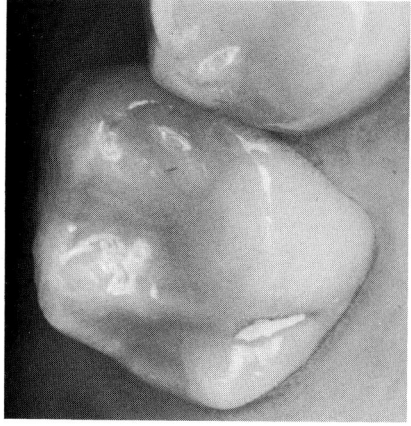

Figure 8-10 Maxillary second primary molar in a child 5 years of age. Note lack of supplementary grooves and fissures.

Figure 8-11 Proximal cavity preparation. A wide flaring of buccal and lingual walls is undesirable, since it results in a thin edge of amalgam.

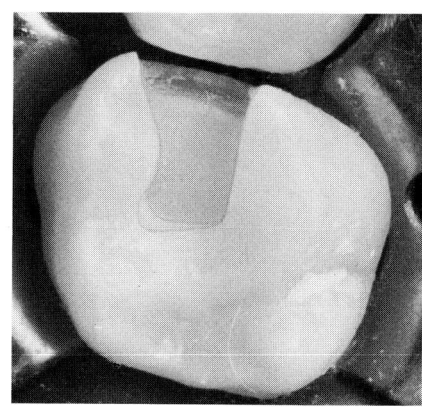

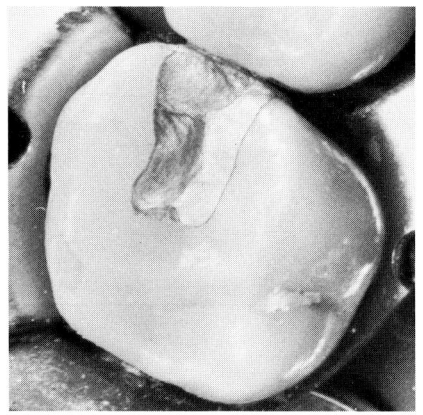

Figure 8-12 Carved amalgam in tooth illustrated in Figure 8-11. Simple anatomical carving is all that is required.

Figure 8-13 Polished restoration. Corrosion and marginal deterioration are held to the minimum if amalgam is properly finished.

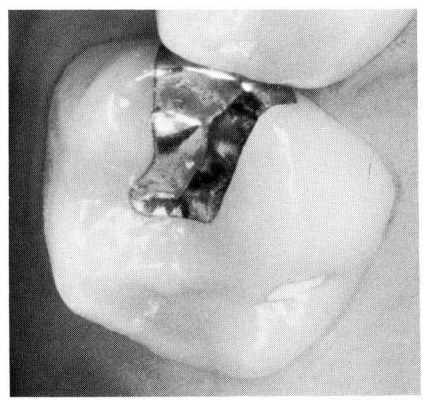

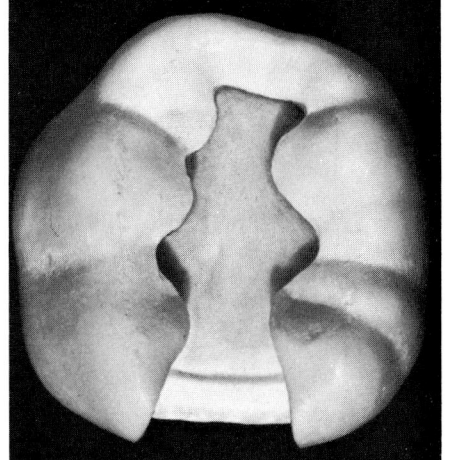

Figure 8-14 Plaster model of mandibular second primary molar showing proximo-occlusal cavity preparation with conservative isthmus.

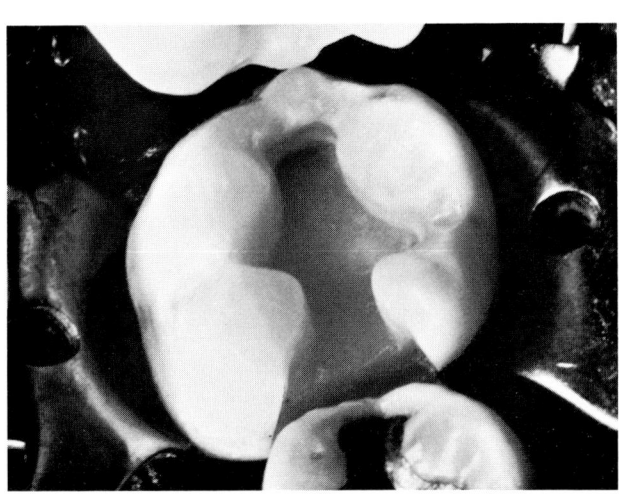

Figure 8-15 Clinical case involving mesio-occlusal cavity preparation in mandibular second primary molar. Note extensions of proximal walls.

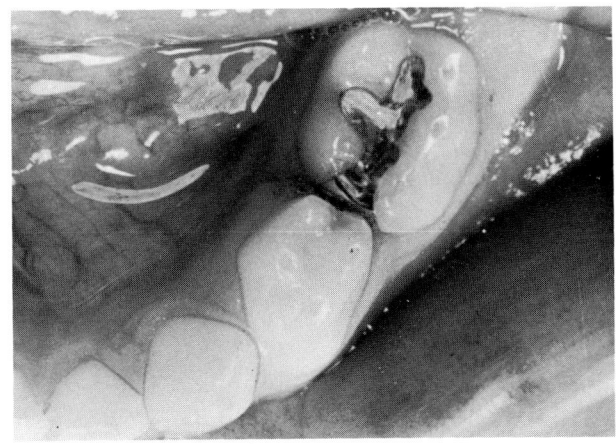

Figure 8-16 Finished mesio-occlusal amalgam restoration in mandibular second primary molar. The opposing cusps should always be checked for traumatic interdigitation and ground off if necessary.

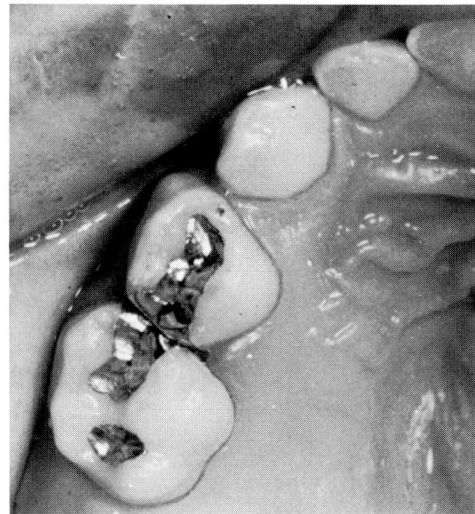

Figure 8-17 Properly finished approximating amalgam restorations.

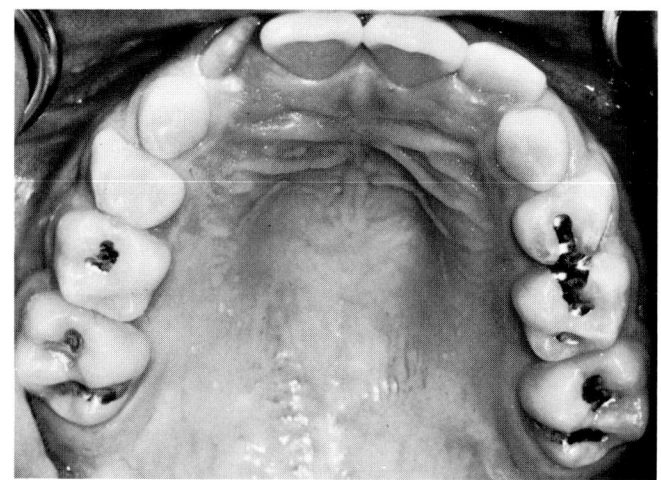

Figure 8-18 Another example of the conservative isthmus in the proximo-occlusal amalgam restoration.

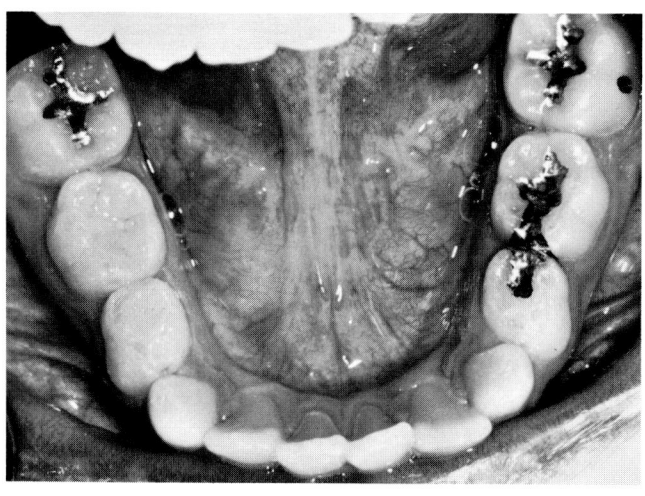

Figure 8-19 Mandibular arch with finished amalgam restorations.

OPERATIVE DENTISTRY 171

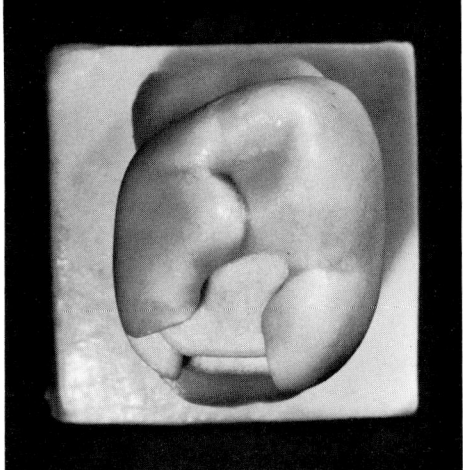

Figure 8-20 Plaster model showing reduction of the distolingual cusp of a mandibular first primary molar. This is frequently necessary if the cavity wall is fragile.

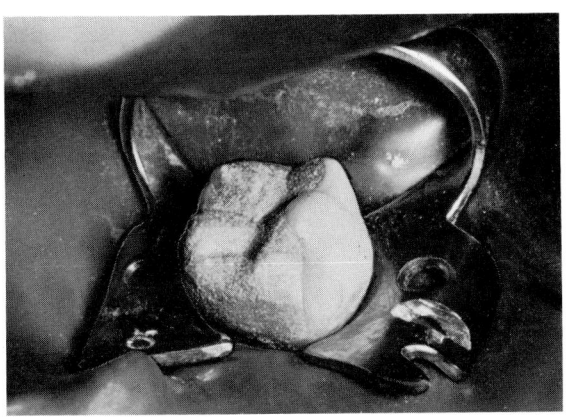

Figure 8-21 A carved amalgam restoration in a mandibular second primary molar illustrating the complete reduction of the mesiobuccal cusp to prevent fracturing.

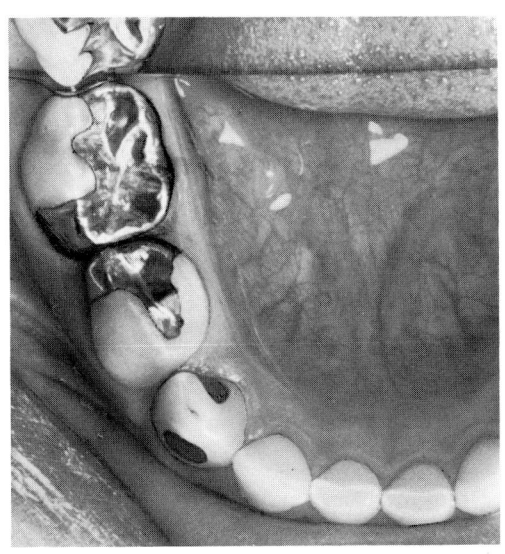

Figure 8-22 A clinical case in which the primary molars have been restored with amalgam. Note the cuspal coverage with amalgam to prevent fracture.

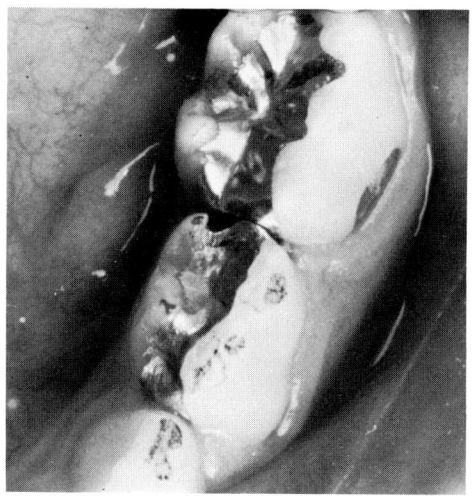

Figure 8-23 Fracture of the marginal ridge of a disto-occlusal amalgam in a mandibular first primary molar. This usually occurs from traumatic interdigitation of the lingual cusp of the maxillary first primary molar.

Figure 8-24 Carbon markings on the mandibular arch prior to beginning operative procedures. Markings on marginal ridge denote need for reduction of opposing cusp.

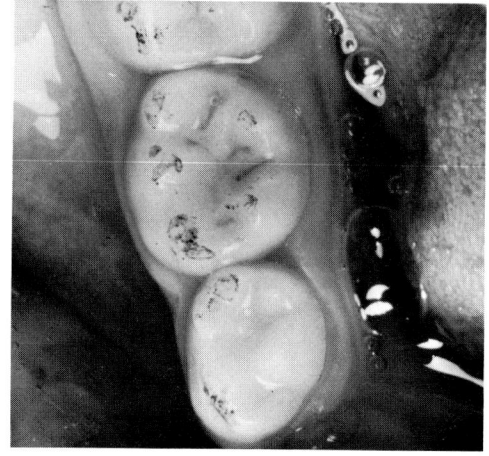

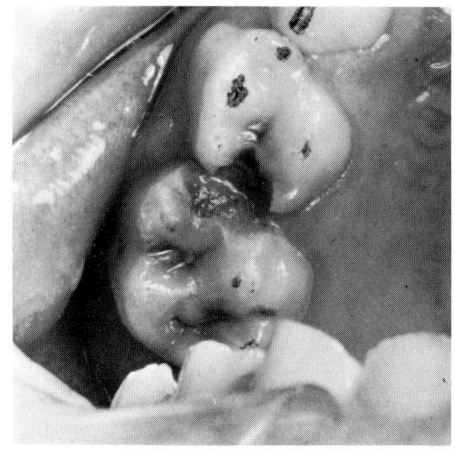

Figure 8-25 Opposing teeth in case illustrated in Figure 8-24. Sharp lingual cusp of first primary molar should be reduced.

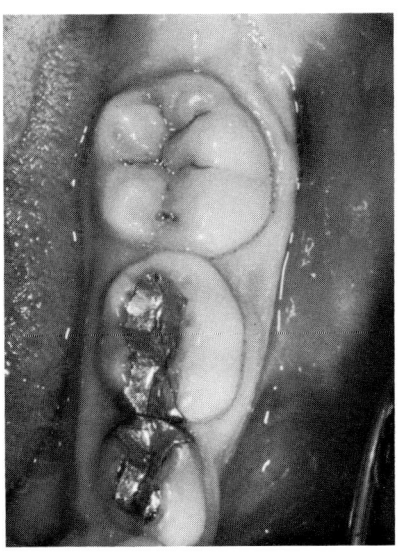

Figure 8-26 Marginal deterioration or ditching in proximo-occlusal amalgam restorations. Overcarving or undercarving can cause this, as can rough enamel walls, or in some cases poor manipulation of alloy and mercury.

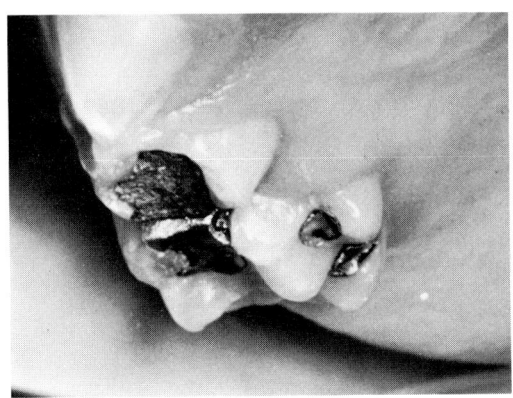

Figure 8-27 Marginal ditching that may be the result of a wide flaring cavity preparation.

Figure 8-28 A mouth restored with cast silver inlays. These have the advantage of superior edge strength and resistance to fracture. (Courtesy Dr. Quentin Williams.)

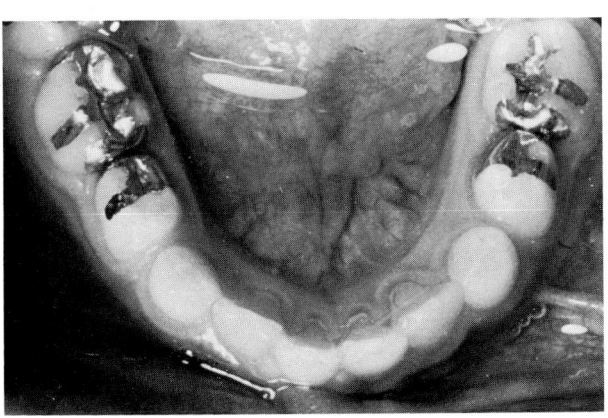

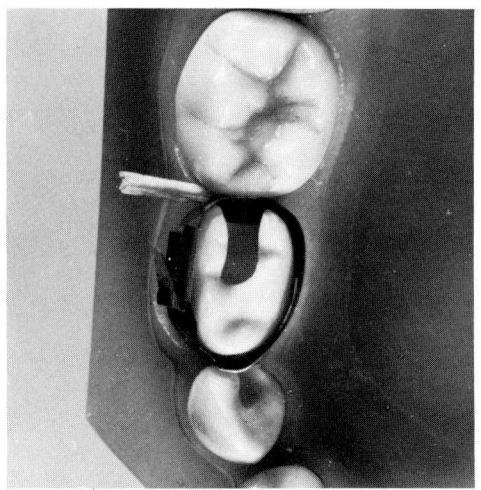

Figure 8-29 Model demonstrating use of a T-band matrix. The proximal surface of the band should be contoured to attain proper contact with the adjacent tooth.

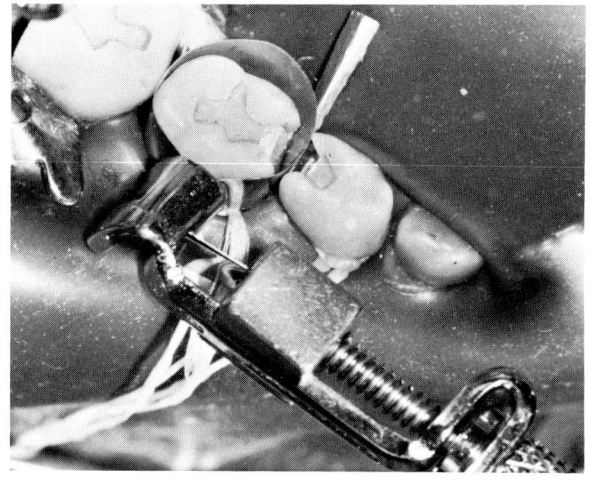

Figure 8-30 Tofflemire matrix holder prior to insertion of amalgam.

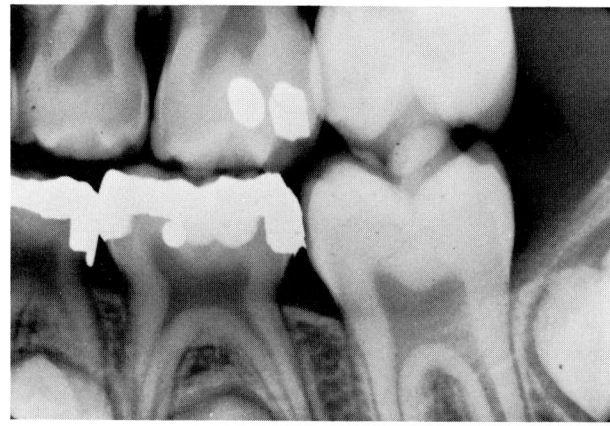

Figure 8-31 Radiograph illustrating result of faulty matrix. Wedging is necessary to prevent overhangs at gingival.

OPERATIVE DENTISTRY   175

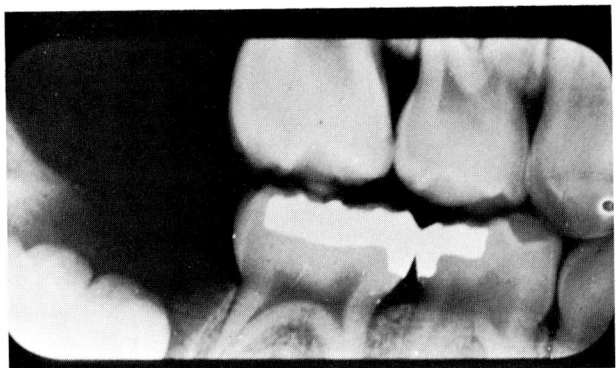
Figure 8-32   Well-contoured amalgam restorations.

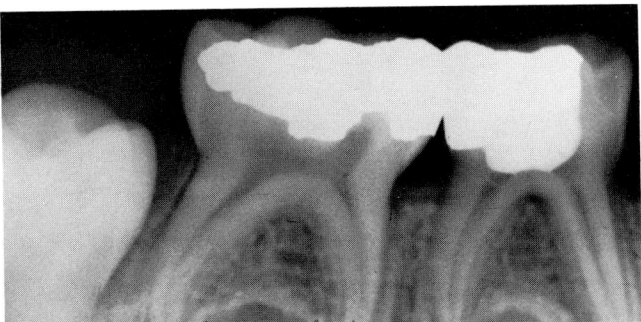
Figure 8-33   Another example of properly contoured approximating amalgam restorations.

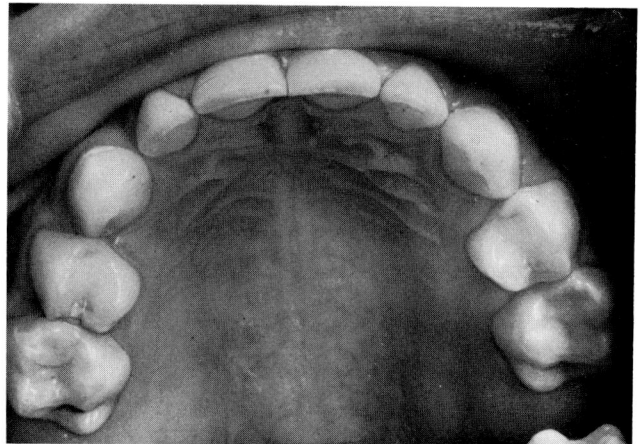

Figure 8-34 A 4-year-old child with multiple interproximal carious lesions. In this case the operator elected to restore the teeth with conventional amalgam restorations.

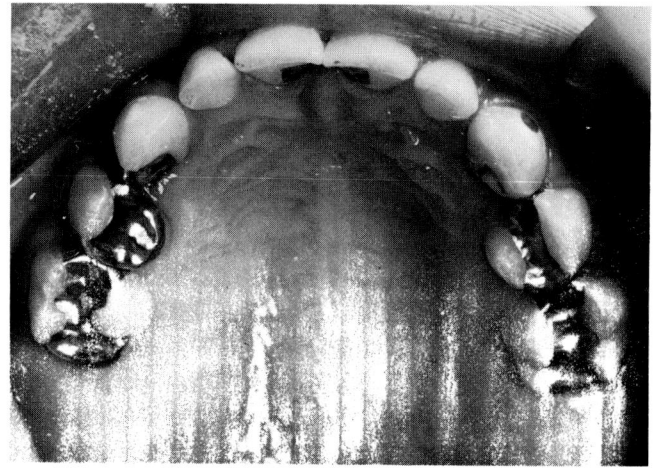

Figure 8-35 Same case illustrated in Figure 8-34 after careful operative work was completed.

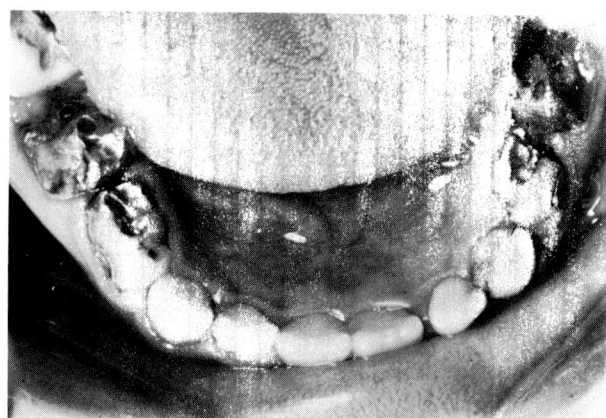

Figure 8-36 Failure of conventional primary molar restorations in a case of rampant caries. Steel crowns are the only recourse in this situation.

OPERATIVE DENTISTRY 177

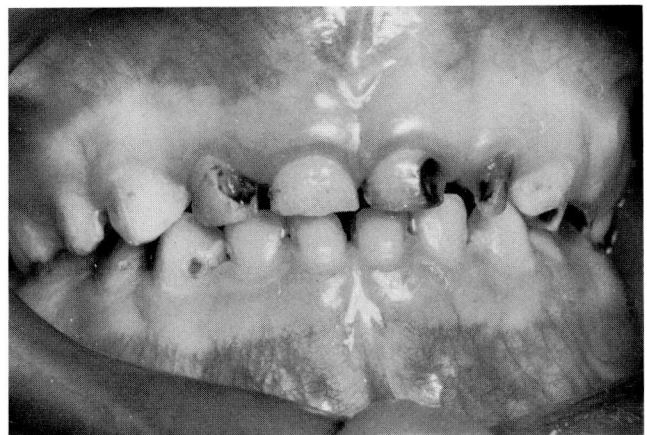

Figure 8-37 Multiple carious lesions involving primary anterior teeth. One practical method of restoring these teeth is with preformed bands.

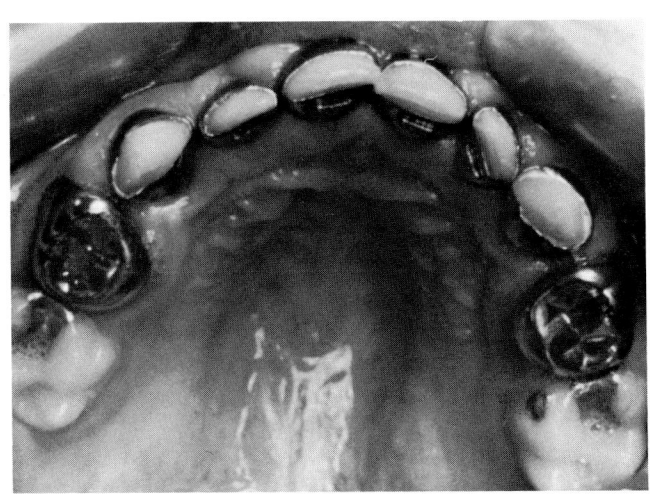

Figure 8-38 Primary incisors restored with preformed bands. Caries is removed from proximal surfaces, a protective pulpal base is placed, and the bands are cemented to position.

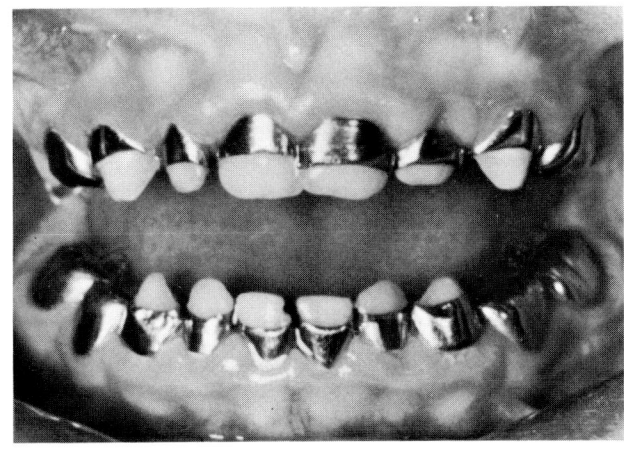

Figure 8-39 Labial view in case involving multiple band restorations.

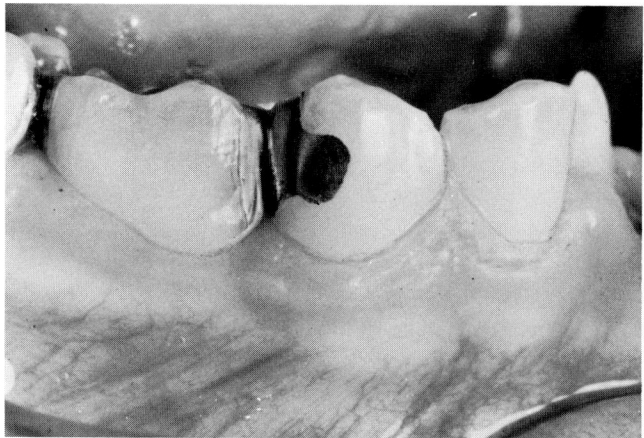

Figure 8-40 Labial dovetail amalgam restoration, restoring the distal surface of the mandibular cuspid.

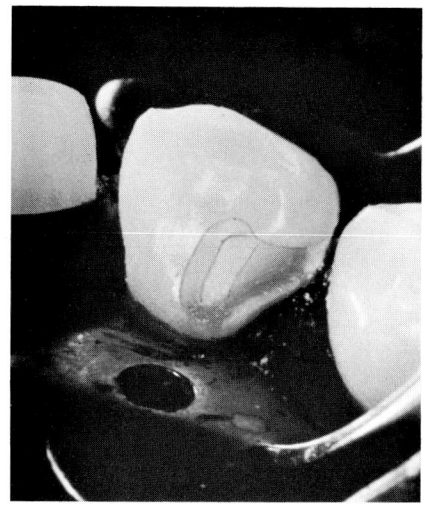

Figure 8-41 Lingual dovetail cavity preparation on a primary cuspid. The incisal edge should not be undercut if later fracture is to be avoided.

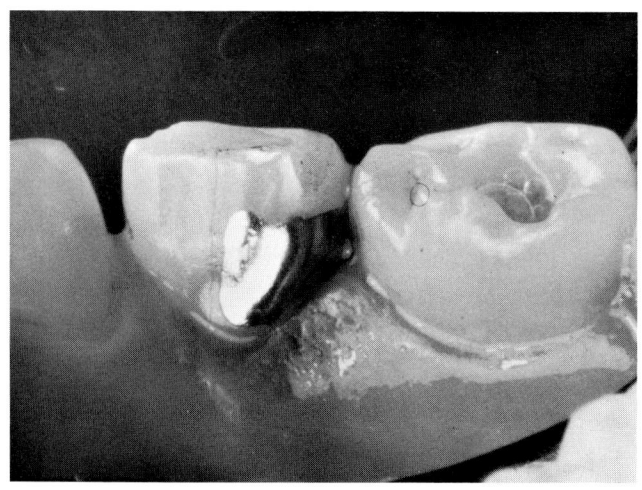

Figure 8-42 Restoration placed. Same tooth as shown in Figure 8-41.

Figure 8-43 Proximal caries on the mandibular incisors in a boy 8 years old. This is an indication of very high caries susceptibility. In this case amalgam restorations were placed. They will later be replaced by a more esthetic material.

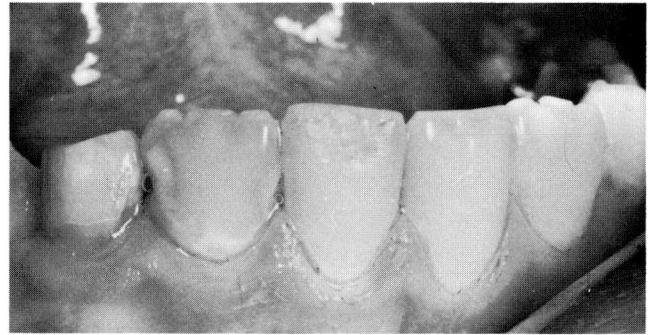

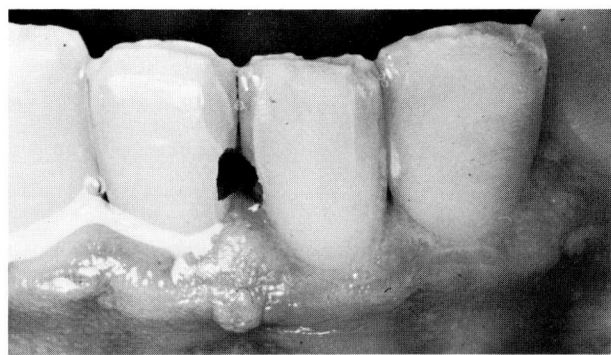

Figure 8-44 Gold foil used to restore proximal carious lesions in the mandibular central incisors of a 12-year-old boy. This material should be used more frequently in restorations in children.

Figure 8-45 Gingival caries in a 4-year-old boy who received amalgam restorations. Other materials may be utilized in this situation but in this case amalgam was chosen for its durability and economy.

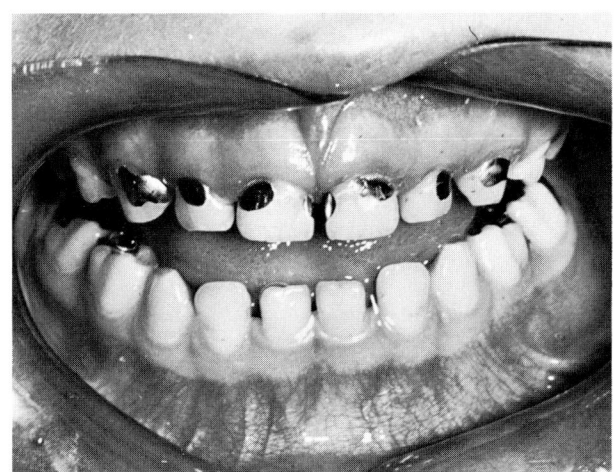

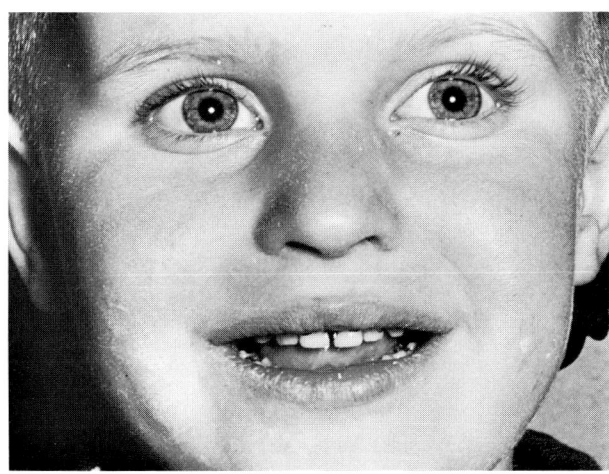

Figure 8-46 Same boy as seen in Figure 8-45. Lip coverage hides the restorative material quite well.

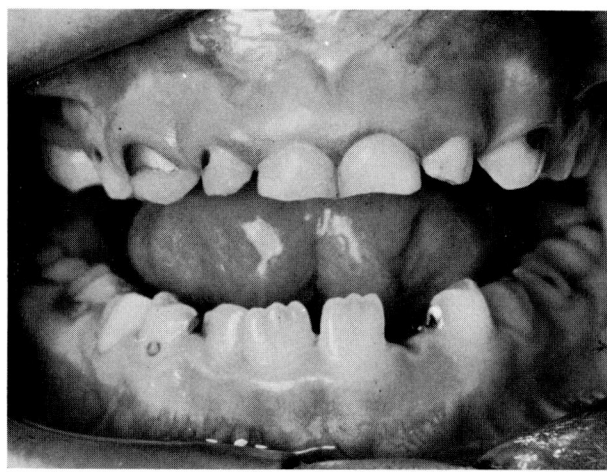

Figure 8-47 Gingival amalgam restorations in a 6-year-old child. If well finished and polished, these restorations will give excellent service.

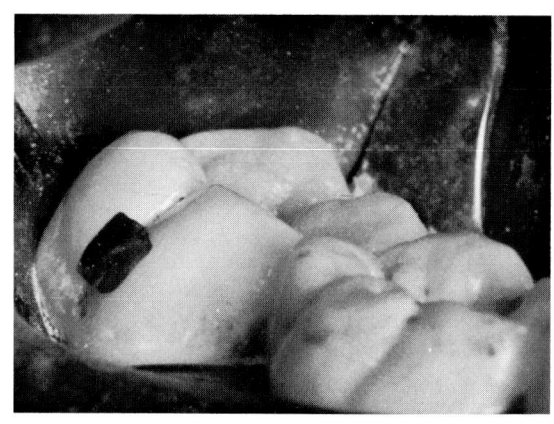

Figure 8-48 Buccal pit in a permanent first molar restored with gold foil. The location and size of this lesion are suitable for the use of gold foil.

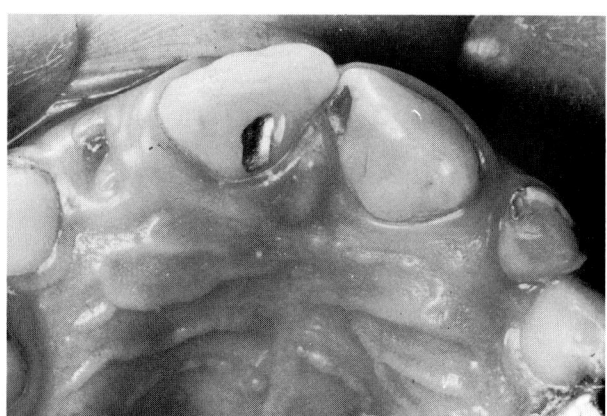

Figure 8-49 Lingual pit on a maxillary permanent incisor restored in gold foil. The location is well suited to the use of this material.

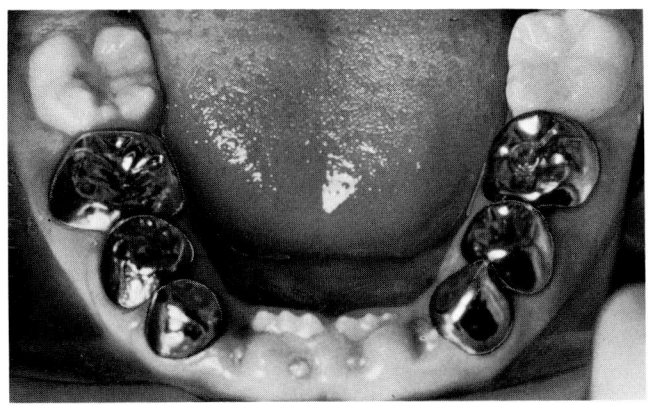

Figure 8-50 Mandibular primary molars and cuspids restored with stainless steel crowns. Constantly gaining in popularity, these crowns make excellent restorations.

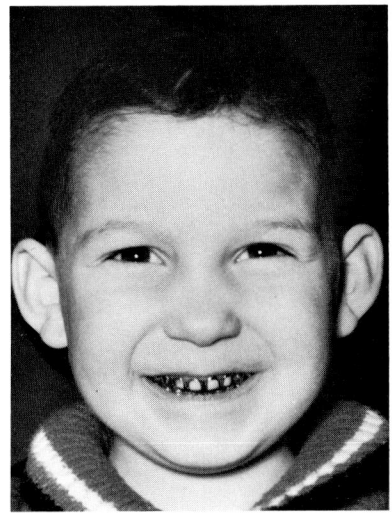

Figure 8-51 A 5-year-old boy with complete stainless steel crown coverage on all primary teeth.

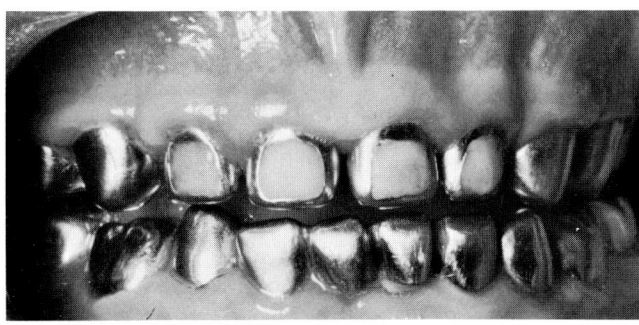

Figure 8-52 Full face view of child seen in Figure 8-51. Maxillary crowns have been cut away on the labial to enhance esthetics. (Courtesy Dr. R. L. Van Derschelden)

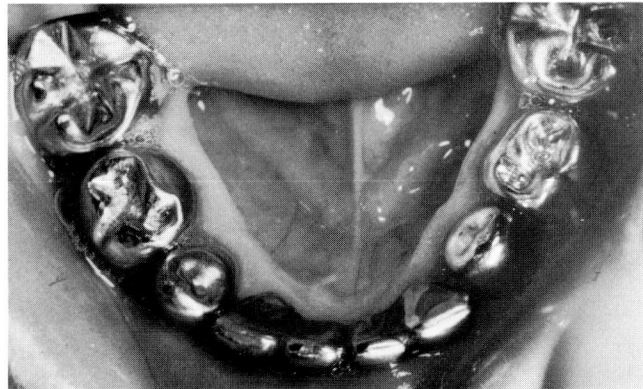

Figure 8-53 Mandibular arch of child shown in Figure 8-51 illustrating crown adaptation.

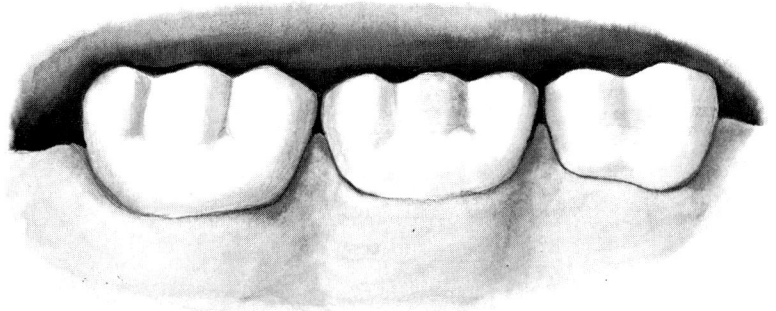

Figure 8-54 Lower right second primary molar prior to preparation for a stainless steel crown. (Modified from Mink, J. R., and Bennett, I. C.: The stainless steel crown. Journ. Dent. Child. 35:186-196, May, 1968.)

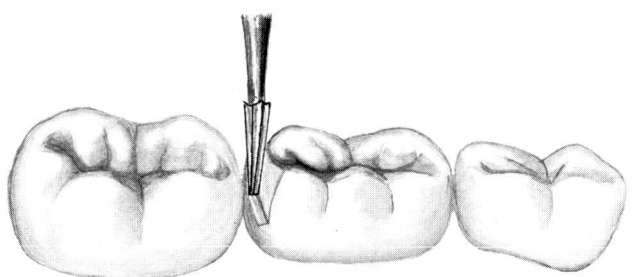

Figure 8-55 Following isolation of the operating area with a rubber dam, the first step is mesial and distal proximal reduction. A No. 69 or 70 friction grip bur is used for this purpose. First a ledge is made on the distal marginal ridge. As the bur cuts gingivally a *slice* preparation is made (see Figure 8-56). There *must not be a ledge* at the gingival of the preparation. Avoid reducing adjacent teeth during this step.

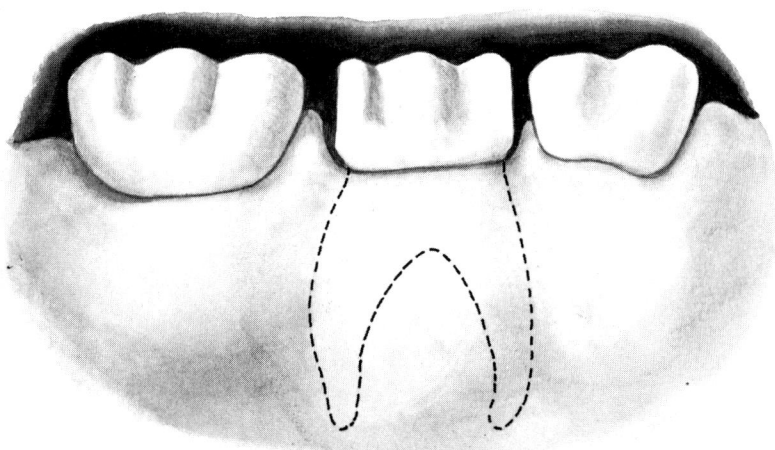

Figure 8-56 Buccal view of the proximal slices. Note: there is *no ledge* at the gingival.

OPERATIVE DENTISTRY 183

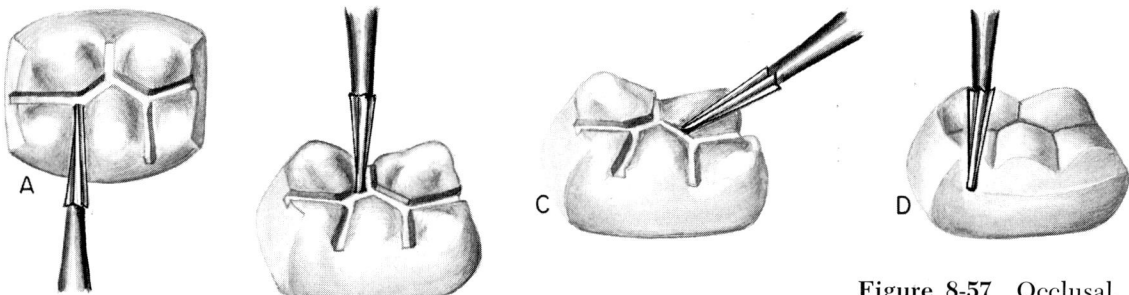

Figure 8-57 Occlusal, occlusobuccal and occlusolingual reductions.

A, Depth cuts established by placing bur on side. Occlusal reduction should be approximately 1 to 1.5 mm. This is easily established by cutting into the tooth slightly deeper than the diameter of the bur.
B, Depth cuts established in occlusal groves.
C, Completion of occlusal reduction by reducing tooth structure between depth cuts.
D, Occlusobuccal reduction. The occlusolingual may be reduced at this time also.
  Note: The buccogingival one-third and the linguogingival one-third of the tooth are not usually reduced. On occasion when a tooth has a large buccal bulge the gingival one-third also is reduced.

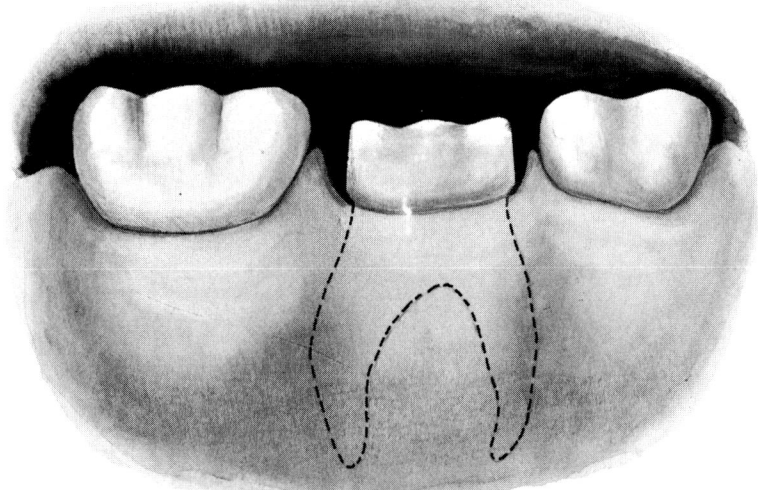

Figure 8-58 Cross-sectional view of proximal and occlusal reductions.

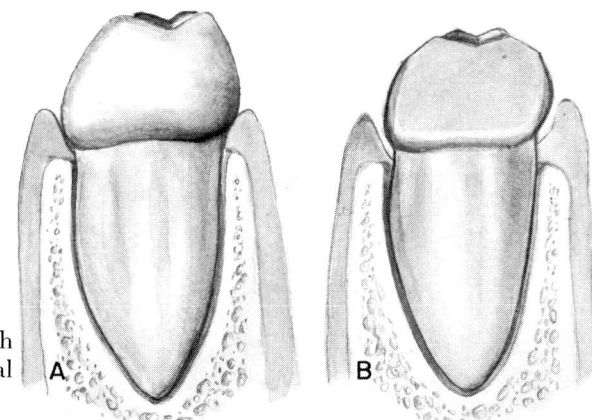

Figure 8-59 Mesial view of tooth before and after proximal and occlusal reductions.
  A, Before reduction.
  B, After reduction. Note that tooth structure was not reduced in buccogingival one-third or linguogingival one-third. The only time tooth structure is reduced below the gingiva is during the proximal slice. There is *no* finish line for this preparation.

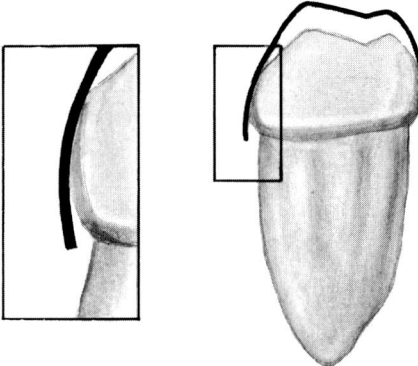

Figure 8-60 Initial placement of stainless steel crown on tooth. In some cases the crown extends too far gingivally, it must then be trimmed.

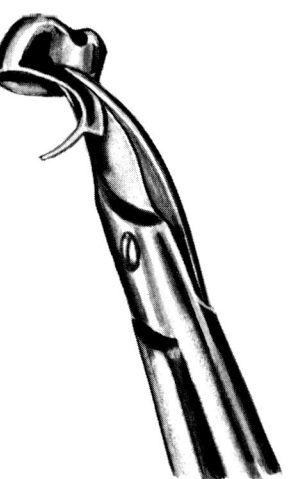

Figure 8-61 Trimming excess material from crown.

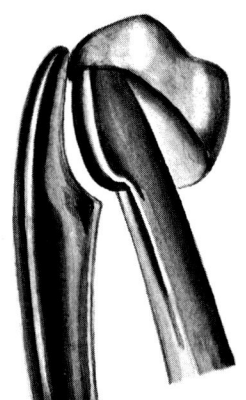

Figure 8-62 Crimping the gingival one-third of the crown in with the No. 114 plier.

OPERATIVE DENTISTRY 185

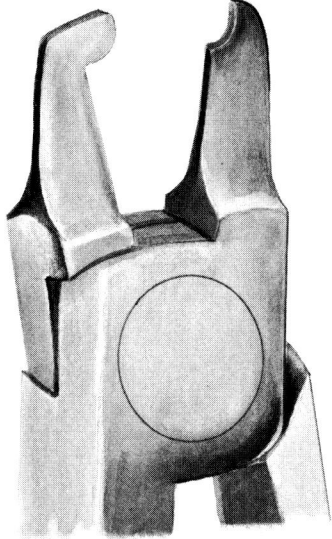
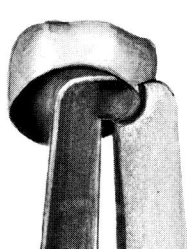

Figure 8-63 Finer crimping of the crown may be accomplished with the No. 109 crown crimping plier.

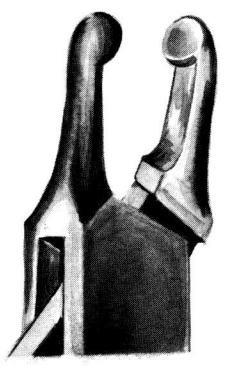
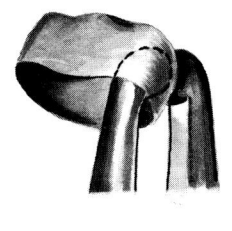

Figure 8-64 The No. 112 plier may be used to increase the mesiodistal dimension of the crown when it is slightly shy of contact with adjacent teeth.

Figure 8-65 Final finishing of the gingival margin of the crown. The gingival margin of the crown should be finished to a knife edge, as shown in the enlarged gingival view in Figure 8-66. The edge should then be polished with a rubber wheel.

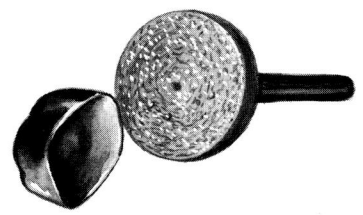

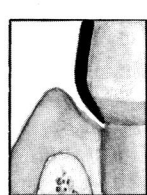
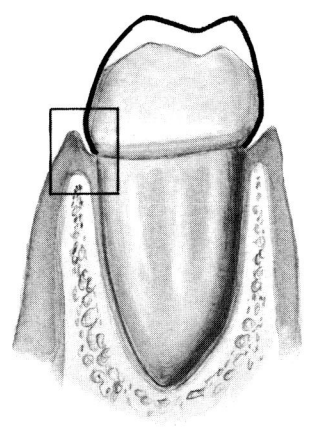

Figure 8-66 Cross-sectional view of finished stainless steel crown in place. The crown may be cemented with a rubber dam in place or with the area isolated with cotton rolls. After the cement has set, all loose pieces should be removed and the gingival one-third of the crown polished with pumice in a prophylaxis cup, to remove any remaining small particles of cement.

REFERENCES

1. Brauer, J. C., Higley, L. B., Lindahl, R. L., Massler, M., and Schour, I.: *Dentistry For Children.* The Blakiston Co., Inc., 1964, New York.
2. Lampshire, E. L.: An evaluation of cavity preparations in primary molars. J. Dent. Child. 22:7, 1955.
3. MacRae, P. D., Zackerl, W., and Castaldi, C. R.: A study of defects in Class II dental amalgam restorations in deciduous molars. J. Canad. Dent. Assoc. 28:491-502, 1962.
4. Nadal, R., Phillips, R. W., and Swartz, M. L.: Clinical investigation on the relation of mercury to the amalgam restorations: II. J.A.D.A. 63:488-496, 1961.
5. Sweet, C. A.: Cavity preparation in deciduous teeth. J.A.D.A. 38:423-430, 1949.
6. Terkla, L. G., and Mahler, D. B.: Clinical evaluation of interproximal retention grooves in Class II amalgam cavity design. Journ. Prosth. Dent. 17:596-602, 1967.

Chapter 9

PULP THERAPY

Conservation of the vitality and health of the dental pulp is one of the most important preventive aspects of the practice of dentistry for children. No space-maintaining appliance can equal the natural tooth during the developmental years, nor can the psychologic value of retention of natural teeth be overestimated. Some differences exist in the approach to clinical management of the exposed or nearly exposed dental pulp in the primary and immature permanent dentition as contrasted to the fully formed adult dentition.

The primary teeth exhibit special morphologic characteristics which make conventional endodontic procedures somewhat difficult. The root canals tend to be more flat and ribbon-like, particularly as the tooth becomes more mature. Root resorption presents problems in obtaining a good apical seal. In spite of these complicating factors there is increased interest in utilizing endodontic procedures in the non-vital primary tooth during the preschool years. By far the most common pulpal problem in children is the carious exposure in the vital primary tooth. This is best treated by pulpal amputation and sealing off at the canal orifices with a suitable agent which will promote healing and maintain viable tissue in the root canal. Thus far the formocresol drugs have proved to be far more successful in this regard than calcium hydroxide in treating the primary teeth. Other agents will undoubtedly be developed that may prove even more effective, but in the long run the prevention of the carious lesion is still the most rewarding approach to the problem.

There is little justification for so-called capping in carious exposures in primary teeth. Pulpotomy has been demonstrated to be much more successful and the extra time required is not significant. Indirect pulp capping has demonstrated considerable usefulness in recent years. In this procedure a drug such as calcium hydroxide or zinc oxide and eugenol is placed over partially excavated carious dentin to inhibit bacterial activity and stimulate dentin calcification. Although it is of greater value in treating doubtful cases in the immature permanent dentition, the operator may elect to utilize this procedure on primary teeth in selected instances.

Special considerations surround the problem of pulp exposure in the young immature permanent tooth. In most cases, the apical foramen is still open, complicating endodontic procedures. Often, too, the dentition is still in a state of adjustment and transition and tooth loss is especially undesirable. Here again the clinician must elect to perform the procedure most likely to conserve and protect the involved tooth. Traumatic injury is one of the most frequent causes of exposure in the immature permanent tooth, and these cases have responded quite successfully to pulpotomy with calcium hydroxide. When apical completion has occurred, endodontics must be weighed against the pulpotomy procedure. The decision remains with the operator to determine which will be most successful over a period of years.

Indirect pulp capping is the sealing in of a suitable drug over partially excavated carious dentin. The purpose is to arrest the existing caries process and stimulate sclerosis and hardening in the remaining vital dentin. Calcium hydroxide has been used successfully as well as zinc oxide and eugenol and also camphorated monochlorophenol. Indications: for deep carious lesions approaching the pulp, especially in young permanent teeth with incompletely formed root ends. Contraindications: history of dental pain, frank dental exposure, or periapical pathology.

Pulp capping is the direct placement of a drug or medication over small pulpal exposures. It is recommended for accidental operative exposures primarily, although it is used by some clinicians for small carious exposures of 1 mm. or less. Numerous different drugs have been suggested for this procedure, calcium hydroxide being currently the most widely utilized. Capping has never been a consistently successful approach to pulp management and should be employed sparingly.

Pulpotomy implies the complete amputation of the vital coronal pulp and the placement of a suitable drug over the remaining exposed tissue. The objective is to maintain the vitality of the pulp remaining in the root canals so that the restored tooth can function as a healthy biological unit. A variety of drugs have been used in the pulpotomy procedure including zinc oxide and eugenol, calcium hydroxide, formocresol, and other combinations. Current research indicates formocresol to be the drug of choice in treating carious exposures in primary teeth, while calcium hydroxide is preferred for the immature permanent tooth such as the traumatically injured incisor.

Pulpectomy or complete extirpation of the pulp tissue from the crown and root canals of teeth may be employed in treatment of necrotic primary teeth. The root canal sealant must be capable of being resorbed. Best results will be achieved in pulpectomy on primary teeth when performed on single rooted teeth or on molars during the preschool years before secondary calcification has taken place. Success can also be attained in pulpectomy on immature permanent teeth. Recent developments indicate an advantage in using calcium hydroxide and camphorated monochlorophenol filling material in these cases to promote root end closure.

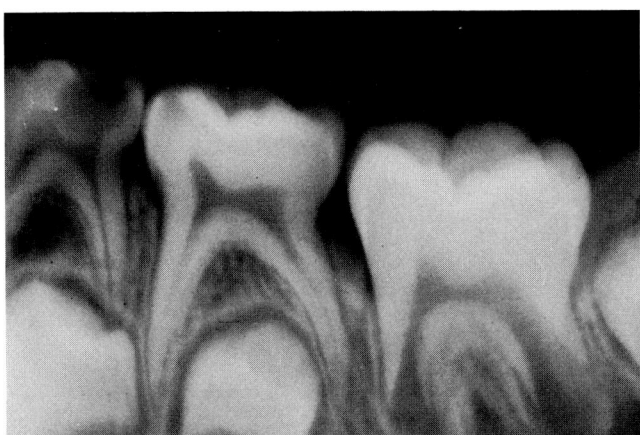

Figure 9-1 Deep carious lesion (almost pulpal exposure) in occlusal surface of the mandibular first primary molar. In a mouth with multiple lesions similar to this the *indirect pulp capping* technique may be used to great advantage. In one visit all severely affected areas may be temporarily treated and caries arrested, and at a later visit permanent restorations may be placed. The procedure is as follows:

A, Remove all soft leathery carious dentin (harder carious dentin is not removed to avoid exposing the pulp).

B, Cover the harder carious dentin with a paste of calcium hydroxide, and place over it a temporary amalgam restoration.

C, In 3 to 6 months remove the amalgam and calcium hydroxide and extirpate any remaining carious dentin. By this time most of the underlying carious dentin has become hard.

This technique enables the dentist to temporarily treat multiple areas in one sitting and usually prevent pulpal exposures when the permanent restorations are placed.

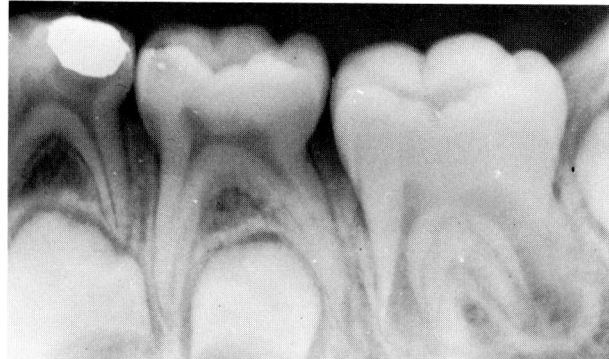

Figure 9-2 Same patient as seen in Figure 9-1 immediately after treatment. Note radiolucency under the amalgam. This is calcium hydroxide, which normally appears radiolucent in a radiograph.

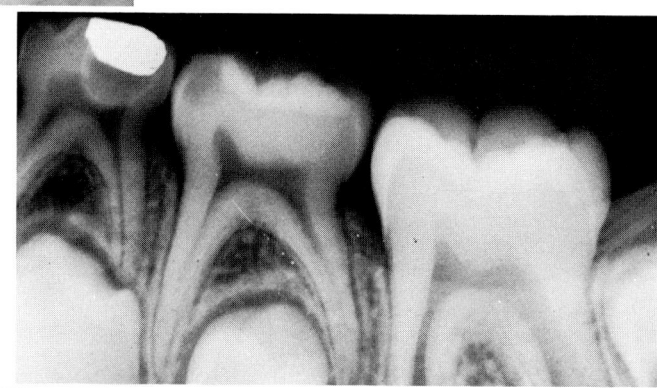

Figure 9-3 Same patient as shown in Figures 9-1 and 9-2, 6 months after *indirect pulp capping*. Note increased radiopacity under the calcium hydroxide. This is a reflection of the increased density of the vital dentin. The tooth is now ready for a permanent restoration.

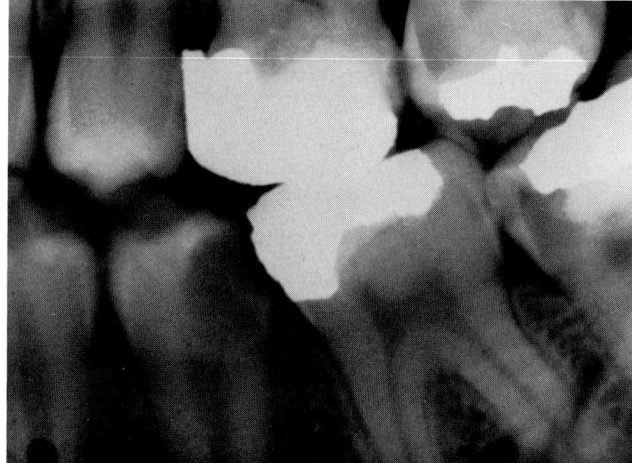

Figure 9-4 Deep carious lesion in a mandibular second bicuspid. Tooth was treated with an *indirect pulp capping*, as described in Figure 9-1.

Figure 9-5 Same patient as seen in Figure 9-4, 6 months after indirect pulp capping. Note increased radiopacity of tooth structure adjacent to calcium hydroxide. Pulpal exposure was avoided and the tooth successfully treated.

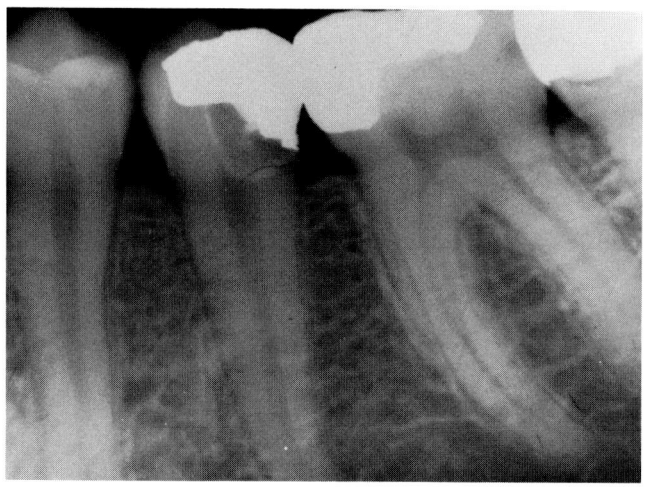

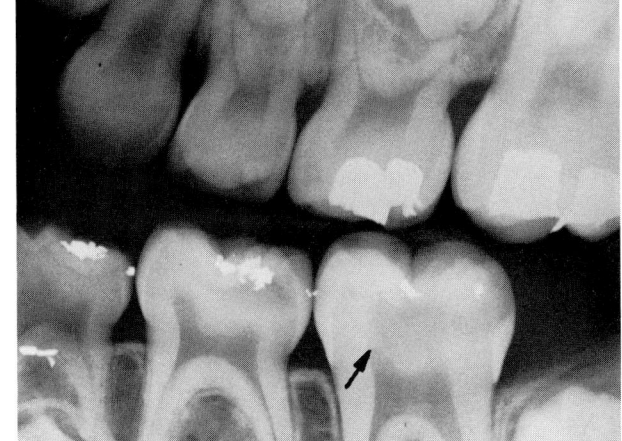

Figure 9-6 A 9-year-old girl with deep occlusal caries encroaching on the pulp. This case is ideal for indirect pulp capping with calcium hydroxide paste.

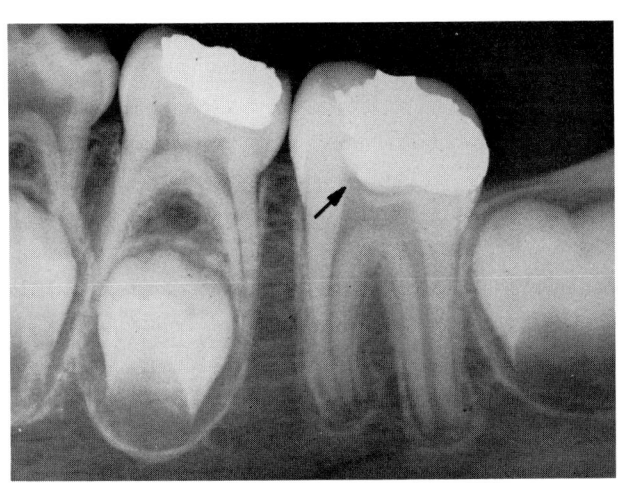

Figure 9-7 Postoperative radiograph of tooth seen in Figure 9-6, showing partial removal of caries and placement of calcium hydroxide under a temporary amalgam restoration. Note incomplete root apices.

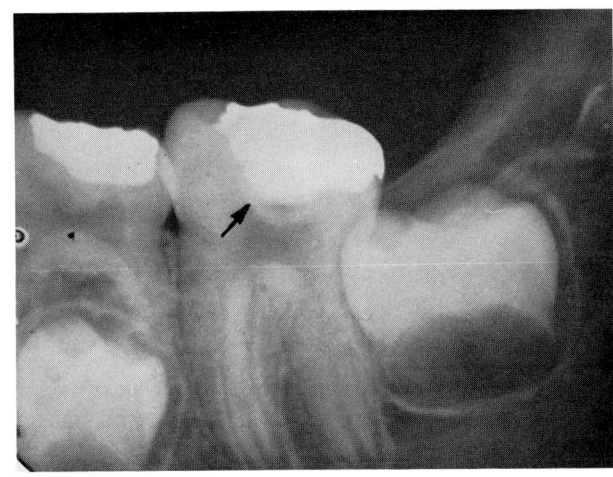

Figure 9-8 Radiograph of tooth shown in Figure 9-6, 7 months postoperatively. Note radiopaque line under calcium hydroxide base. This represents a layer of sound dentin of increased density. Note continued development of root ends.

PULP THERAPY

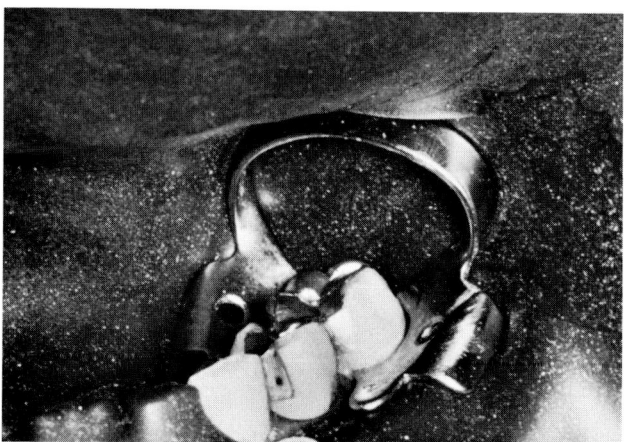

Figure 9-9 A minute surgical exposure on the mesial surface of a mandibular primary molar. Small *surgical* exposures may be capped with a paste of calcium hydroxide.

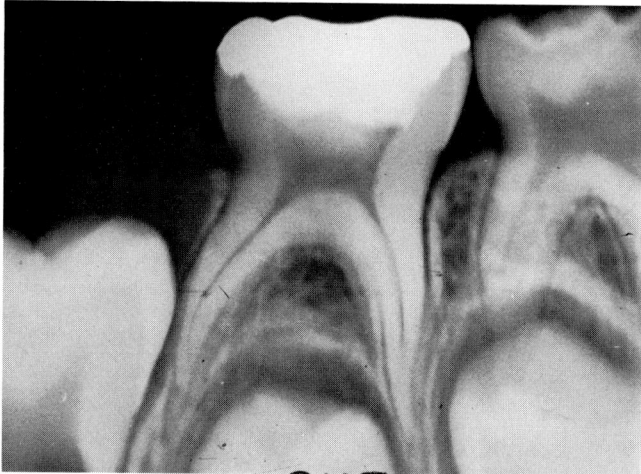

Figure 9-10 Radiograph of successful calcium hydroxide capping on mesial horn of mandibular second primary molar.

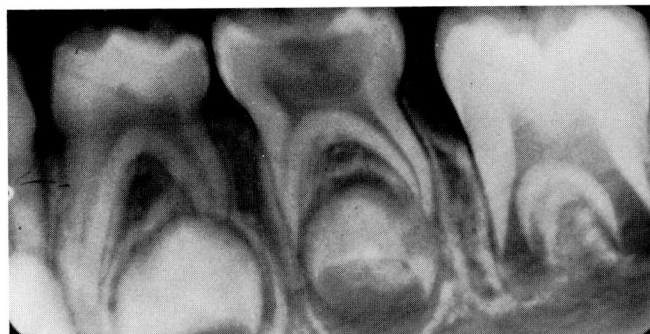

Figure 9-11 A large carious exposure in a primary second molar. A *formocresol pulpotomy* is the treatment of choice for this tooth. Contraindications for the formocresol pulpotomy are the following:
  A, On clinical evaluation
    1. History of spontaneous pain.
    2. Pain from percussion.
    3. Suppuration.
  B, On radiographic evaluation
    1. Calcified globules in the pulp.
    2. Internal resorption.
    3. Pathologic bifurcation radiolucency.
    4. Pathologic periapical radiolucency.

None of the contraindications listed were observed in this case, so the formocresol pulpotomy was performed with success. Formocresol pulpotomy is done on primary teeth only.

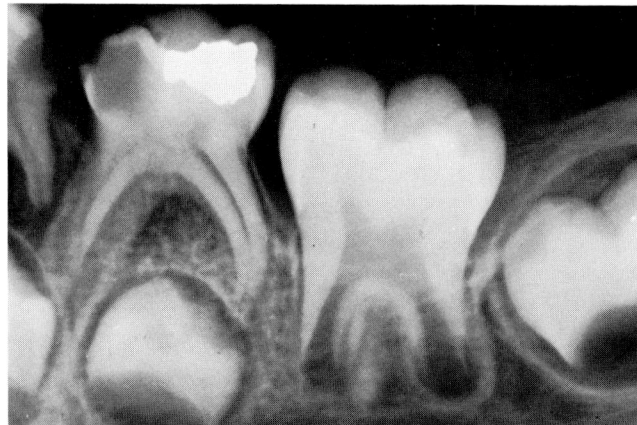

Figure 9-12 Primary second molar with a carious exposure on the mesial surface. Clinical and radiographic findings were normal. Formocresol pulpotomy was the treatment of choice.

Figure 9-13 Pulp exposures in adjacent primary molars. Hyperplasia of the pulp is not a contraindication for pulp treatment so long as the clinical and radiographic findings are normal. (See contraindications listed in Figure 9-11.)

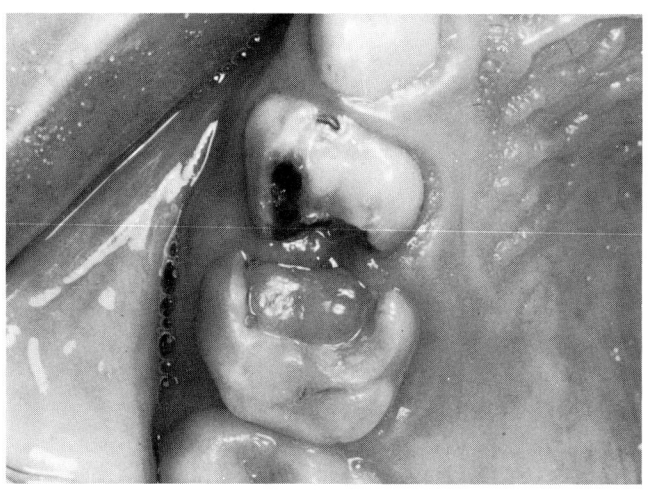

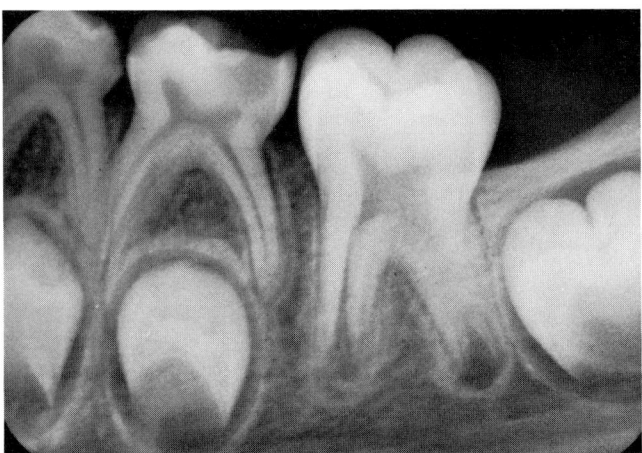

Figure 9-14 Radiograph of a carious exposure in a primary second molar. Formocresol pulpotomy is the treatment of choice.

Figure 9-15 Two primary molars with pulp exposures resulting from deep interproximal caries. There is questionable radiolucency in the bifurcation area and possible beginning internal resorption in the distal root of the second molar. In such cases additional films should be taken varying the exposure time. It is also helpful to examine comparable radiographs from the opposite side to determine what is normal for the patient.

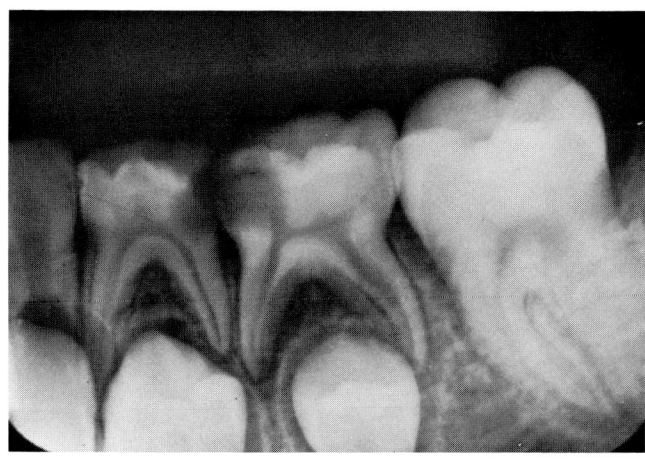

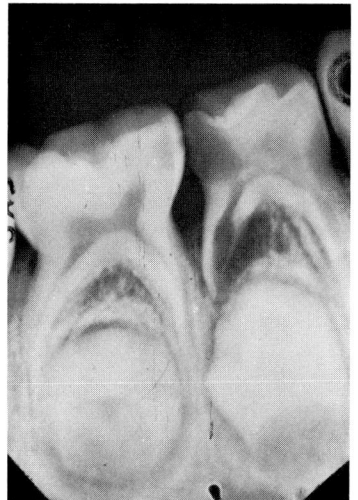

Figure 9-16 Radiograph of a primary first molar with a large carious exposure. Note the internal resorption in the distal canal and the radiopaque calcific body lying just above the orifice of the distal canal. These are indications of advanced degenerative changes of the pulp. Successful pulpotomy therapy is dependent upon proper selection of cases; with these degenerative changes it is definitely contraindicated.

Figure 9-17 A 5-year-old child with advanced caries in both first and second primary molars. Note the pathologic calcification above the distal canal of the first primary molar (a contraindication for pulp therapy).

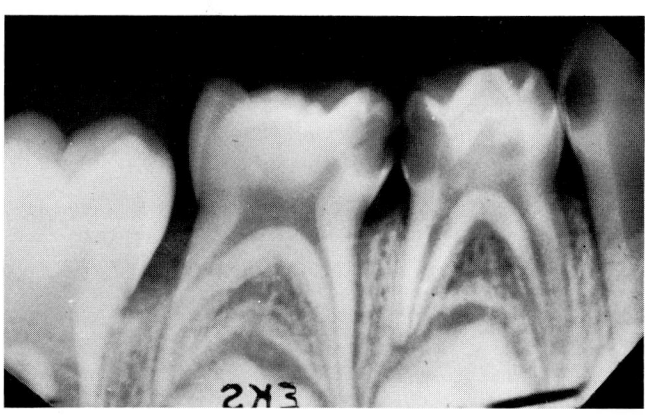

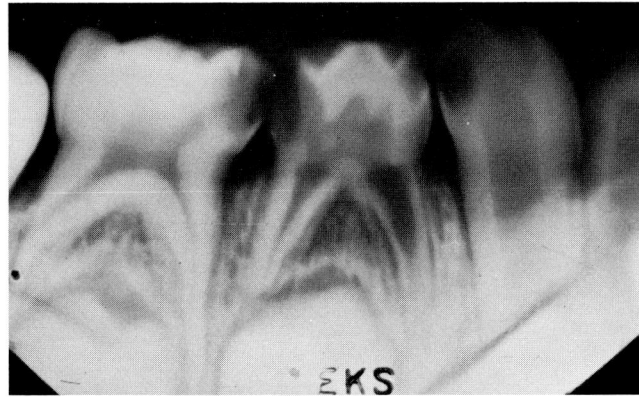

Figure 9-18 Same patient as seen in Figure 9-17, 6 weeks later. There is marked internal resorption of the first primary molar indicating advanced degenerative changes. These changes were forecast in the earlier radiographs.

PULP THERAPY

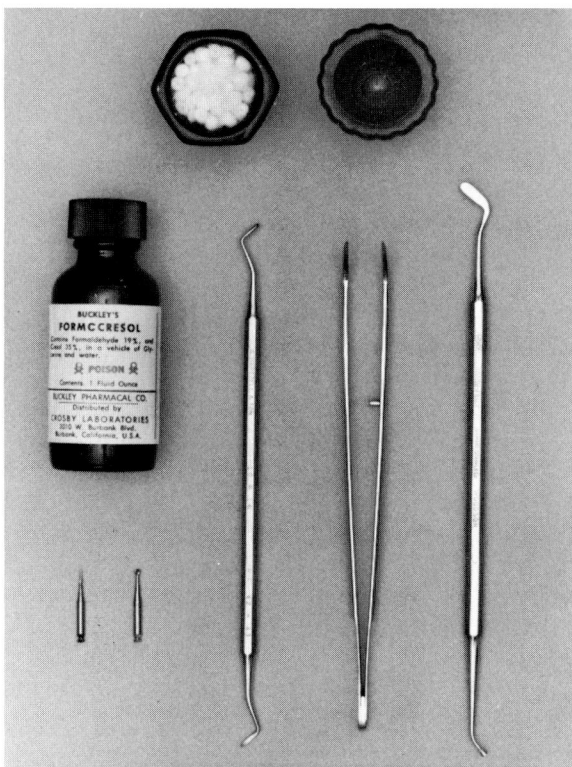

Figure 9-19 Tray setup for a formocresol pulpotomy; small cotton pellets, dish for formocresol liquid (Dappen dish), formocresol liquid (19 per cent formaldehyde, 35 per cent tricresol in a vehicle of 15 per cent glycerin plus water), fissure bur (high or low speed), round bur (low speed No. 4 or No. 6), excavator, cotton plier, applicating instrument. The procedure for treatment of primary teeth with the 5-minute formocresol pulpotomy is described in Figures 9-20 to 9-24.

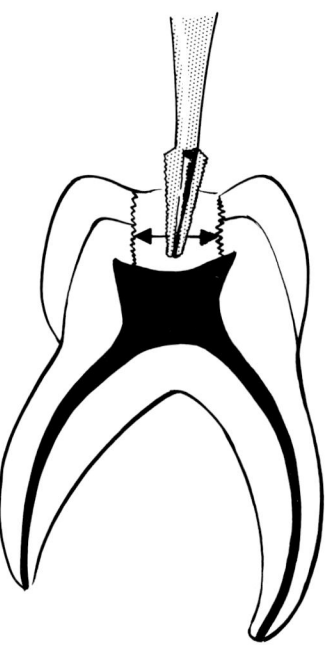

Figure 9-20 After the tooth is anesthetized, rubber dam is placed and the roof of the pulp chamber is removed with a fissure bur.

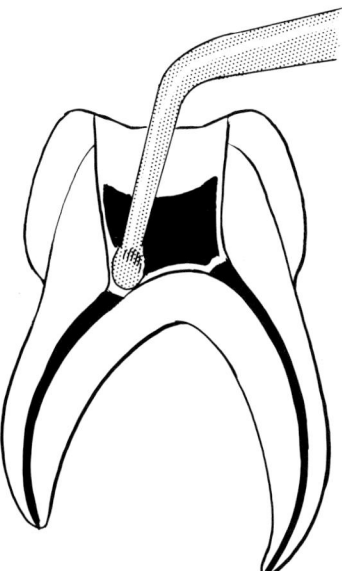

Figure 9-21 Excavator used to remove coronal portion of dental pulp. A round bur may also be used to remove the coronal pulp, however, extreme care must be taken to avoid perforating floor of pulp chamber with the round bur. Be sure walls of pulp chamber are exposed and that no dentin hangs over to constrict the chamber. Pulp chamber is then flushed with sterile water.

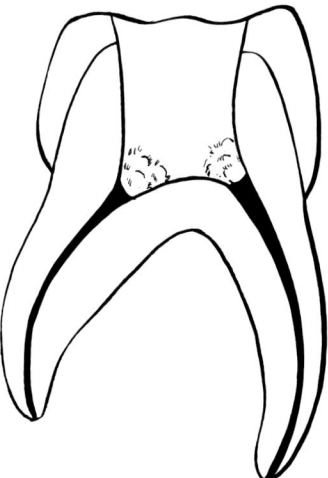

Figure 9-22 Hemorrhage is stopped with dry cotton pellets or a cotton pellet moistened with epinephrine. Hemorrhage must be stopped before placing cotton pellets impregnated with formocresol over pulp stumps.

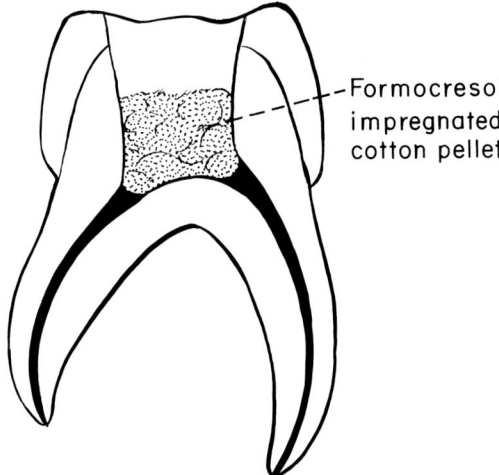

Figure 9-23 Cotton pellets moistened with formocresol are placed over pulp stumps and left in place for 5 minutes. Cotton pellet must not be so thoroughly saturated with formocresol that excess liquid might leak out under the dam onto the tissue. Formocresol is a caustic liquid and will cause tissue necrosis (see Figure 9-26). Excess liquid in the pellet should be absorbed by another pellet before it is placed in the pulp chamber. If hemorrhage has stopped after the formocresol impregnated cotton pellet has been in place for 5 minutes, then proceed to Figure 9-24, for the final step in the one-stage formocresol pulpotomy treatment. If, however, hemorrhage has not stopped after 5 minutes or time is lacking to complete the restoration of the tooth, a two-stage formocresol pulpotomy may be performed. The formocresol impregnated cotton pellets are sealed in over the pulp stumps with a zinc oxide and eugenol temporary filling. The patient is then scheduled for completion of treatment within 5 to 7 days. On the second visit the cotton pellets are removed and treatment is completed as described in Figure 9-24.

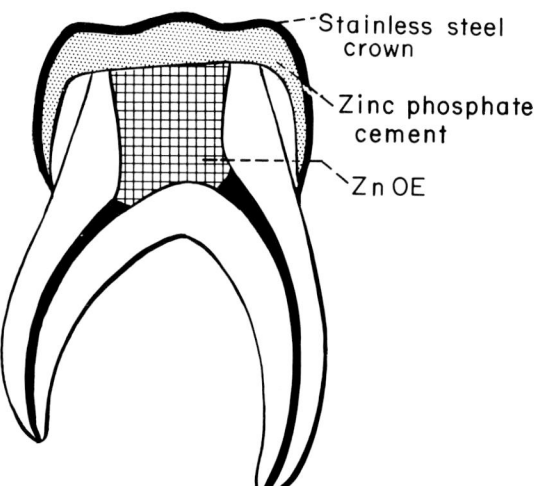

Figure 9-24 Remove formocresol pellet and leave area slightly moist with the drug. Slightly overfill pulp chamber with a paste consisting of zinc oxide powder and a liquid prepared by mixing equal parts of formocresol and eugenol. Finish preparation for a stainless steel crown.

Figure 9-25 Graph depicting yearly success rate in two clinical studies of 434 formocresol pulpotomies performed on primary teeth. Teeth treated with formocresol pulpotomy should be evaluated clinically and radiographically on the recall visit for success or failure. (From Law, D. B., and Lewis, T. M.; Formocresol pulpotomy in deciduous teeth. J.A.D.A. 69:601-607, Nov., 1964.)

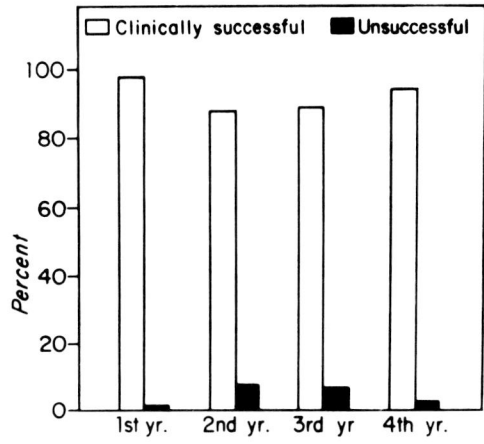

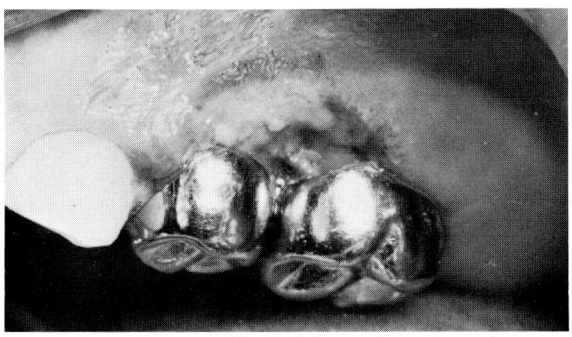

Figure 9-26 Formocresol burn from liquid which leaked out onto the tissue during pulpotomy procedure.

Figure 9-27 Radiograph of a mandibular second primary molar 2½ years after formocresol pulpotomy. This tooth was restored with a stainless steel crown. These teeth will often fracture because of the brittleness of the dentin from dehydration. Therefore, a stainless steel crown is the restoration of choice.

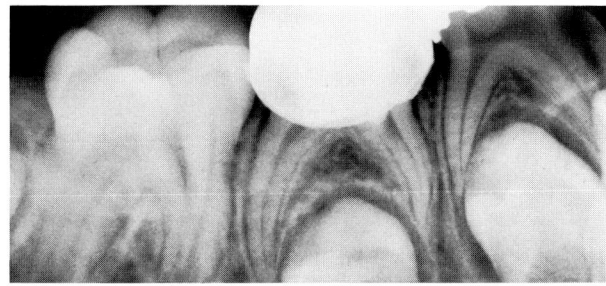

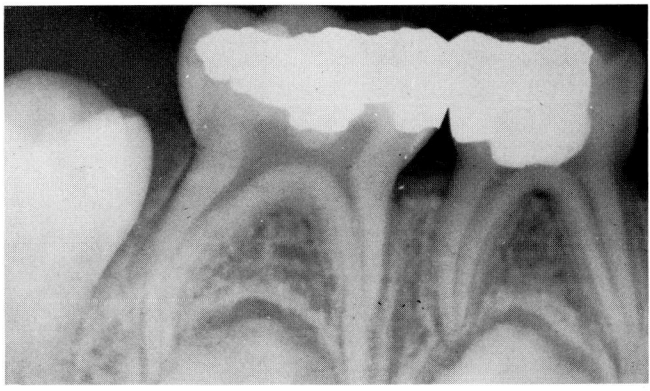

Figure 9-28 A first primary molar which exhibits a dentin bridge in the distal canal. This tooth underwent formocresol pulp therapy. Usually this drug does not stimulate calcification at the site of pulpal amputation.

Figure 9-29 An obvious formocresol pulpotomy failure of the mandibular first primary molar caused by degenerative changes around the distal root. Tooth had to be extracted.

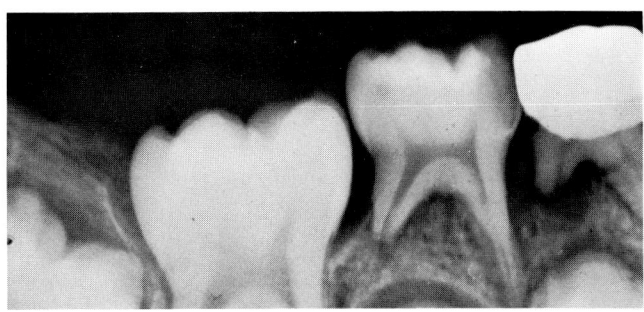

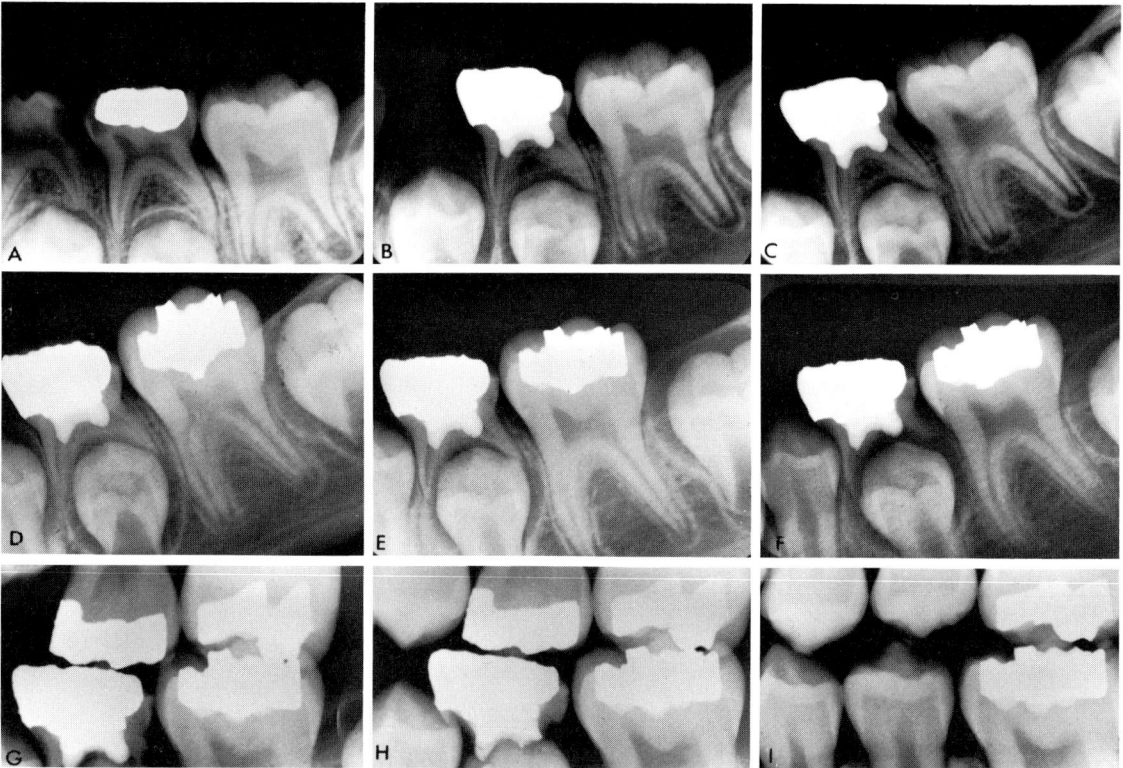

Figure 9-30 Radiographic series of a successful formocresol pulpotomy on a second primary molar over a 5-year period. Pulpotomy was performed when the child was 7 years of age. (Courtesy Dr. Donald R. Dietz.)

- A, Preoperative radiograph of a 7-year-old child prior to formocresol pulpotomy of the second primary molar.
- B, Six months after pulpotomy.
- C, One year after pulpotomy.
- D, Two years after pulpotomy.
- E, Three years after pulpotomy.
- F, Three and one-quarter years after pulpotomy.
- G, Three and one-half years after pulpotomy.
- H, Four years after pulpotomy.
- I, Five years after pulpotomy.

PULP THERAPY 201

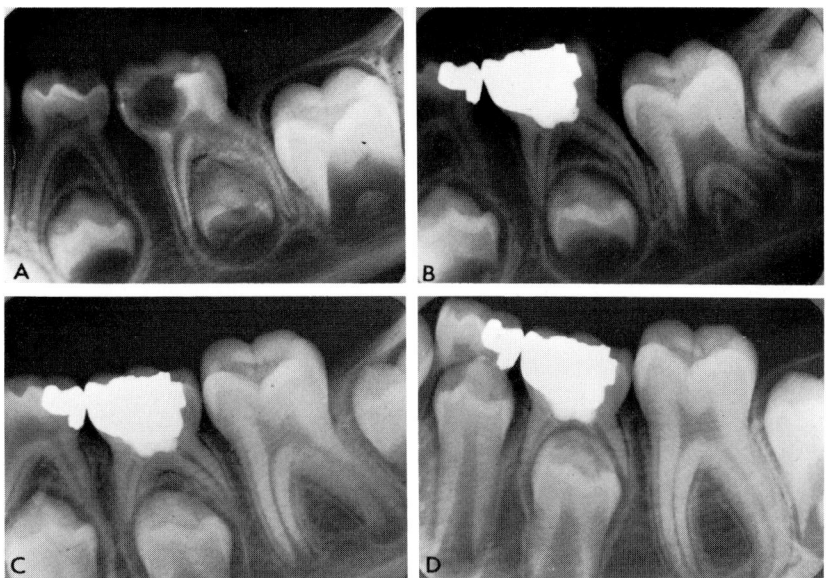

Figure 9-31 Radiographic series of a successful formocresol pulpotomy on a second primary molar. (Courtesy Dr. Donald R. Dietz.)
   A, Preoperative radiograph of a 4½-year-old child prior to formocresol pulpotomy of the second primary molar.
   B, One year after pulpotomy.
   C, Three years after pulpotomy.
   D, Five years after pulpotomy.

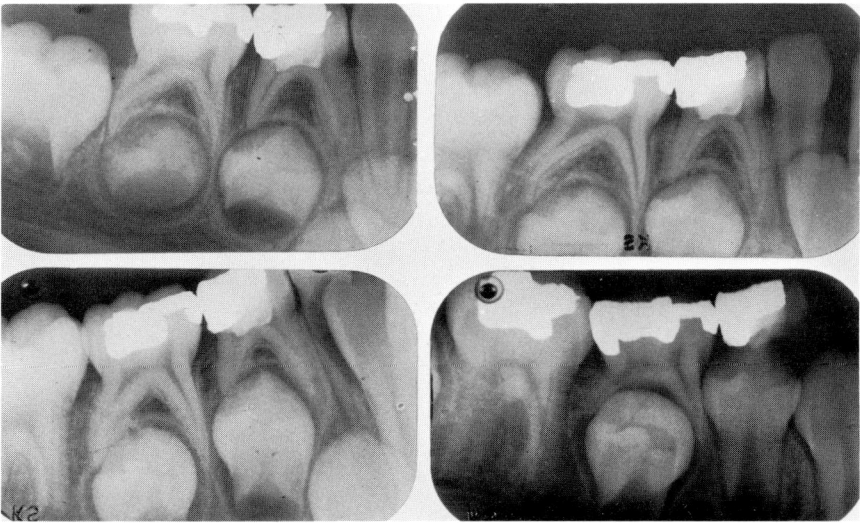

Figure 9-32 The first primary molar illustrated here received a formocresol pulpotomy when the child was 4 years of age. The tooth has remained healthy and exfoliated at the usual time.

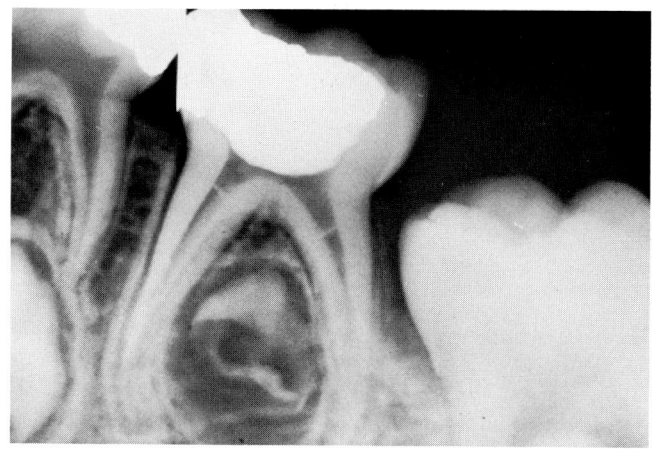

Figure 9-33 Successful pulpotomy using calcium hydroxide in a second primary molar. Dentin bridging can be seen in roots. Such bridging may not always be present in a calcium hydroxide pulpotomy.

Figure 9-34 Internal resorption in the mesial canal of a second primary molar following calcium hydroxide pulpotomy. This is frequently the cause of failure in calcium hydroxide pulpotomies.

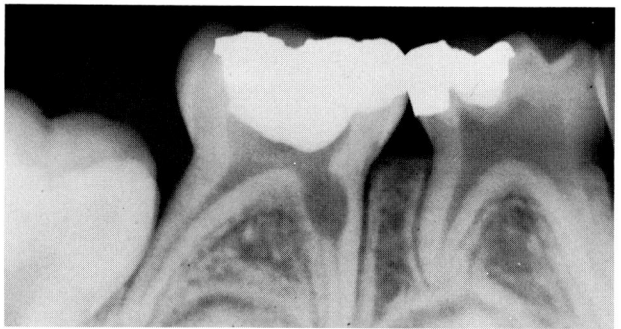

PULP THERAPY 203

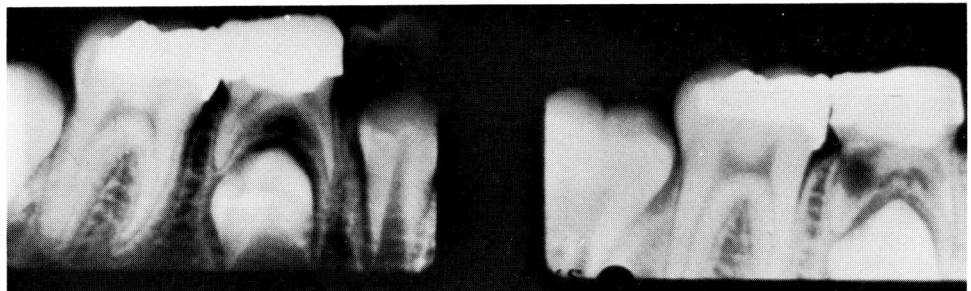

Figure 9-35 Rapid internal resorption in the distal canal of a second primary molar following calcium hydroxide pulpotomy. This occurred in less than 9 months. The tooth had to be extracted.

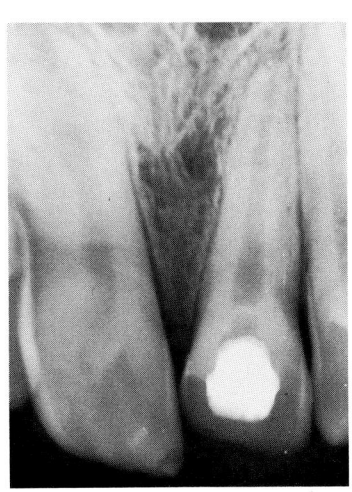

Figure 9-36 Radiograph of a fractured maxillary incisor showing a dentin bridge formed 3 months after a calcium hydroxide pulpotomy. See Chapter 14, page 289, for calcium hydroxide pulpotomy procedure on permanent incisors with pulpal exposures.

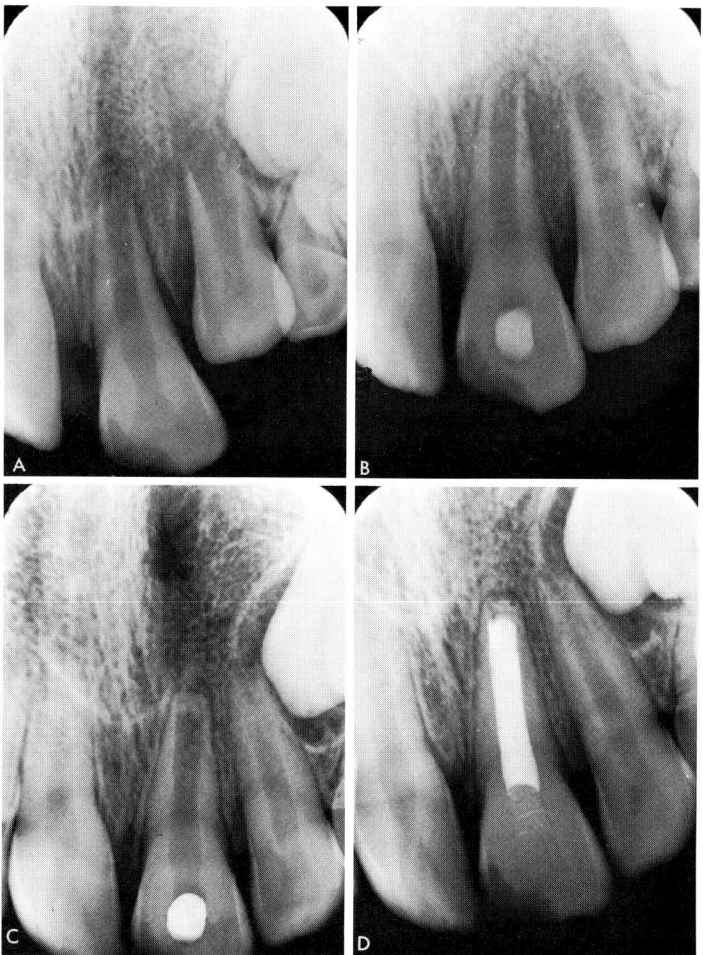

Figure 9-37 Treatment of a *nonvital* maxillary left central incisor with an incompletely formed apex in an 8-year-old boy (From Steiner, J. C., Dow, P. R., and Cathey, G. M.: Inducing root end closure of non-vital permanent teeth. J. Dent. Child. 35:47-54, Jan., 1968).

A, Fractured maxillary left central incisor with periapical lesion.
B, Fractured incisor filled temporarily with calcium hydroxide and camphorated monochlorophenol (CMCP).
C, Note root end closure of fractured incisor with calcium hydroxide and CMCP temporary filling.
D, Permanent root canal filling with gutta percha 13 months later.

Treatment Procedure for Inducing Root End Closure of Non-Vital Permanent Teeth

Acute symptoms of the involved tooth must first be controlled before beginning root end induction procedures. For example, if an acute abscess is present the tooth must be opened for drainage, antibiotics prescribed if necessary, and root end induction procedures postponed until the tooth is clinically asymptomatic.

First Appointment
1. After access to the root canal is established the coronal half of the canal is debrided with large reamers or files.
2. The canal is thoroughly irrigated and dried.
3. A cotton pellet moistened with CMCP is placed in the pulp chamber and sealed with Cavit.

Second Appointment (7 days later)
1. Cavit is removed and the canal irrigated.
2. An approximation is made of tooth length in order to avoid any instrumentation of the thin apical dentinal walls. All instrumentation should be 3 mm. short of the radiographic apex. The dentinal walls are cleaned by peripheral filing. The apical portion of the canal should be avoided to preserve tooth structure and prevent disturbance of any apical cellular organization that may be present.
3. The canal is then irrigated, dried, and filled with a paste of calcium hydroxide U.S.P. and CMCP. The calcium hydroxide and CMCP are mixed together on a sterile glass slab to a consistency resembling that of silicate cement which is ready for placement. A small plunger type amalgam carrier may be used to insert the paste into the canal. The paste is then forced down into the canal with the blunt end of a large gutta percha cone or plugger. Overfilling does not seem to be a cause for concern, since the excess is apparently absorbed. The primary objective is to completely fill and obturate the canal with paste.
4. A radiograph is taken to determine how well the canal has been obturated. Any adjustments to the root canal filling should be made at this time.
5. The excess paste is then removed from the pulp chamber. A small cotton pellet is placed over the canal orifice and the remainder of the pulp chamber is filled with silicate. Cavit should not be used as a temporary filling since an effective seal must last for six months to one year or longer.

Recall Appointment
The patient should be seen in 6 months and a radiograph taken to check for any evidence of root end closure. If closure is occurring, but is incomplete and the coronal seal is adequate, the paste should not be disturbed. If no evidence of closure is seen, the old paste should be removed and new material inserted into the canal. The patient should be continually supervised in this manner until the root end has closed sufficiently to permit placement of a conventional endodontic filling. This may take 12 to 16 months.

Final Appointment
When the apex appears to be closed on the radiograph, the paste is removed from the root canal. The walls are freshened with peripheral filing and the root canal is prepared 1 mm. short of the radiographic bridge. It is then irrigated, dried, and filled with gutta percha using the lateral condensation technique. The patient should be followed every 6 months to make sure of continued success. It has been observed that failure with this technique has resulted when the paste of calcium hydroxide U.S.P. and CMCP was not left in the tooth long enough.

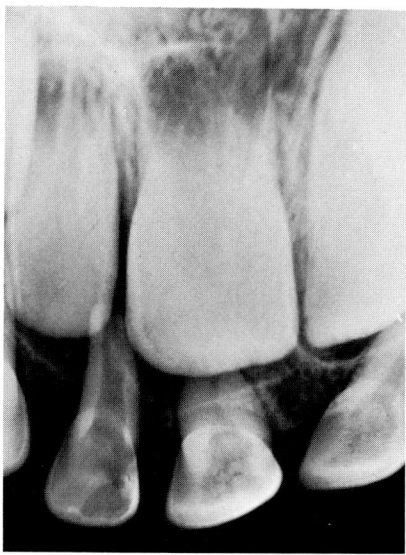

Figure 9-38 Maxillary primary lateral with cariously involved pulp. Anterior deciduous teeth are the most likely candidates for endodontic treatment. Being straight and single rooted for the most part, they frequently have root canals that are of sufficient size to be readily treated.

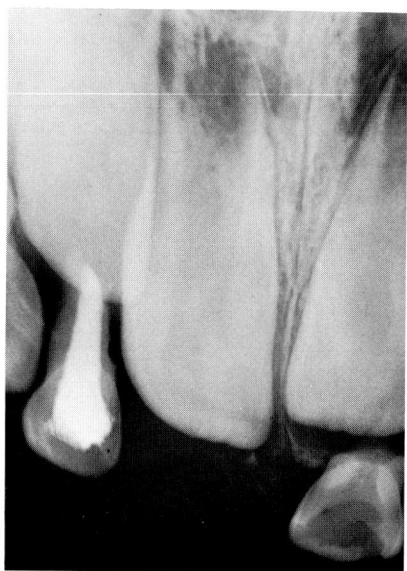

Figure 9-39 Maxillary primary lateral 6 months after successful endodontic therapy (see Figure 9-38). A paste of zinc oxide and eugenol was used as the filling material. Tooth will be exfoliated in normal manner. Several important points should be kept in mind when endodontic treatment is performed on primary teeth.
  A, Care should be observed not to penetrate past the apical ends of the tooth when reaming out the canal or canals. To do so might injure the permanent tooth bud which is developing.
  B, A resorbable compound such as zinc oxide and eugenol paste should be used as the filling material. Silver points or gutta percha should be avoided as they will not be resorbed and can act as irritants.
  C, The filling material should be introduced into the canal with light pressure so that little, if any, is extruded through the apex of the root.
  D, Apicoectomy should not be performed except in the absence of a developing permanent tooth.

PULP THERAPY   207

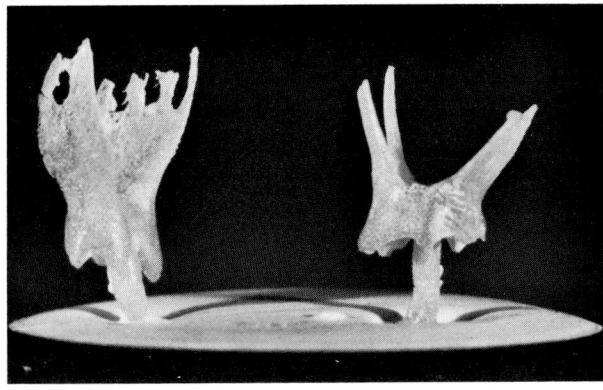

Figure 9-40 Plastic models of pulps of primary molars acquired by injecting extracted teeth.

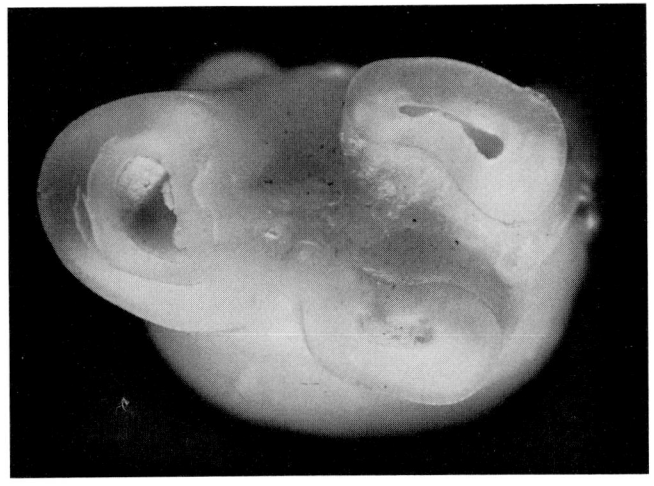

Figure 9-41 Apices of a maxillary primary molar cut off to show the flat shape of the root canals.

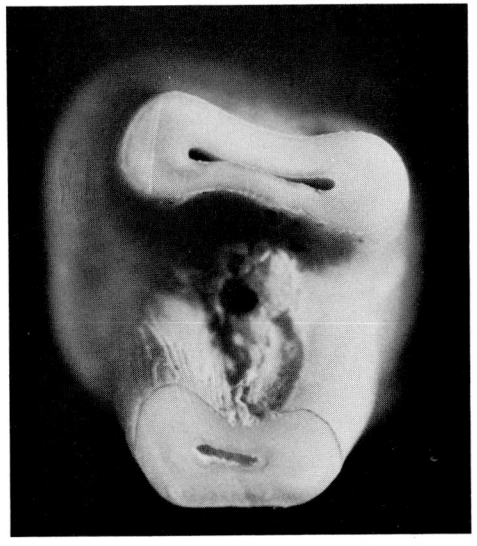

Figure 9-42 Apices of a mandibular primary molar cut off to show the flattened contour of the root canals.

Figure 9-43 Successful endodontic therapy in a mandibular second primary molar. (Courtesy Dr. Paul E. Starkey.)

A simplified technique for performing endodontics on primary teeth consists of filing out the root canals as thoroughly as possible at the first appointment and flushing with sodium hypochloride. A paper point impregnated in a suitable anesthetic agent such as camphorated monochlorophenol or formocresol should be placed in each canal and the tooth sealed. At the second appointment the tooth is reopened and the paper point removed. Canals are then filled with a material that can be resorbed such as zinc oxide and eugenol or Oxpara* paste.

*Ranson and Randolph Company, Toledo, Ohio.

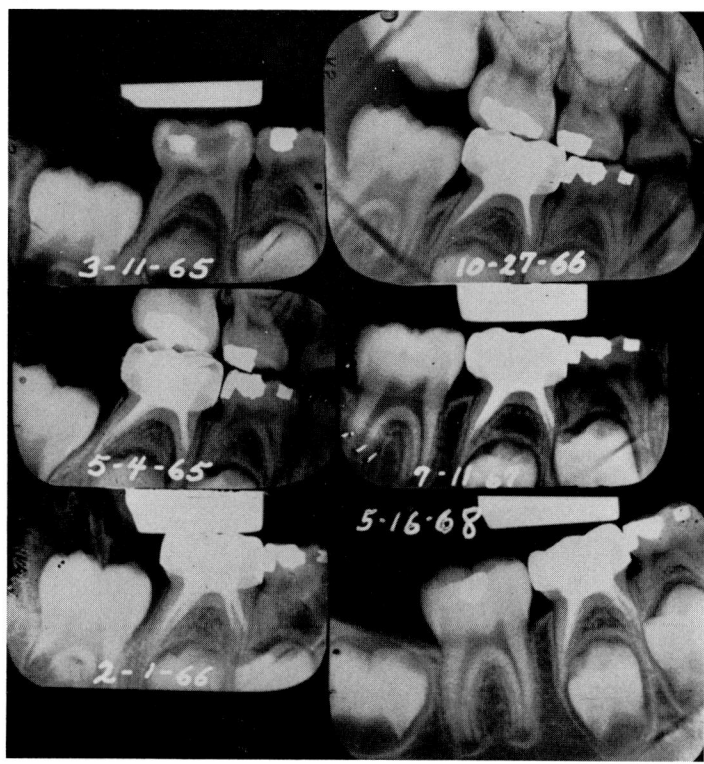

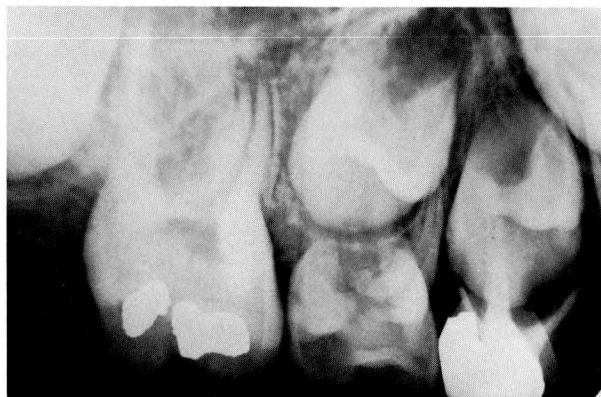

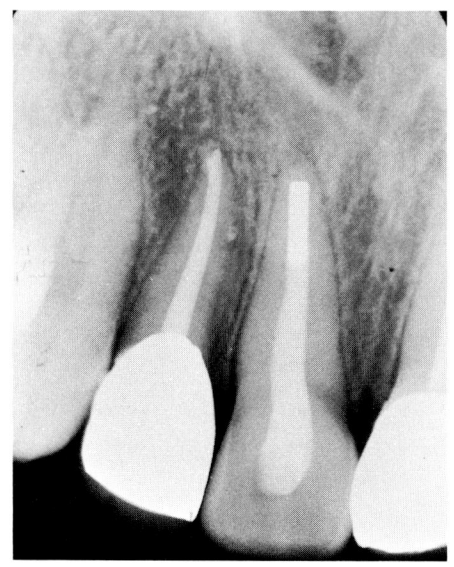

Figure 9-44 A primary first molar that underwent root canal treatment. It is good practice to place a stainless steel crown over primary molars treated endodontically. Endodontic treatment of nonvital or putrescent primary molars should be carefully considered and the plan evaluated in light of the possibilities of success, the number of appointments necessary, and the cost of treatment.

Figure 9-45 Root canal filling of a maxillary permanent central incisor. With root end development completed, conventional endodontic technique may be used with great success on permanent teeth. (Courtesy Dr. Eugene Natkin.)

EXODONTIA IN THE PRIMARY DENTITION

Chapter 10

    The extraction of primary teeth is an integral part of any dental practice which includes children. Fear, the main deterrent for seeking dental care, reaches its maximum in a child anticipating any form of oral surgery. For this reason alone it is very desirable that the dentist who has successfully carried the youngster through many previous experiences (the first visit to the dental office, dental x-ray examinations, prophylaxis, and operative procedures) be the person to perform the extraction. Whenever possible, the child should always be informed several days in advance that he has an appointment for extraction of teeth. If this is not done, he will be apprehensive of every visit to the dental office. Baldwin has indicated that a period of 4 to 7 days prior notice of impending surgery is adequate for children, and that such a period of advance warning is a deterrent to adverse psychological reactions.

    Recognition of an abnormality and diagnosis of the condition is a prerequisite to the correct resolution of any oral surgical problem. Good dental radiographs, therefore, are of prime importance before any surgery is undertaken. They are also essential for protection against medicolegal action.

    The most frequent oral surgical problem in children is the extraction of one or more carious teeth. Good radiographs will determine if the roots of the primary molars are still fully formed and encircle the developing tooth bud. If so, extra care must be taken to separate the roots and prevent dislodgment of the succedaneous tooth. If a carious tooth is to be extracted whose roots are partially resorbed, the radiographs will denote the areas of resorption and potential areas of root fracture.

    Dentists frequently see children when they are in pain from a toothache. If so, the offending tooth is generally easy to identify because of its mobility and sensitivity to percussion. Lymphadenopathy often exists along with soft tissue swelling and reddening around the affected area. Radiographs are essential as part of the diagnosis and should be retained as a permanent record.

    The use of antibiotics in children needing dental extractions is an important consideration. A good rule to follow is that if the dental abscess is well resolved and a fistulous tract established, and if the patient is asymptomatic and in good general health, then an antibiotic is not mandatory. If, however, there is pain or fever or periapical swelling and adenopathy and the infection apparently has not reached its maximum limit or if the child has a chronic debilitating condition such as congenital heart disease, then proper antibiotic therapy should be instituted.

One of the tenets of good surgery is profound anesthesia. Inasmuch as good operative dentistry is based on the same premise, the dentist should be able to provide this quite readily. Chapter 6 illustrates the procedures for local anesthesia. In some cases, especially with the very young child, extraction of teeth is best performed under general anesthesia. It should be pointed out that the decision to perform more complex operations such as frenectomies, removal of impacted teeth, and the like, will depend entirely on the dentist's training and feeling of competency. He should, however, be able to diagnose these conditions, understand their implications, relate them to the parent, and render acceptable judgments as to when surgery should take place.

In all procedures with children, slow, smooth, and graceful movements as opposed to fast, jerky, and awkward movements are the most desirable. This is particularly true during extractions. Not only will such actions be conducive to good patient management, but they also will minimize breaking the roots of primary teeth which are frequently thin and fragile. If one should be fractured, it is advisable to be cautious in removing the root tips, so that the permanent tooth bud will not be jeopardized. Frequently, the better part of valor is to leave the embedded root tip and let it be exfoliated or resorbed. In such a case, the parent should be advised that the root tip remains. This should be recorded in the patient's chart, and the area rechecked at periodic intervals.

Postoperatively, young children seldom have any problems with healing of extraction sites. So-called dry sockets are rarely encountered. Some discomfort, however, may be experienced from the wearing off of the local anesthetic. It is good procedure to have children bite on a gauze pack for at least ½ hour following surgery. In addition, children should keep their head elevated and avoid eating or drinking for several hours. Soft diets are recommended for the first day avoiding such foods as peanuts and popcorn so that food debris will not be trapped in the sockets. The prevention of lip biting can be a problem, but with the use of short-acting anesthetic agents and an appropriate warning to the child and the parent, trauma to the cheeks and lips should be infrequent.

EXODONTIA IN THE PRIMARY DENTITION 211

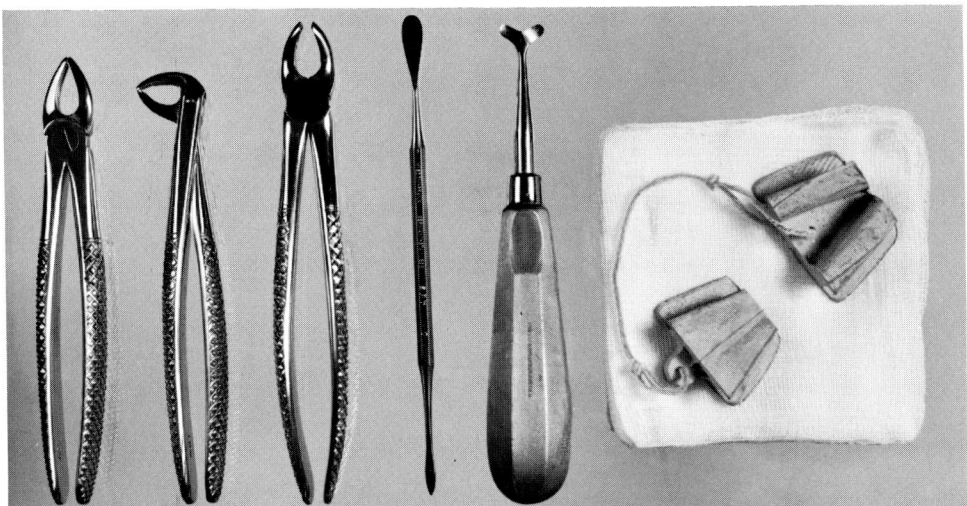

Figure 10-1 Suggested tray for routine extractions of primary teeth:
Ash 37, universal maxillary pedodontic forceps; Ash 123, universal mandibular pedodontic forceps; Ash 157 forceps; periosteal elevator; Forsyth elevator (optional); 4 x 4 gauze sponges; two rubber mouthprops.

A mouthprop should be used during extraction of mandibular primary molars when excessive stress is applied to the opposite mandibular condyle.

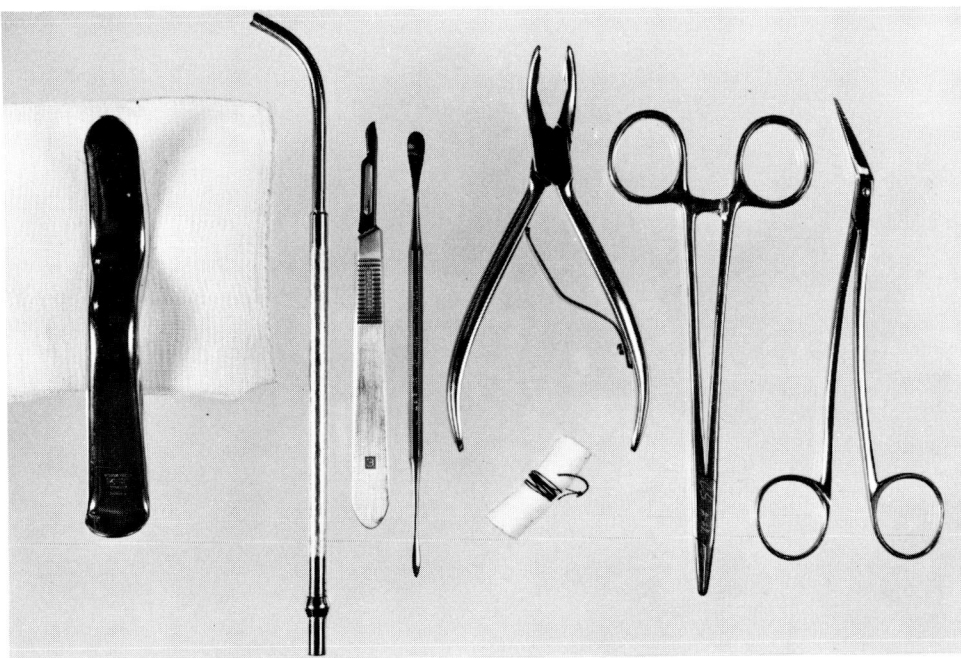

Figure 10-2 Suggested tray for tissue flap procedures:
lip retractor, suction tip, scalpel and blade, periosteal elevator, rongeur, suture material with needle, hemostat, scissors, and 4 × 4 gauze sponges.

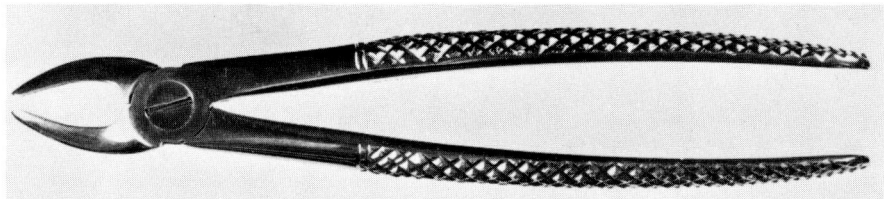

Figure 10-3 Ash 37 forceps used in extraction of maxillary primary centrals, laterals, and cuspids.

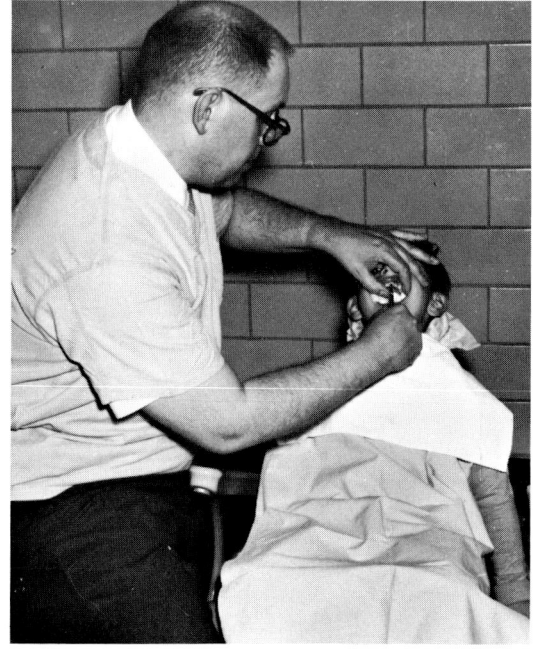

Figure 10-4 Position of dentist and patient for extraction of maxillary primary anterior teeth.

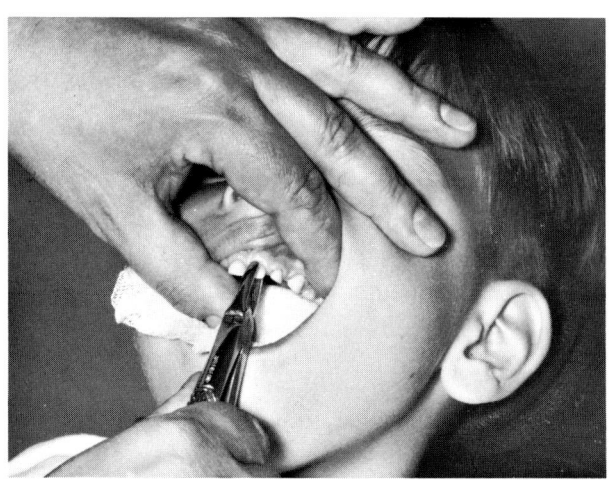

Figure 10-5 Placement of forceps for extraction of maxillary primary anterior teeth. Note position of dentist's fingers.

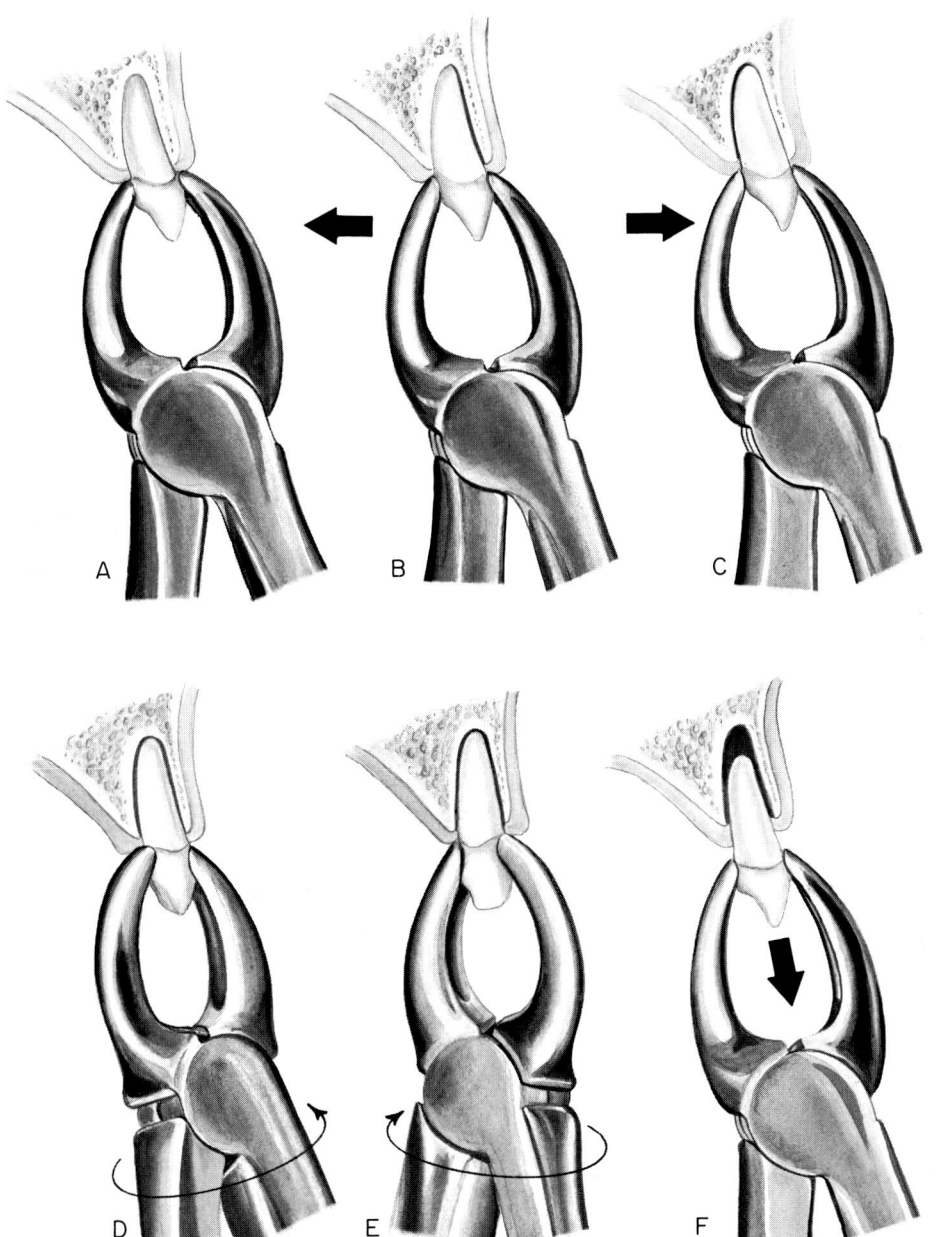

Figure 10-6 Movements used in extracting maxillary primary centrals, laterals, and cuspids.
  A, Placement of forceps.
  B, Movement to lingual and hold.
  C, Movement to labial and hold.
  D, Rotary movement.
  E, Rotary movement reversed.
  F, Extraction of tooth in path of least resistance.

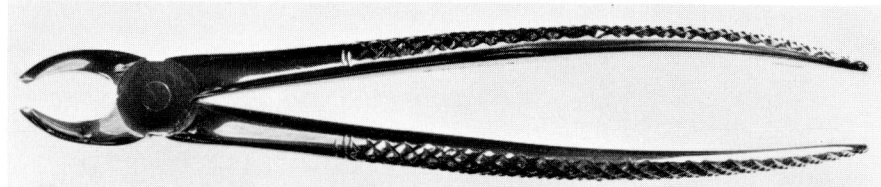

Figure 10-7 Ash 157 forceps used in extraction of maxillary primary molars.

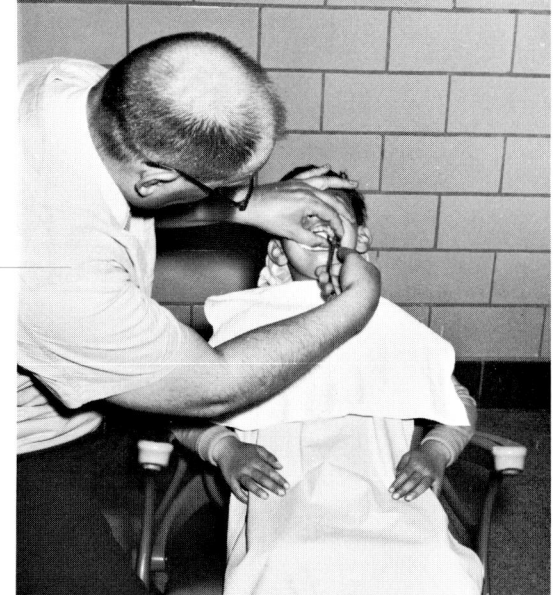

Figure 10-8 Position of dentist and patient for extraction of maxillary primary molars.

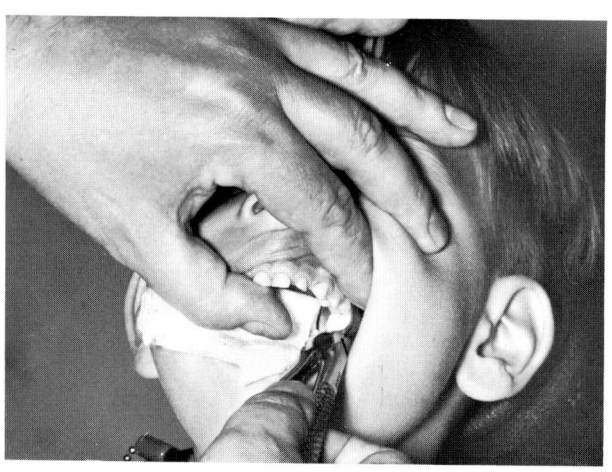

Figure 10-9 Placement of forceps for extraction of maxillary primary molars. Note position of dentist's fingers.

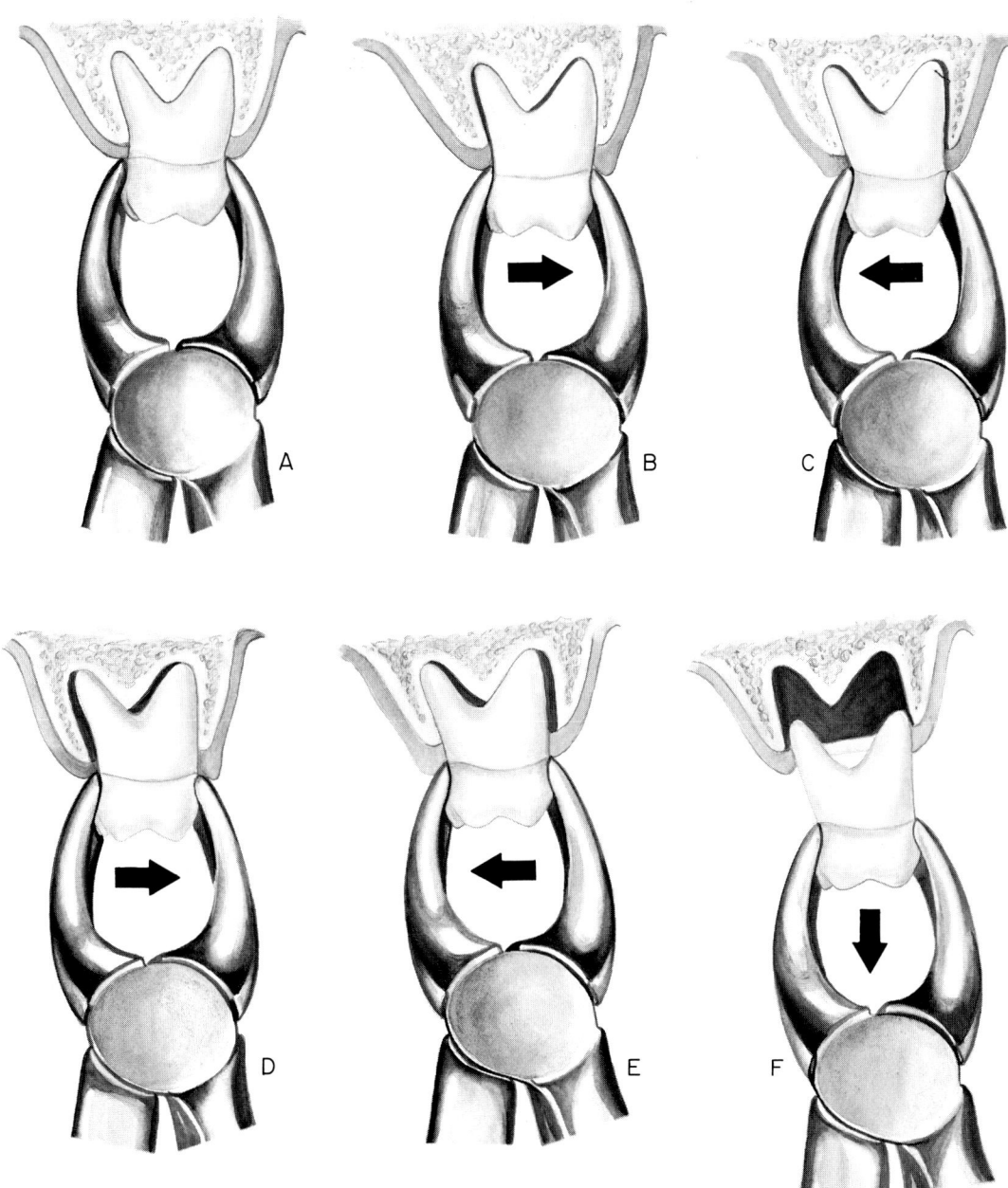

Figure 10-10 Movements used in extracting maxillary primary molars.
A, Placement of forceps.
B, Movement to buccal and hold.
C, Movement to lingual and hold.
D, Stronger movement again to buccal.
E, Stronger movement again to lingual.
F, Extraction of tooth in path of least resistance.

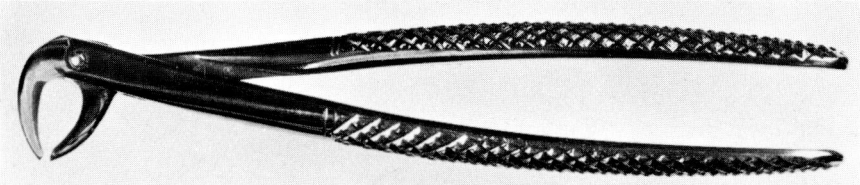

Figure 10-11 Ash 123 forceps used in extraction of mandibular primary centrals, laterals, and cuspids.

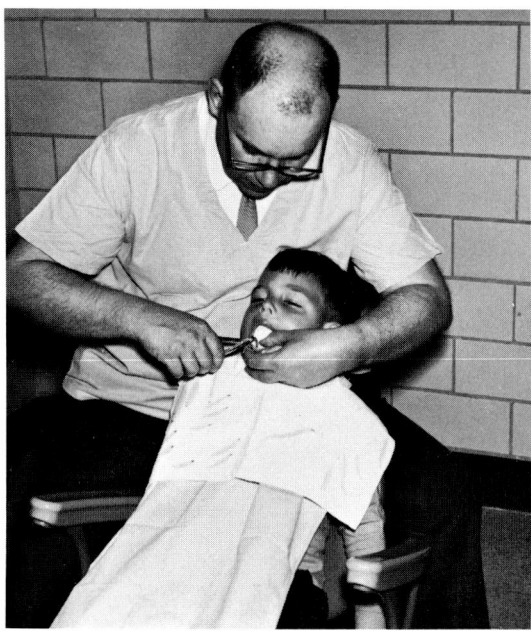

Figure 10-12 Position of dentist and patient for extraction of mandibular primary anterior teeth.

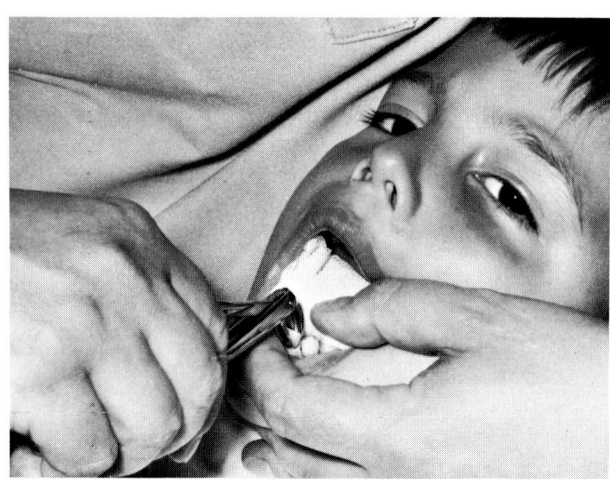

Figure 10-13 Placement of forceps for extraction of mandibular primary anterior teeth. Note position of dentist's fingers.

EXODONTIA IN THE PRIMARY DENTITION 217

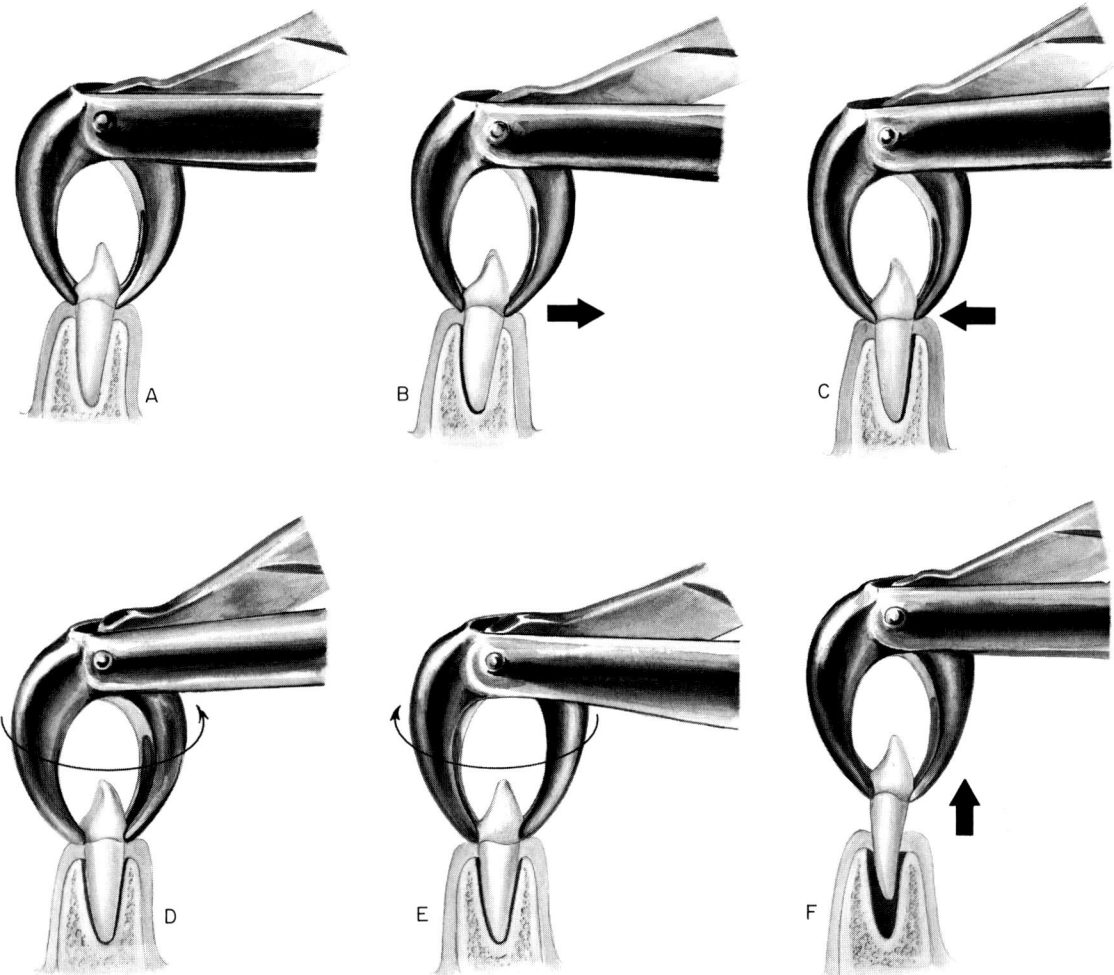

Figure 10-14 Movements used in extracting mandibular primary centrals, laterals, and cuspids.
A, Placement of forceps.
B, Movement to labial and hold.
C, Movement to lingual and hold.
D, Rotary movement.
E, Rotary movement reversed.
F, Extraction of tooth in path of least resistance.

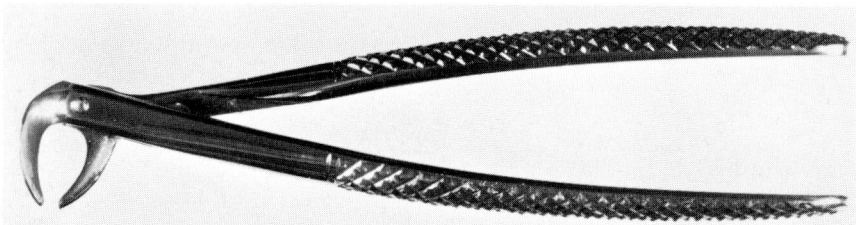

Figure 10-15 Ash 123 forceps used in extraction of mandibular primary molars.

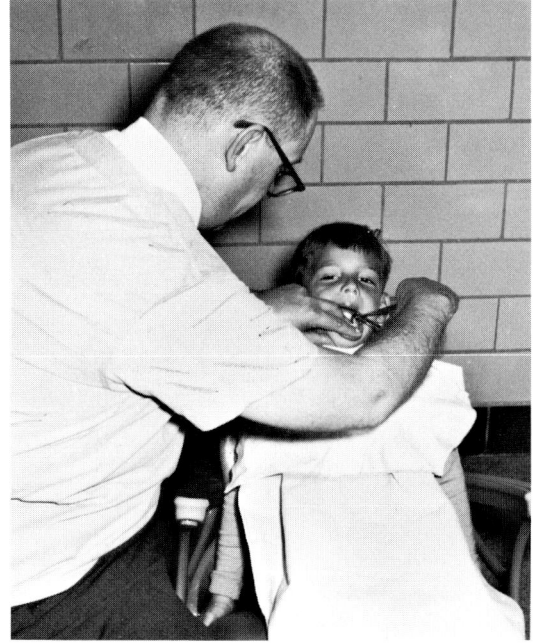

Figure 10-16 Position of dentist and patient for extraction of mandibular primary molars.

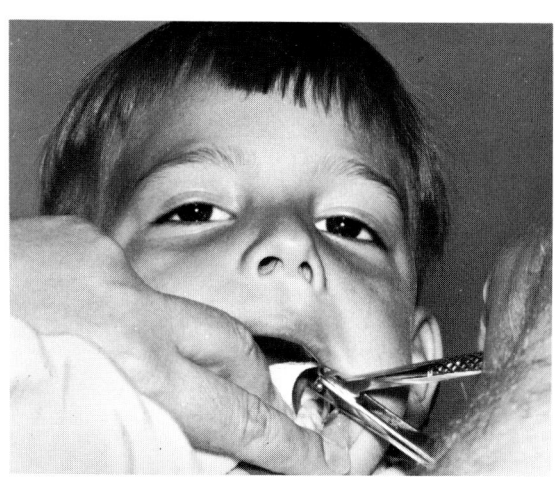

Figure 10-17 Placement of forceps for extraction of mandibular primary molars. Note position of dentist's fingers.

EXODONTIA IN THE PRIMARY DENTITION 219

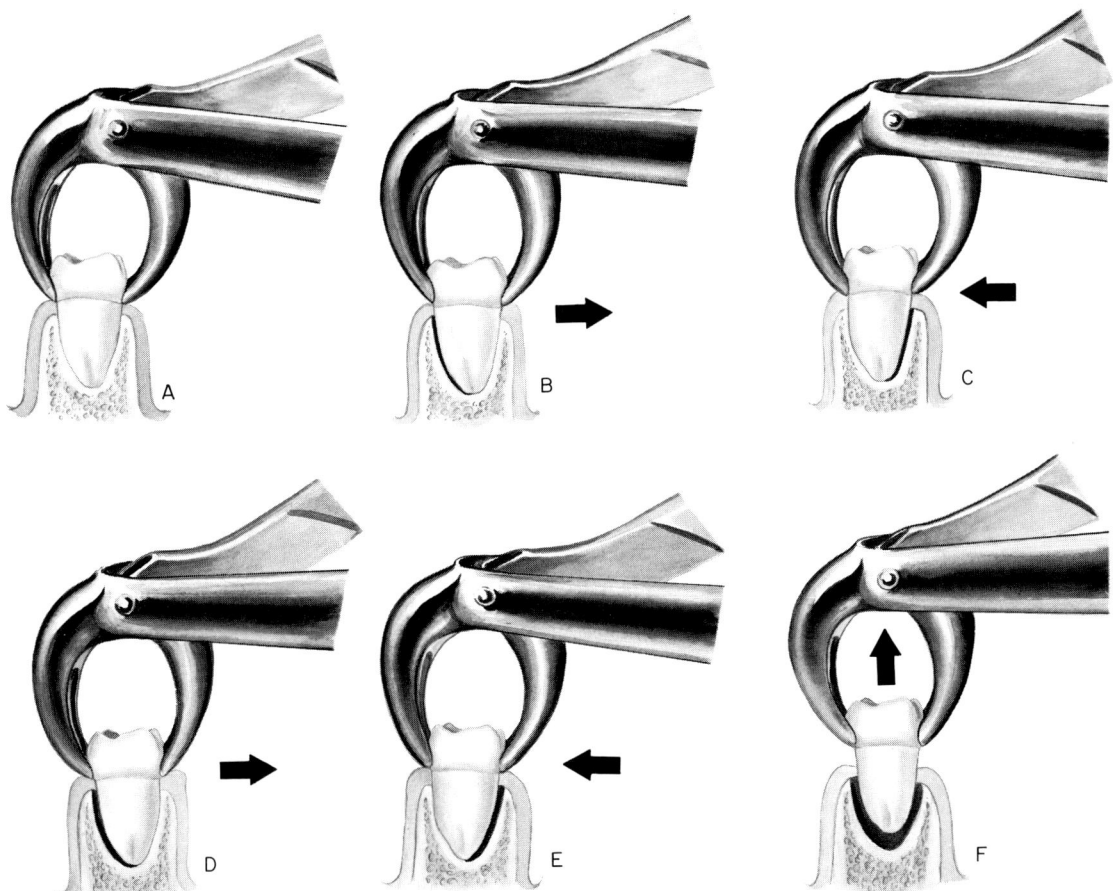

Figure 10-18 Movements used in extracting mandibular primary molars.
A, Placement of forceps.
B, Movement to buccal and hold.
C, Movement to lingual and hold.
D, Stronger movement again to buccal.
E, Stronger movement again to lingual.
F, Extraction of tooth in path of least resistance. Slight rotary movement may be used; however, when solid resistance is felt this movement should be diminished.

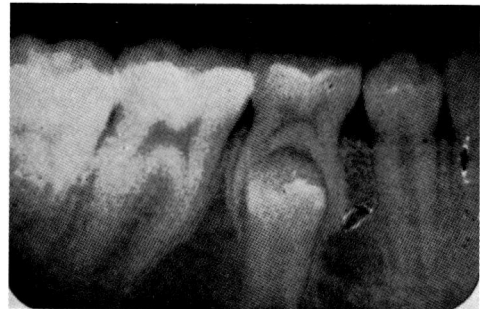

Figure 10-19 Radiograph of primary molar with roots enclosing crown of bicuspid. (From Thoma, K. H.: *Oral Surgery*. 3rd ed., C. V. Mosby Company, St. Louis, 1958, p. 204.)

Figure 10-20 Radiograph of tooth shown in Figure 10-19 being sectioned prior to extraction. Sectioning a tooth with unresorbed roots which encloses a developing bicuspid prevents extraction of the bicuspid along with the primary molar. (From Thoma, K. H.: *Oral Surgery*. 3rd ed., C. V. Mosby Co., St. Louis, 1958. p. 204.)

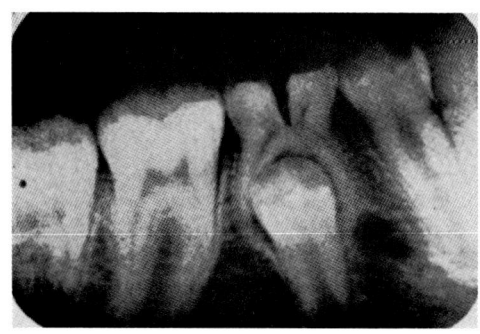

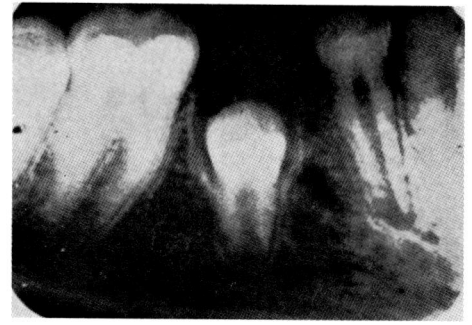

Figure 10-21 Same patient as seen in Figures 10-19 and 10-20, with primary molar extracted. (From Thoma, K. H.: *Oral Surgery*. 3rd ed., C. V. Mosby Co., St. Louis, 1958, p. 204.)

Reference

Baldwin, D. C. Jr.: An investigation of psychological and behavioral responses to dental extraction in children. J. Dent. Res. 45:1637-51, Nov.-Dec., 1966.

SPACE MAINTENANCE AND INTERCEPTIVE ORTHODONTICS

Chapter 11

The preservation of arch length is the function of the space maintainer, a fixed or removable appliance is usually placed following premature loss of a primary tooth resulting from caries or other causes. The term "interceptive orthodontics" as used in this chapter refers to simple procedures involving minor tooth movement, the purpose of which is to improve the occlusion. It can be differentiated from orthodontics per se by defining its scope and limitations. It does not imply the treatment of skeletal disharmonies in occlusion. It does not include the full banding of all the teeth in either arch to accomplish its objectives. It is usually limited to space regaining by tipping of teeth, to correction of anterior and posterior crossbites as well as ectopic eruptions, and to retraction of protruding anteriors on patients with Class I molar occlusion.

Since the child's dentition undergoes many changes in the process of growth and development, it is the responsibility of the dentist to be alert to any situations which lend themselves to intermediate treatment to prevent more serious malocclusion. A good example is the extraction of a primary molar with an indeterminate time before the eruption of the bicuspid. Here, a simple appliance will maintain space; sometimes a second appliance is required. It is seldom good judgment to "watch" or "observe" such spaces since too often time slips by and the patient is seen after collapse has occurred, creating a far more difficult problem than existed originally.

Considerable difference of opinion exists among clinicians concerning the desirability of fixed versus removable appliances for the purpose of space maintenance. If a fixed appliance can be constructed, however, it is preferable since it minimizes such problems as breakage and patient cooperation. In some cases suitable abutment teeth are not present and the removable appliance is the only recourse. Intensive parent and patient education is necessary in these cases if disappointment and failure are to be avoided.

It is not the purpose of this chapter to treat exhaustively the complete subject of interceptive orthodontics and the construction of appliances for active tooth movement. The more common problems that may be encountered by the practicing dentist and which are within the scope of treatment by simple means will be described.

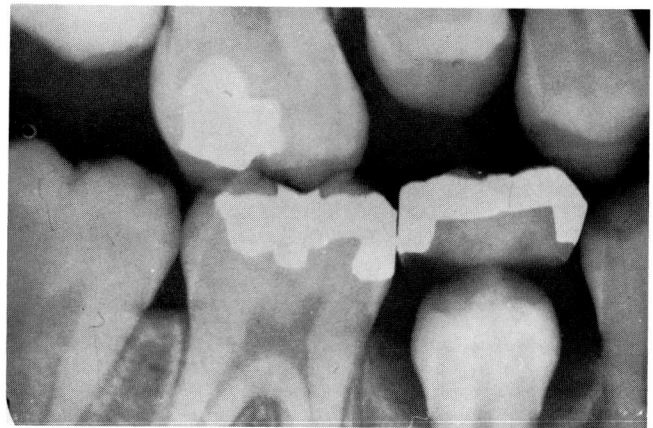

Figure 11-1 Radiograph demonstrating the most efficient space maintainer, the natural tooth.

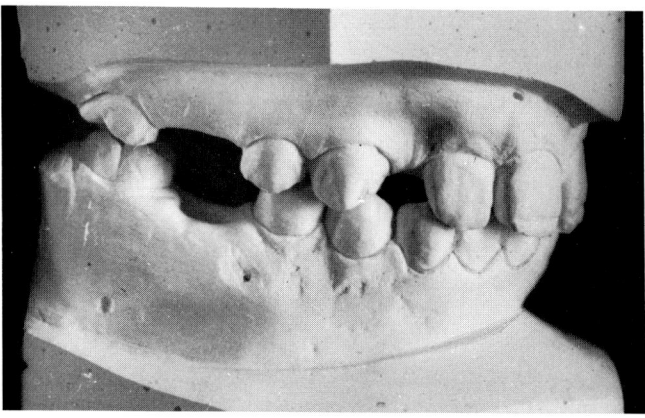

Figure 11-2 Study models in occlusion. Note space created by extraction of maxillary right second primary molar. No space maintainer was placed.

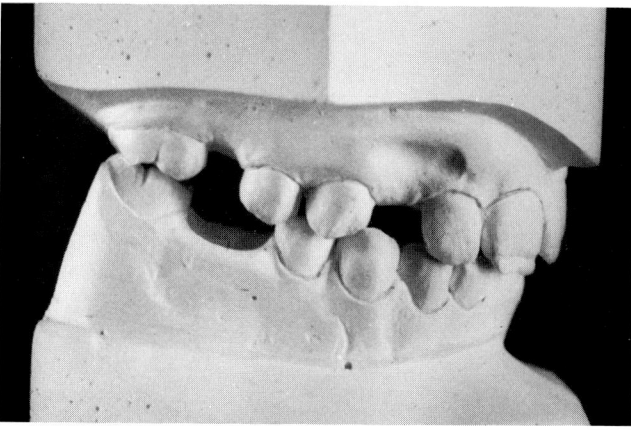

Figure 11-3 Study models of same patient as shown in Figure 11-2, 6 months later. Note space closure in this area. A space maintainer obviously should have been placed.

SPACE MAINTENANCE AND INTERCEPTIVE ORTHODONTICS   223

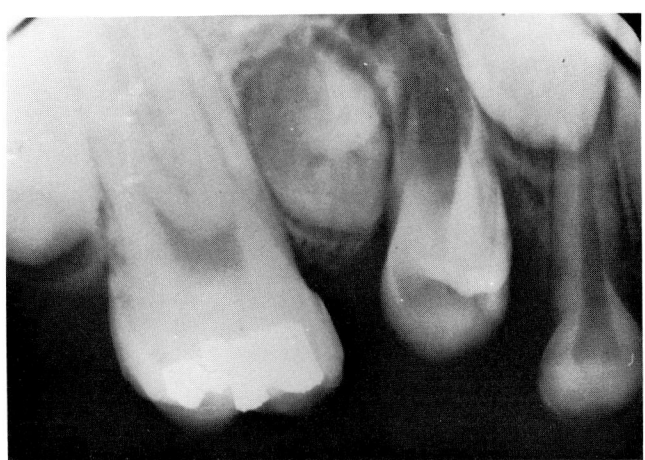

Figure 11-4 Radiograph showing effect of premature extraction of primary molar and failure to use a space maintainer. Maxillary second bicuspid is almost completely blocked out. It may lie dormant, become cystic, or erupt in a lingual position.

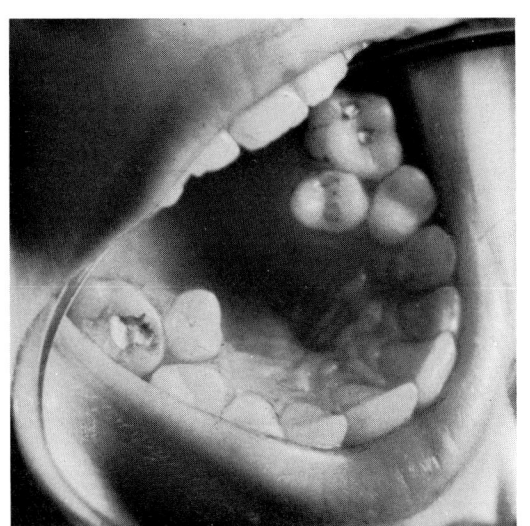

Figure 11-5 Mirror view of maxillary arch showing right and left second bicuspids erupting in a lingual position as a result of premature extraction of both second primary molars. No provision was made for space maintenance.

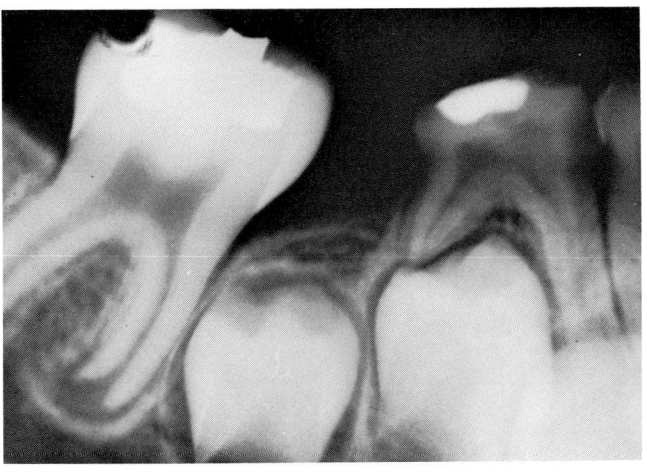

Figure 11-6 Radiograph showing premature loss of mandibular second primary molar. Note how the first permanent molar has tipped mesially, causing a loss in arch length; consequently the second bicuspid is blocked out from its natural path of eruption. A space maintainer should have been placed.

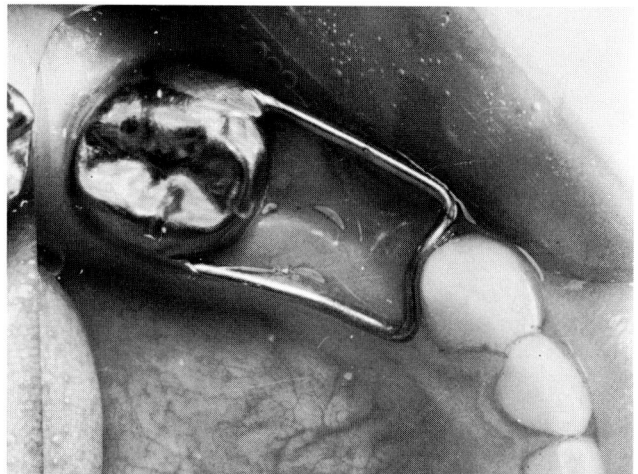

Figure 11-7 Stainless steel crown and loop unilateral space maintainer. This appliance is relatively inexpensive and may be completed during one appointment.

Figure 11-8 Stainless steel unilateral space maintainer. Female unit is spot welded to crown in desired position. Male unit is then inserted and adjusted to desired length. Buccal and lingual female attachments are then crimped to secure position of male unit. Female unit is spot welded mesial to the crimp.

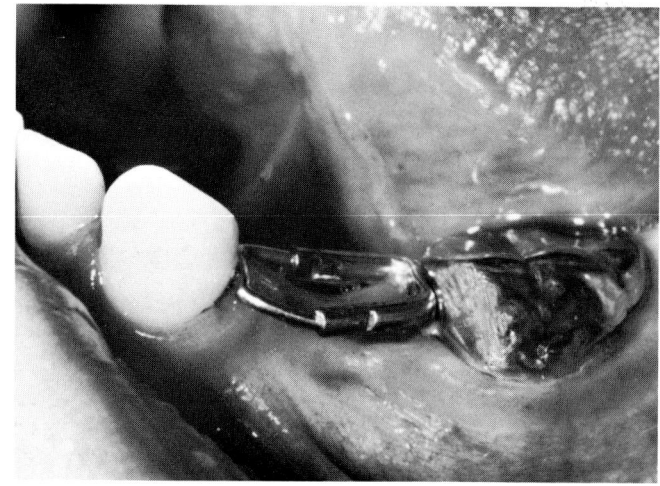

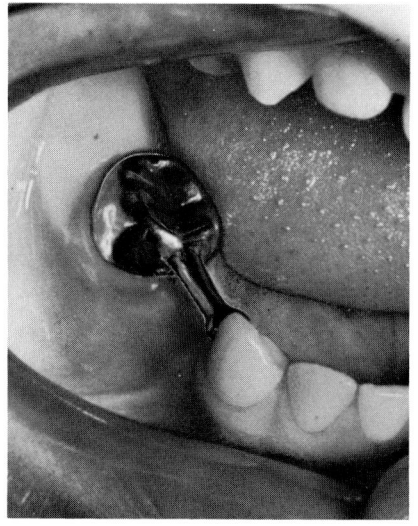

Figure 11-9 Cast gold crown and bar unilateral space maintainer. The bar may be cut away from the gold crown upon eruption of mandibular first bicuspid.

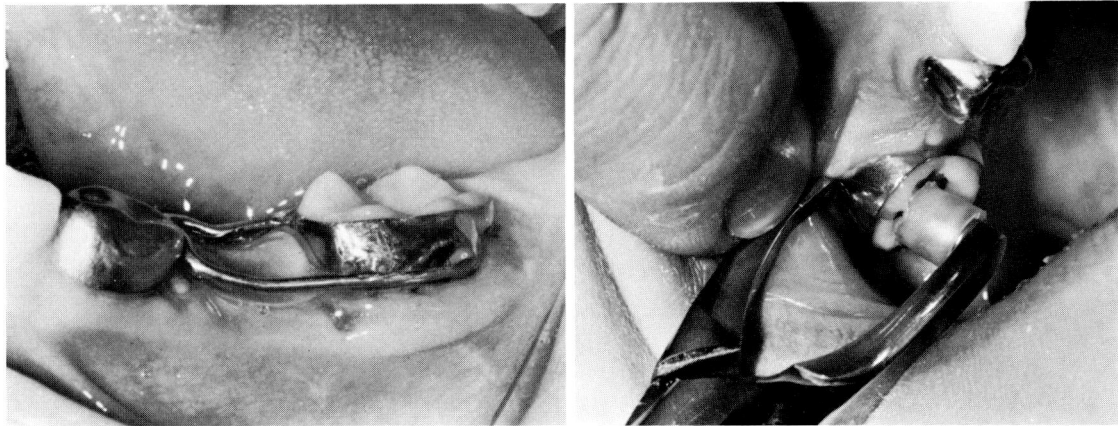

Figure 11-10 *Left,* band and loop stainless steel unilateral space maintainer. When a band is placed on a young permanent molar which has incomplete root formation, it is important not to overmanipulate it. Removal of a band with an excavator by forcefully pulling the band from the tooth may cause severe trauma to the periodontal membrane with resultant ankylosis of the tooth. *Right,* proper use of a band remover on a maxillary first permanent molar.

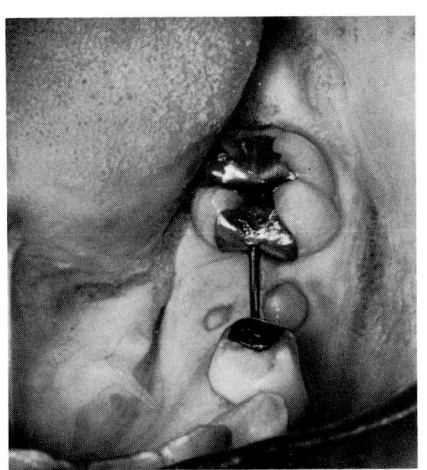

Figure 11-11 Fixed unilateral spacer made by anchoring a heavy gauge stainless steel wire in the adjacent amalgam restorations. A disadvantage of this technique is that the amalgam frequently fractures from the occlusal force exerted on the wire.

Figure 11-12 Band and loop space maintainer designed to allow eruption of the bicuspids.

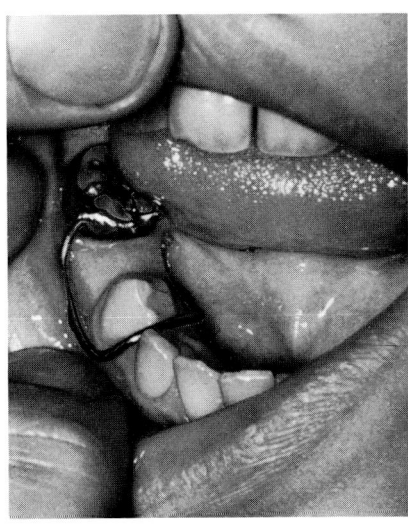

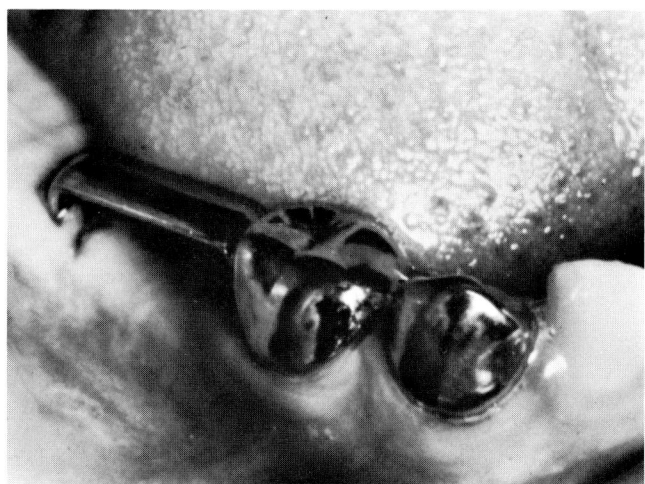

Figure 11-13 Unilateral stainless steel distal shoe appliance. Cuspid and molar crowns are soldered together with gold or silver solder. This appliance is used when the first permanent molar has not erupted and the second primary molar is prematurely lost. It prevents the first permanent molar from drifting mesially into the space formerly occupied by the second primary molar. Appliance is seated after incision is made for distal extension. Distal extension of spacer should be similar to that shown in Figures 11-16 through 11-18. The distal shoe appliance may be used in either the maxillary or mandibular arch, and made of gold or stainless steel.

Figure 11-14 Failure of a mandibular distal shoe appliance. Any prosthetic appliance should be periodically checked for effectiveness.

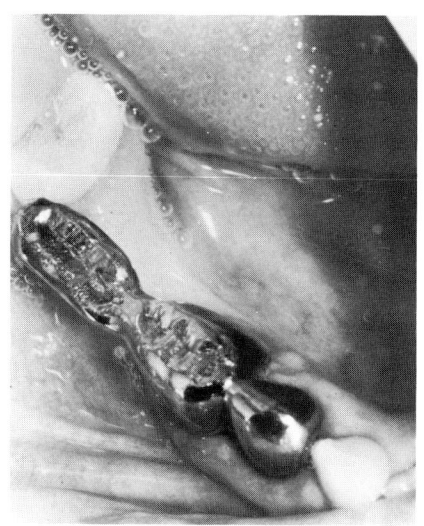

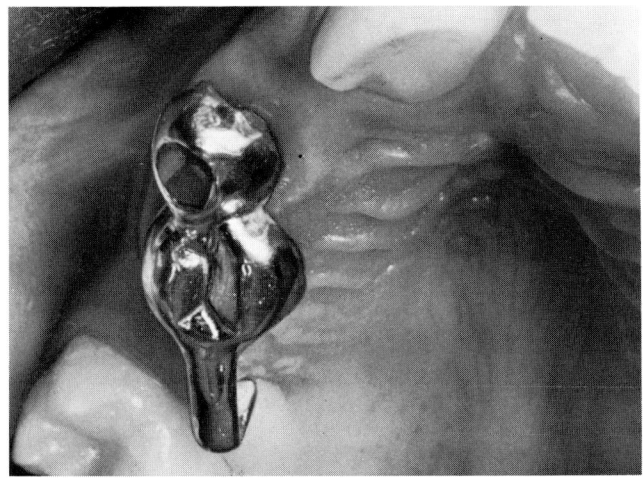

Figure 11-15 Failure of a maxillary distal shoe appliance. This space loss could have been avoided if the child had been seen periodically by the dentist.

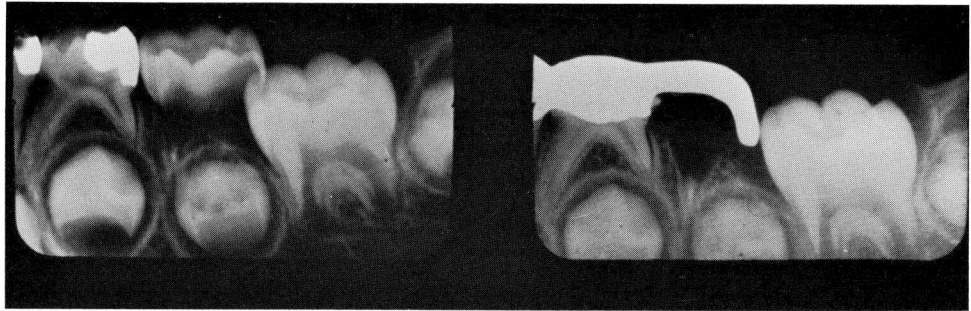

Figure 11-16 Radiograph on left showing an ectopically erupting mandibular first permanent molar. Radiograph on right showing the first step in correction of this situation. The mandibular second primary molar was extracted and a distal shoe appliance immediately cemented to place. (See Figure 11-17.)

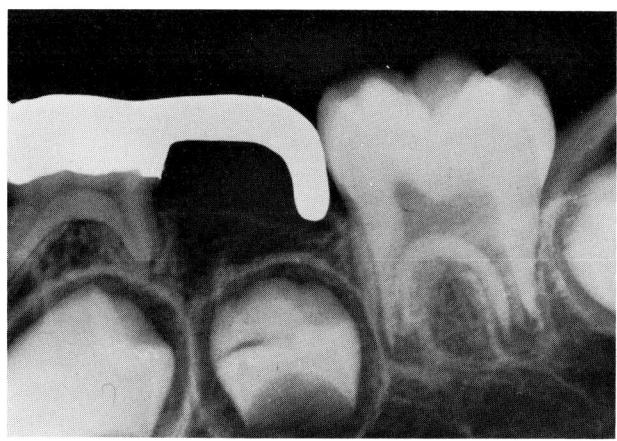

Figure 11-17 Radiograph of distal shoe appliance after eruption of mandibular first permanent molar. Note how space has been maintained for erupting bicuspid. In this case the distal extension of metal at the gingivae is too thick. It should have been tapered more. At the periodic check one should be alert for signs that the appliance is blocking eruption of the second bicuspid.

Figure 11-18 Radiograph of distal shoe space maintainer in position. Such a film is necessary prior to cementation in order to insure proper location of distal shoe. If adjustments are necessary, they may be conveniently made at this time.

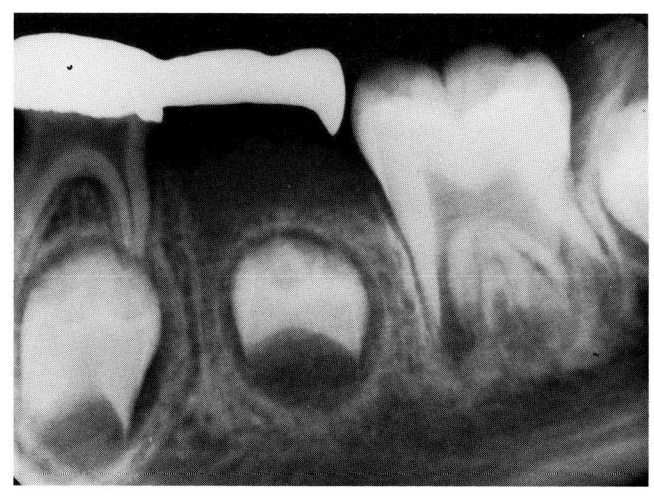

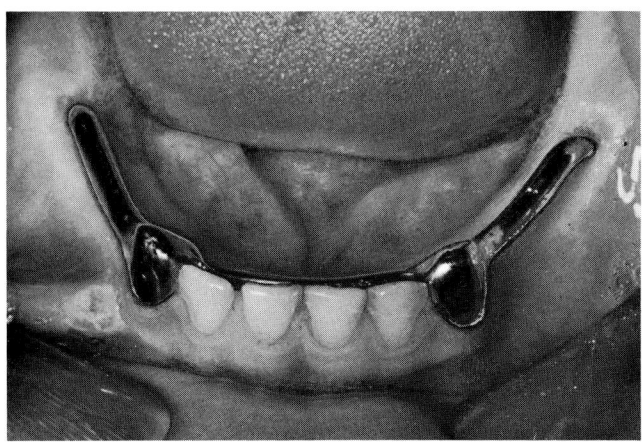

Figure 11-19 A bilateral distal shoe space maintainer with cuspids used as abutments and joined with a lingual bar.

Figure 11-20 Patient seen in Figure 11-19, with first permanent molars erupting successfully into occlusion. At this stage, a new appliance should be considered. Either a lingual arch space maintainer or a removable spacer should be considered at this time.

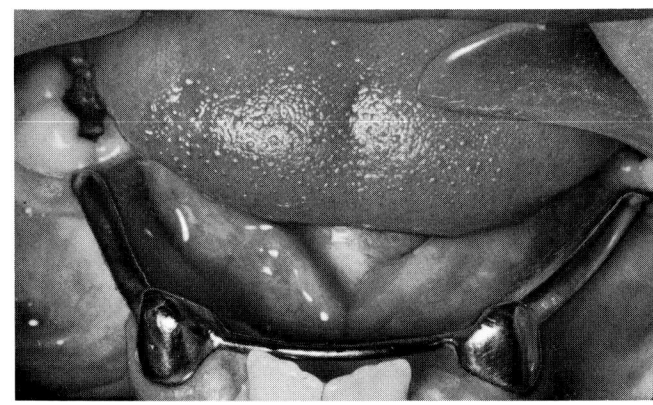

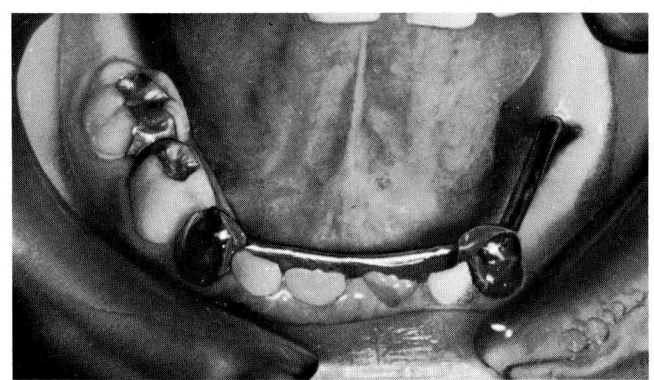

Figure 11-21 Unilateral distal shoe space maintainer. Note that both primary molars on the left side have been extracted. The distal extension reaching back to the unerupted left first permanent molar was cast with the left primary cuspid crown.

Figure 11-22 Mandibular lingual arch space maintainer. This is a convenient means of bilateral space maintenance when first permanent or second primary molars are present. However, whenever bands are placed on teeth, the patient must be *carefully* watched. Caries will progress rapidly under a loose band. It is, therefore, *imperative* to check the patient frequently, and if a loose band is found it must be removed and recemented immediately.

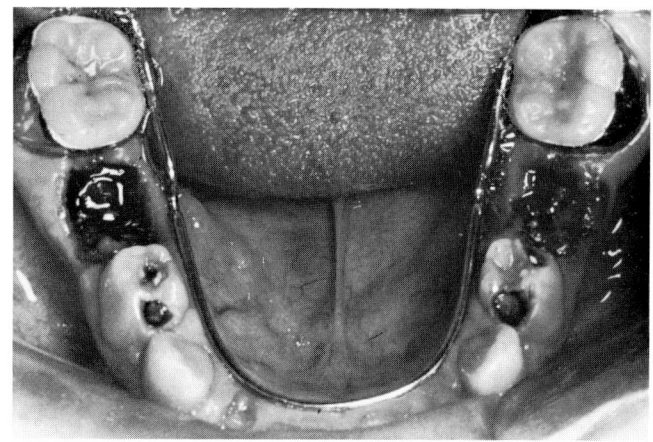

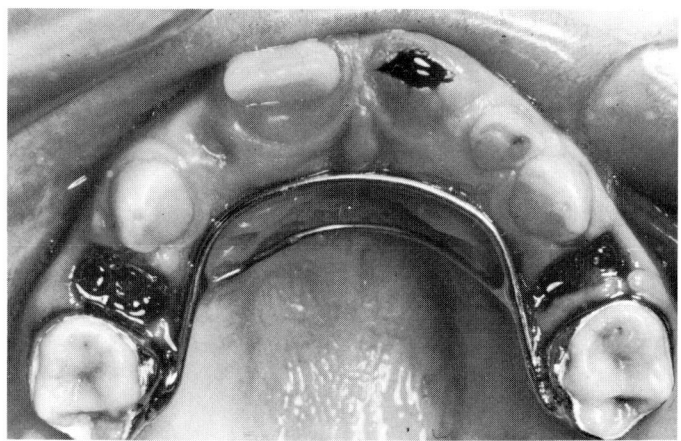

Figure 11-23 Maxillary lingual arch space maintainer. An auxiliary wire is soldered on to this appliance to prevent the wire from digging into the palatal mucosa. The same thing may be accomplished by adding a small button of acrylic in the same area. (See Figure 11-24.) It is imperative to check this appliance periodically. A loose band must be immediately removed and recemented.

Figure 11-24 Maxillary lingual arch space maintainer using a button of acrylic to add stability and prevent the wire from traumatizing the palatal mucosa.

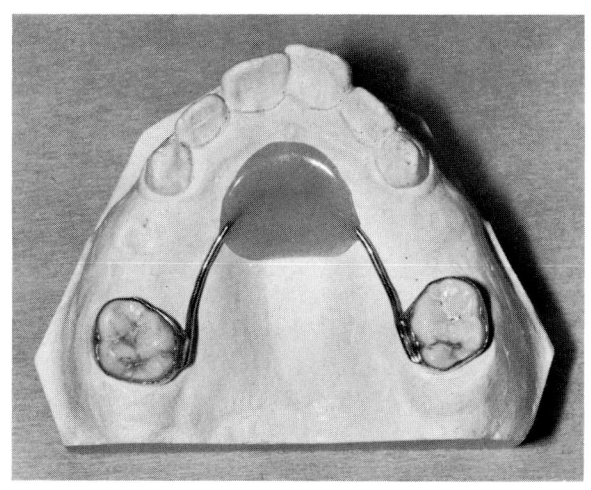

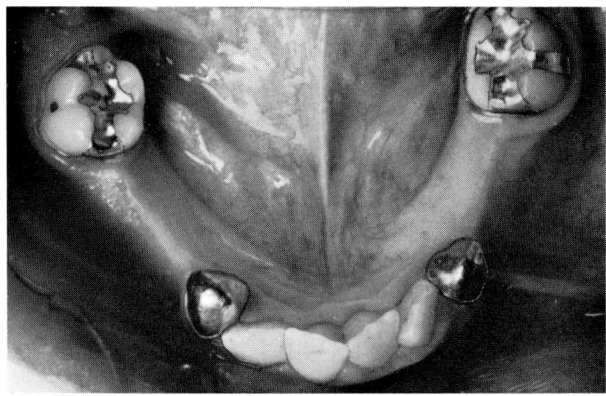

Figure 11-25 Patient with bilaterally missing first and second primary molars. Immediate treatment for space maintenance is critical. Either a fixed (lingual arch) or removable (acrylic) appliance could be used in this case. (See Figure 11-26.)

Figure 11-26 A bilateral acrylic space maintainer used for patient shown in Figure 11-25. Such an appliance is particularly useful when teeth are missing bilaterally.

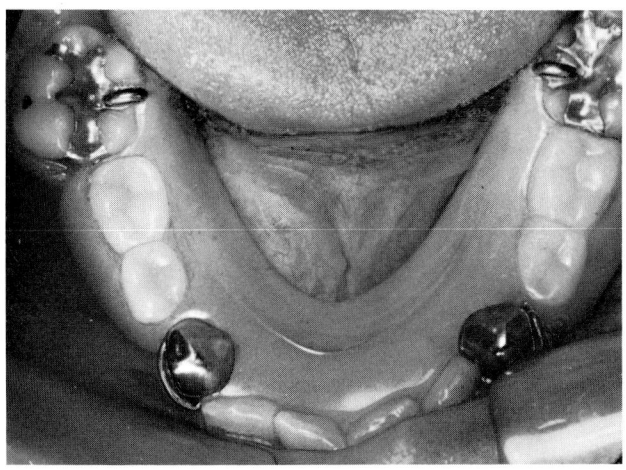

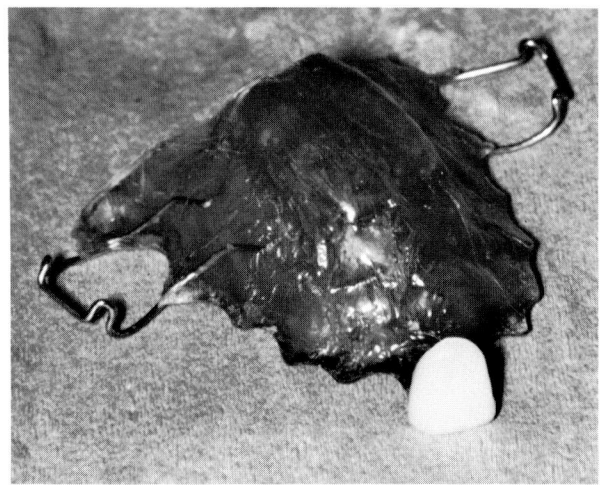

Figure 11-27 Temporary partial denture replacing a maxillary central incisor. This appliance prevents mesial migration of teeth into the area of the lost incisor and also restores esthetics in this area for the patient. A fixed bridge will eventually be placed. (See Figure 11-63.)

SPACE MAINTENANCE AND INTERCEPTIVE ORTHODONTICS

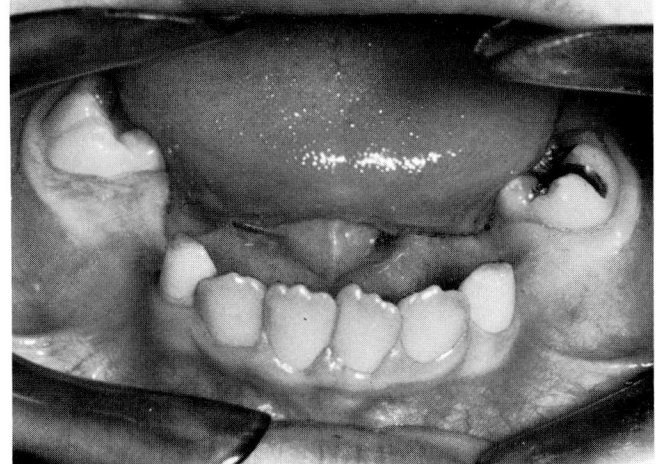

Figure 11-28 Child with bilaterally missing first and second primary molars. (See Figures 11-29 and 11-30.)

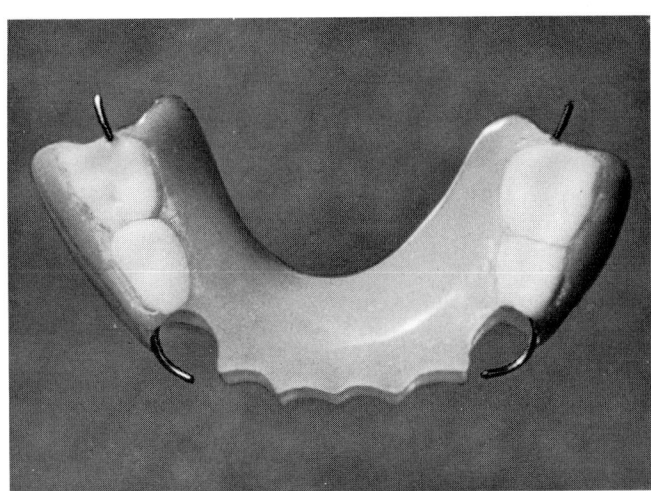

Figure 11-29 Removable acrylic spacer with teeth and wire clasps. This appliance will increase masticatory effectiveness for several years.

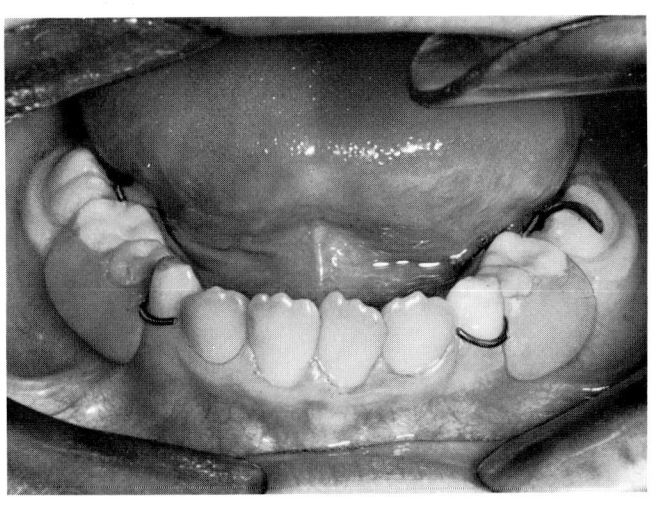

Figure 11-30 Removable acrylic spacer in place.

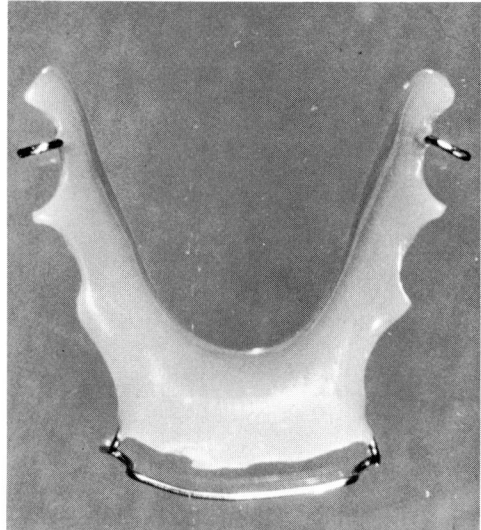

Figure 11-31 Mandibular removable acrylic spacer. Note that in this case teeth were not used on the appliance. (See Figure 11-32.)

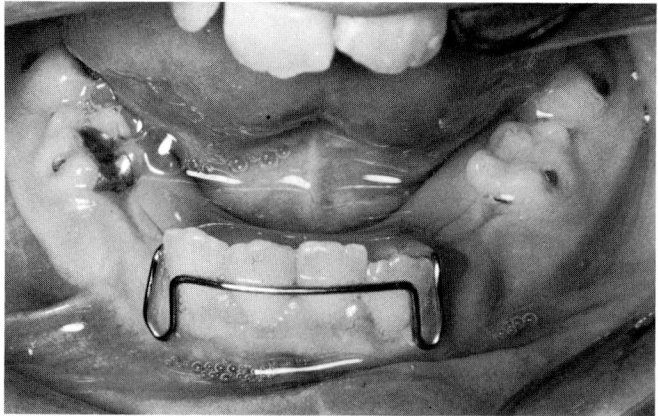

Figure 11-32 Mandibular removable appliance in place. Note the use of a labial extension of wire to add to the retention of this spacer. Occlusal wire rests were used on the molars to prevent the appliance from moving gingivally.

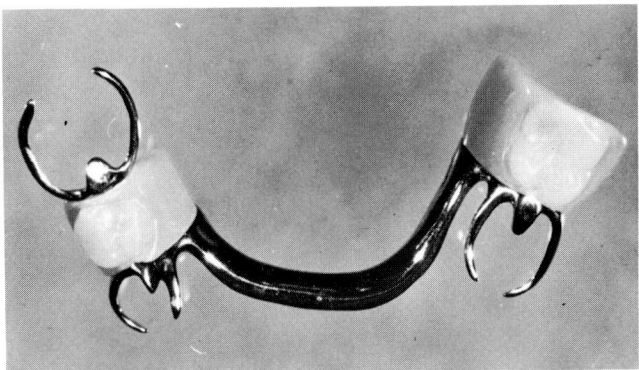

Figure 11-33 A chrome-cobalt lower partial denture used to prevent the mandibular left first permanent molar from drifting mesially. This was used instead of a distal shoe appliance. The distal extension of acrylic is beaded lightly to compress the tissue mesial to the future site of the erupting first permanent molar. (See Figures 11-34 through 11-36.)

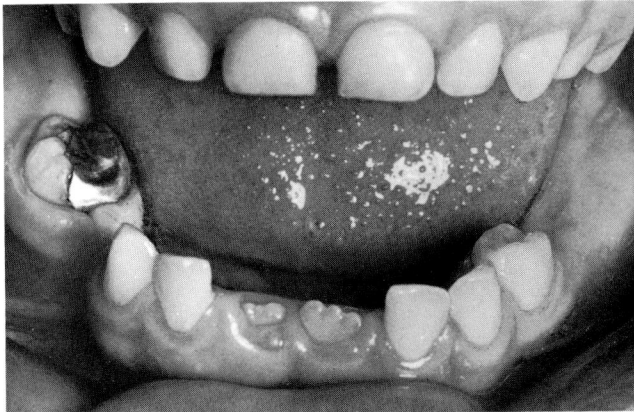

Figure 11-34 Six-year-old child in whom mandibular left second primary molar and right first primary molar are missing. Note that the first permanent molars have not yet erupted.

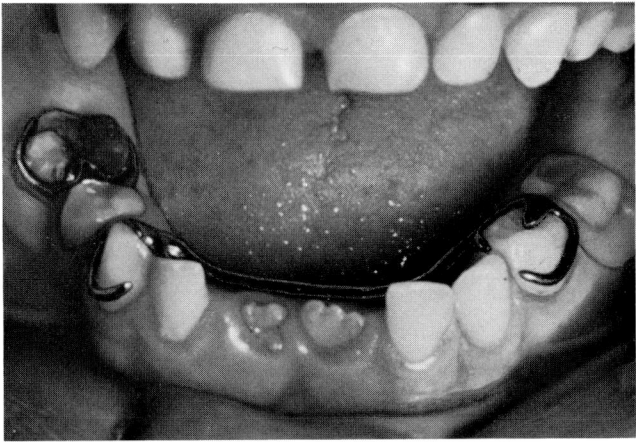

Figure 11-35 Six-year-old child with partial denture in place.

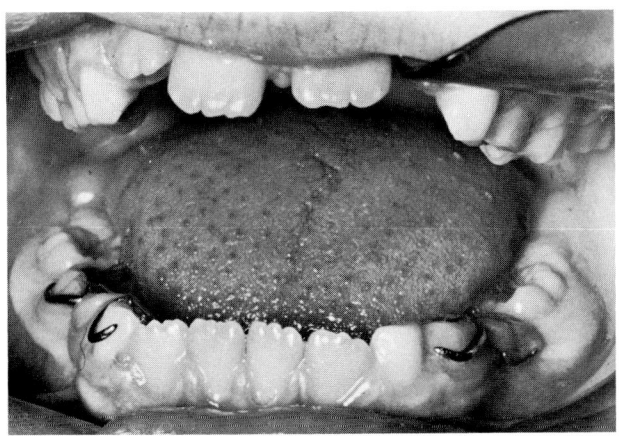

Figure 11-36 Patient shown in Figures 11-34 and 11-35, 2 years later at age 8. Note how the mandibular left first permanent molar has erupted posterior to the distal extension of the partial denture.

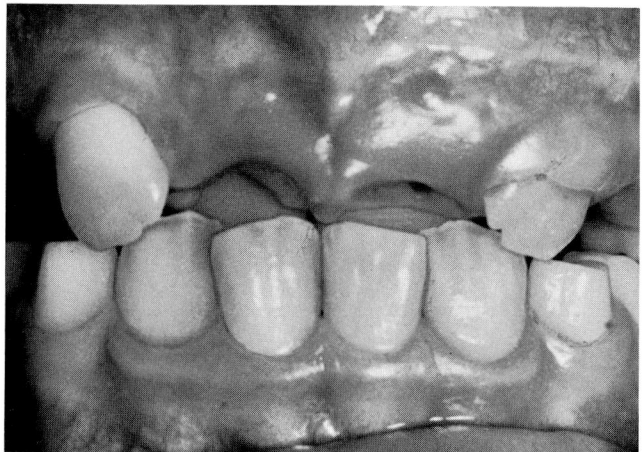

Figure 11-37 Anterior crossbite of maxillary central incisors. Such a condition may be overlooked unless occlusion is checked during examination of each patient.

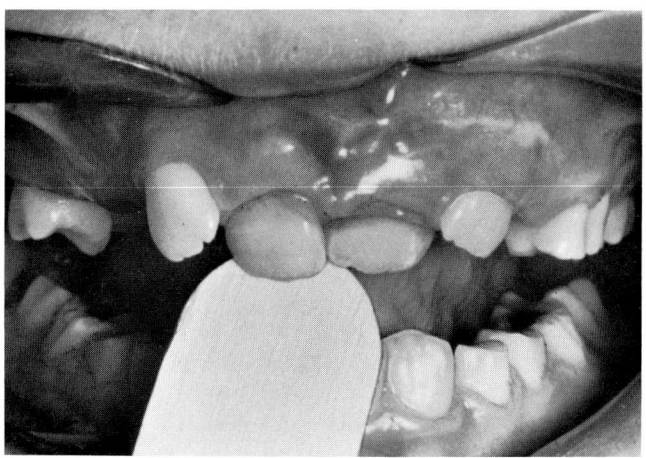

Figure 11-38 Tongue blade or popsicle stick used to correct anterior crossbite (patient shown in Figure 11-37). This technique is usually successful when the overbite is not more than 3 to 5 mm. and the patient is conscientious in the use of the tongue blade. A pressure causing slight blanching of the labial mucosa of the tooth in crossbite is applied in a direction 90 degrees to the long axis of the tooth. The mandibular incisors are used as a fulcrum. Pressure must be applied for 5 to 10 minutes, at least six times per day.

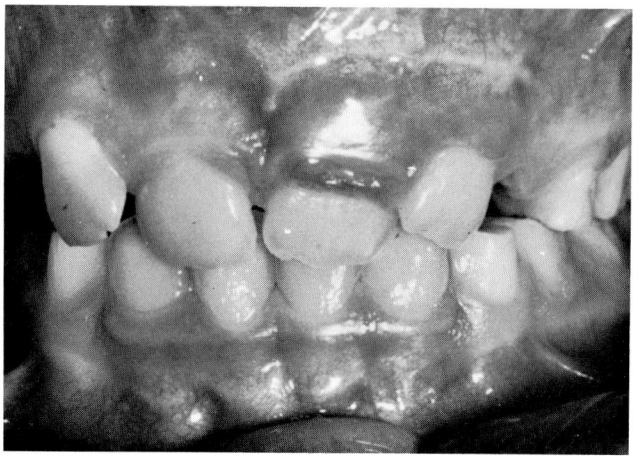

Figure 11-39 Patient shown in Figures 11-37 and 11-38, with anterior crossbite corrected. Temporarily irritated condition of labial tissues around the maxillary left permanent central incisor should return to normal. Following correction of the crossbite, the patient should be seen every 2 weeks for 2 months to assure that the teeth do not relapse.

SPACE MAINTENANCE AND INTERCEPTIVE ORTHODONTICS 235

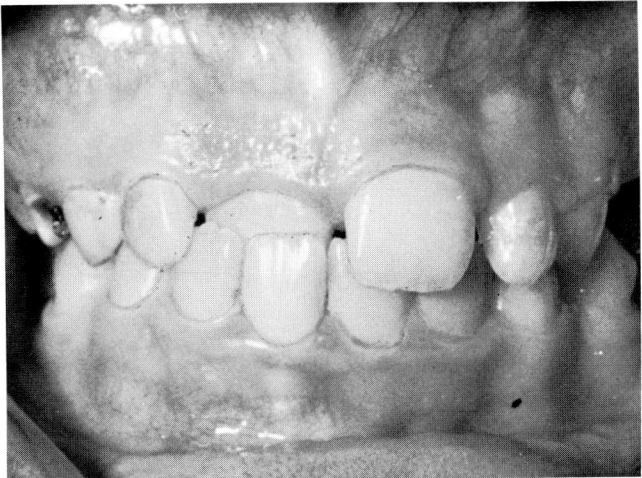

Figure 11-40 Maxillary right permanent central incisor in a crossbite relation.

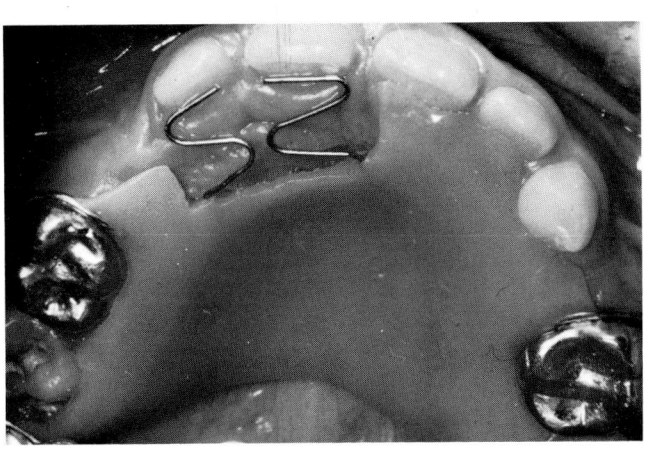

Figure 11-41 Use of a removable acrylic appliance with "Z" springs to correct an anterior crossbite.

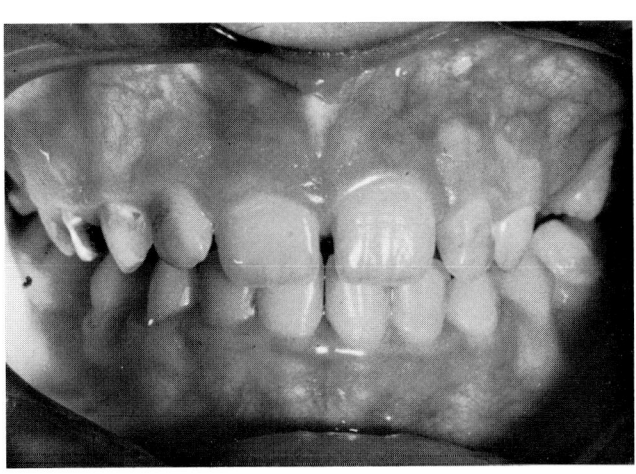

Figure 11-42 Patient shown in Figure 11-40, following correction of anterior crossbite using an acrylic appliance with a "Z" spring.

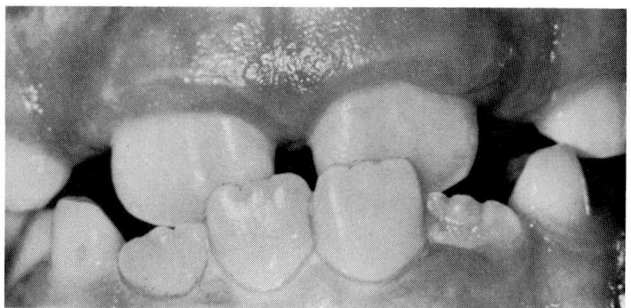

Figure 11-43 Maxillary permanent central incisors erupting in crossbite. An acrylic guide plane was used to correct this condition.

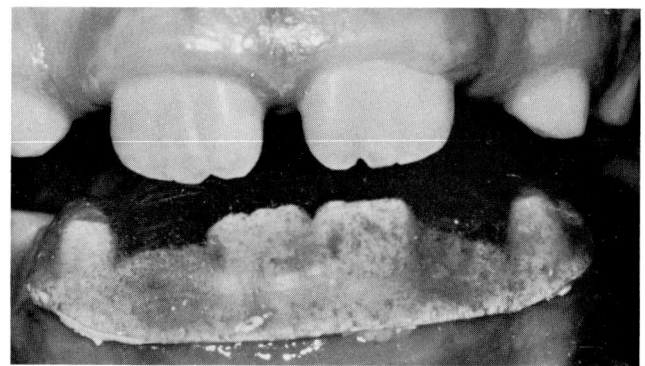

Figure 11-44 Acrylic guide plane cemented on lower incisors with zinc oxide and eugenol. Note how the maxillary incisors contact the acrylic guide plane. The bite should not be opened more than 4 to 5 mm. The appliance should be checked in 1 week. The crossbite should be corrected in 7 to 14 days.

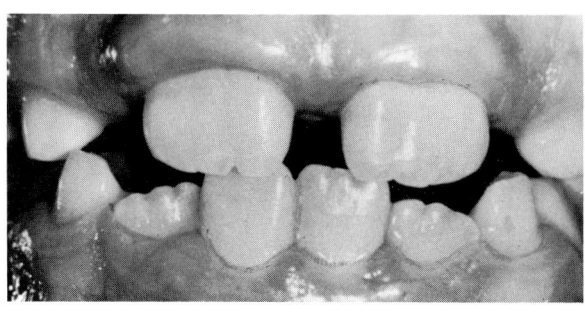

Figure 11-45 Patient 2 weeks after placement of acrylic guide plane with crossbite corrected.

SPACE MAINTENANCE AND INTERCEPTIVE ORTHODONTICS 237

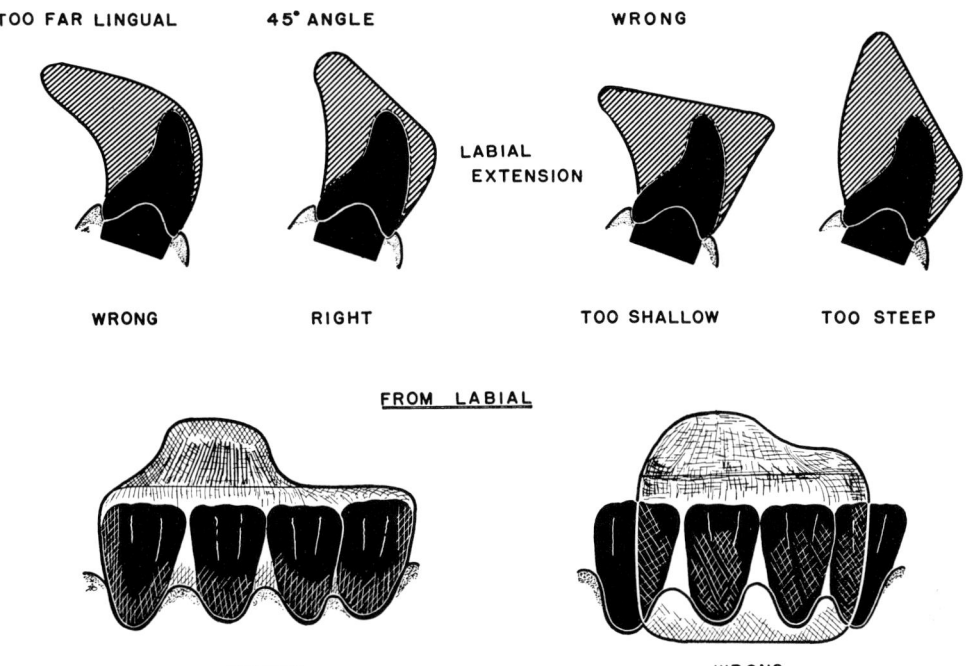

Figure 11-46 Relationship of tooth in crossbite to inclined plane. Only the tooth in crossbite contacts the guide plane. (From Graber, T. M.: *Orthodontics.* 2nd ed., 1966, p. 808.)

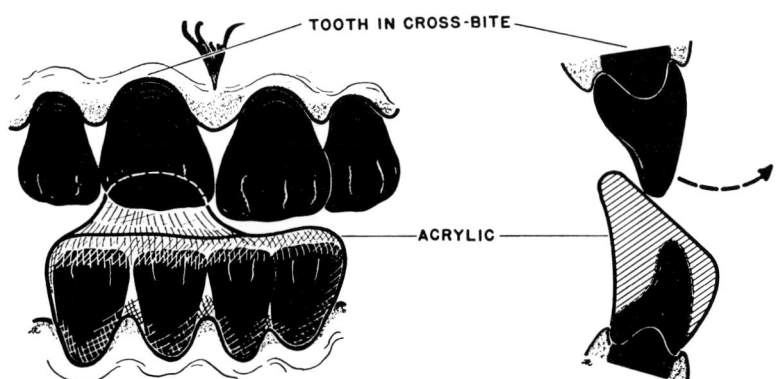

Figure 11-47 Acrylic guide plane. Design, coverage, and inclination of plane are important. A plane that is too shallow is as likely to cause failure as a plane that is too steep. (From Graber, T. M.: *Orthodontics.* 2nd ed., 1966, p. 808.)

238 SPACE MAINTENANCE AND INTERCEPTIVE ORTHODONTICS

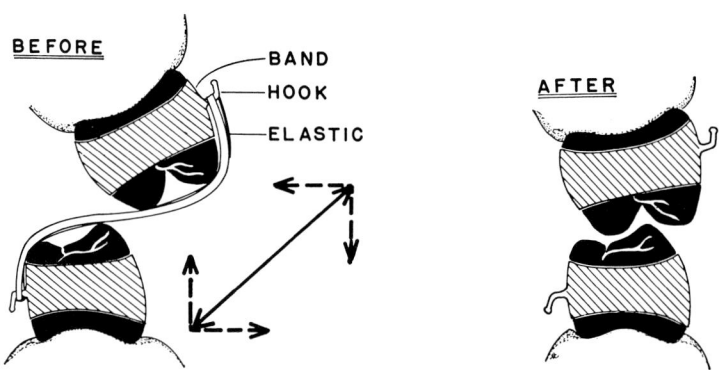

Figure 11-48 Correction of a unilateral posterior crossbite. The involved teeth are banded and rubber elastics used to correct the crossbite. (From Graber, T. M.: *Orthodontics*, 2nd ed., 1966, p. 823.)

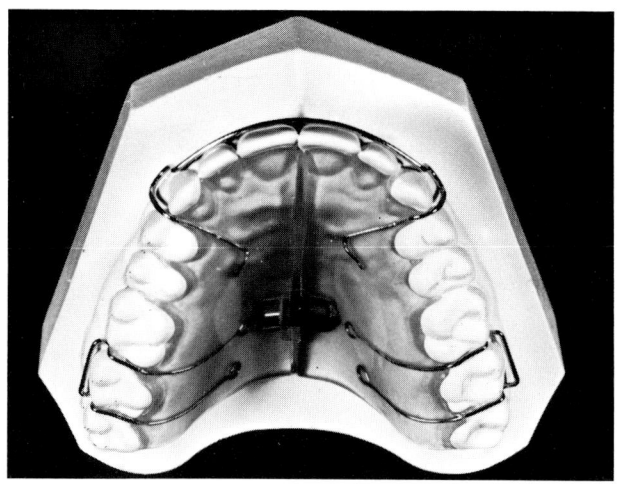

Figure 11-49 Correction of a bilateral posterior crossbite with a removable acrylic appliance and palatal expansion screw. Parent is given an expansion screw key (see Figure 11-50) and told to rotate the screw one-quarter of a turn each day. The patient should be checked at least every other week until the crossbite is corrected. (Appliance courtesy Rocky Mountain Dental Products Co.)

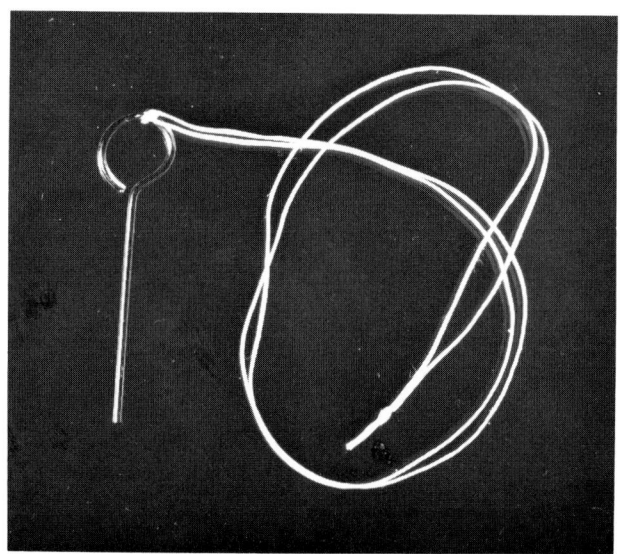

Figure 11-50 Expansion screw key for appliance shown in Figure 11-49 is a piece of heavy gauge stainless steel wire, either straight or bent 45 degrees on the working end. The dental floss on the handle end reduces the possibility of mislaying the key.

SPACE MAINTENANCE AND INTERCEPTIVE ORTHODONTICS 239

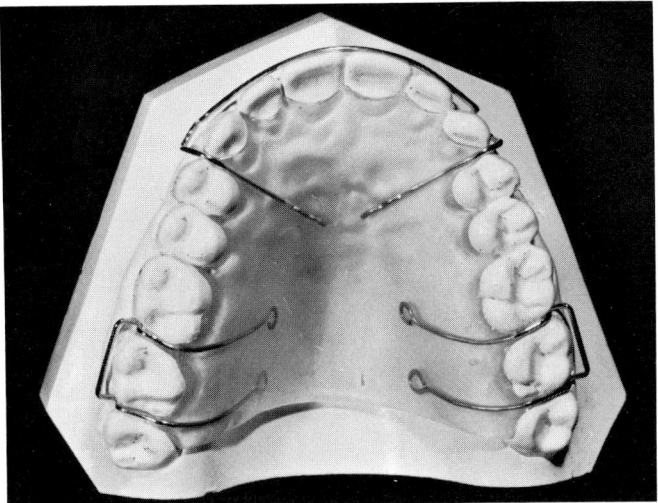

Figure 11-51 Hawley appliance used to correct protruding incisors when adequate room for retraction is available and when a Class I molar relation exists. Appliance is activated by periodically closing the wire loops in the cuspid area. Retraction of protruding incisors is an excellent method of reducing susceptibility to dental trauma. (Appliance courtesy Rocky Mountain Dental Products Co.)

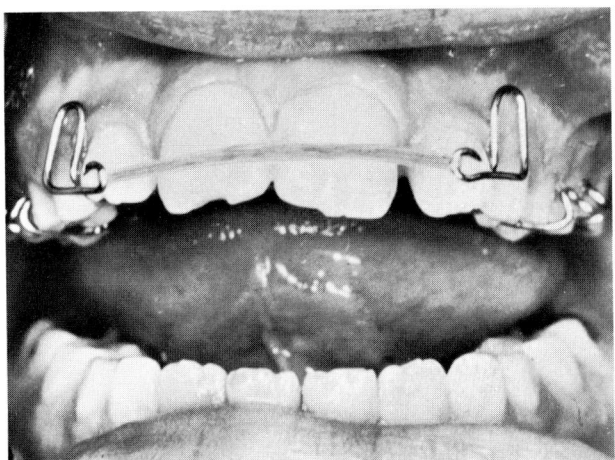

Figure 11-52 Removable appliance similar to that described in Figure 11-51 for retraction of protruding incisors. This appliance is activated by an attached rubber elastic stretched across the maxillary incisors. Note how the maxillary right permanent central incisor has been chipped.

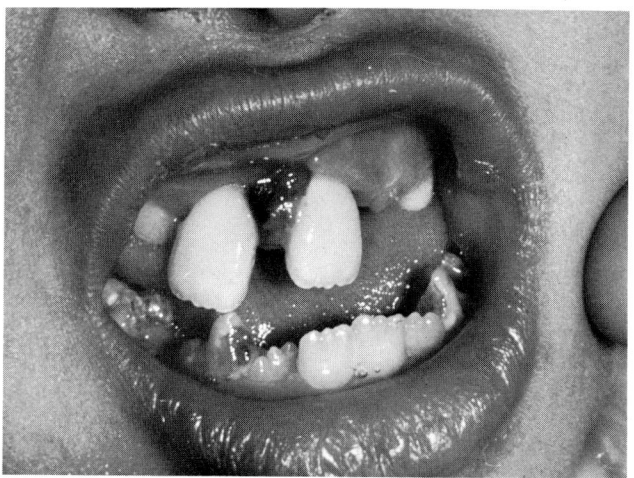

Figure 11-53 Appearance of maxillary central incisors following an attempt to correct a diastema between the incisors by stretching a rubber elastic around them. The elastic slipped apically and stripped the periodontal membrane almost entirely from the teeth.

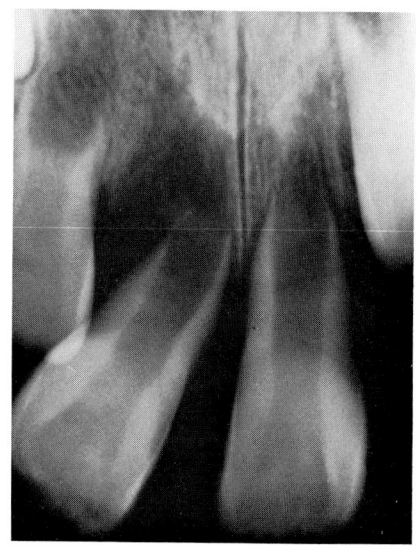

Figure 11-54 Radiographic appearance of teeth following rubber elastic therapy *only*, designed to correct the diastema. (See Figure 11-53.) The central incisors were lost, obviously because of destruction of the supporting structures.

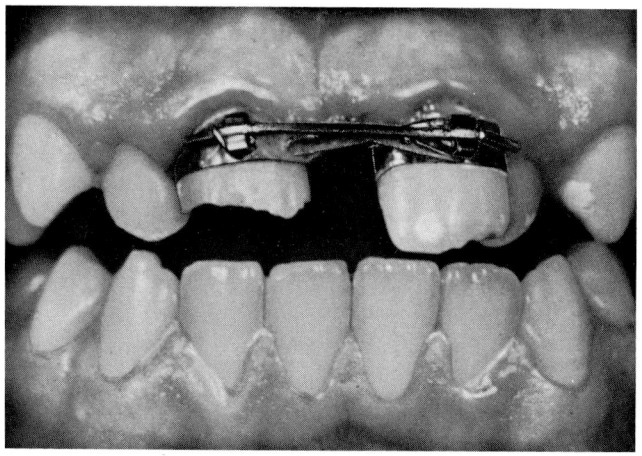

Figure 11-55 Correction of a diastema between central incisors. A well-controlled method for correcting this condition is to place bands with edgewise brackets on the incisors and connect both teeth with an edgewise wire. A rubber elastic is then wrapped in a figure eight around the wire. Patient should be checked every week until the diastema is eliminated.

Figure 11-56 Ectopic eruption of a maxillary first permanent molar. Before a particular method of treatment is decided on, a radiograph of the erupting ectopic molar should be carefully evaluated. If the entire distal root of the primary second molar has been resorbed and the first permanent molar occupies this area, then use of the brass wire technique will likely be ineffective.

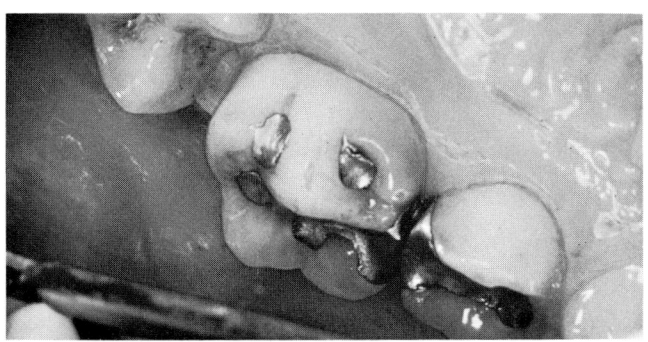

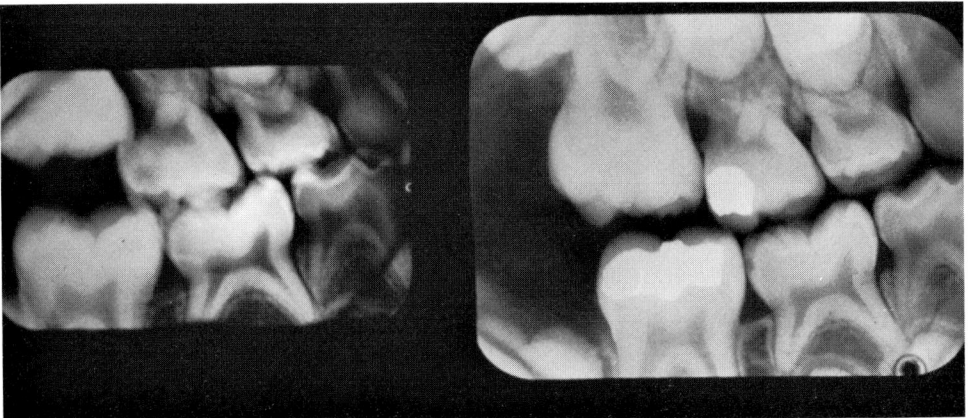

Figure 11-57 Radiograph at left of an ectopically erupting maxillary first permanent molar. Radiograph at right of the maxillary first permanent molar, following correction of the path of eruption with a twisted interproximal brass wire. The wire was placed between the maxillary second primary molar and the maxillary first permanent molar. (See Figure 11-58.)

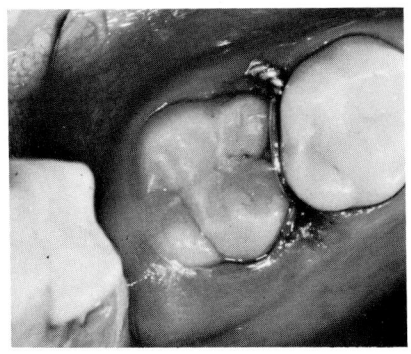

Figure 11-58 Use of a soft brass wire to correct ectopically erupting maxillary first permanent molar. Patient should be seen every week to tighten wire until the eruption is normalized.

Figure 11-59 Correction of ectopically erupting maxillary first permanent molars. Bands are fitted to the second primary molars and a stainless steel wire is soldered to the distal surface of each band. The bands are then cemented in place and each wire is activated by opening the palatal loop. The end of the wire is then cemented with zinc phosphate cement into a small occlusal preparation in the first permanent molar.

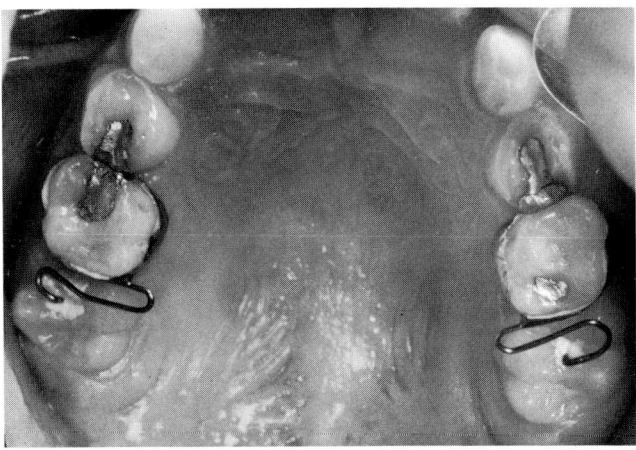

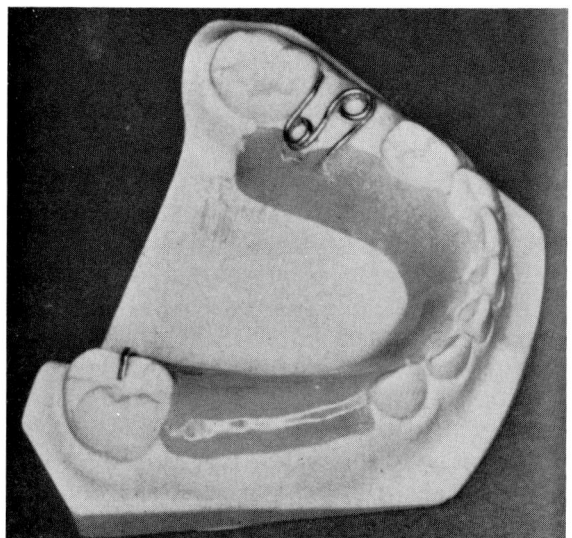

Figure 11-60 Acrylic space regainer with recurved helical finger spring. The action of the wire finger spring (made from 0.025 inch stainless steel wire) is similar to that of a safety pin. No more than 3 to 4 mm. of movement should be expected from this appliance. (From Norton, L. A., and Proffit, W. R.: Molar uprighting as an adjunct to fixed prostheses. J.A.D.A. 76:312-315, Feb., 1968.)

Figure 11-61 Adaptation of 0.025 inch stainless steel wire for a split acrylic space regainer. (From Norton, L. A., and Proffit, W. R.: Molar uprighting as an adjunct to fixed prostheses. J.A.D.A. 76:312-315, Feb., 1968.)

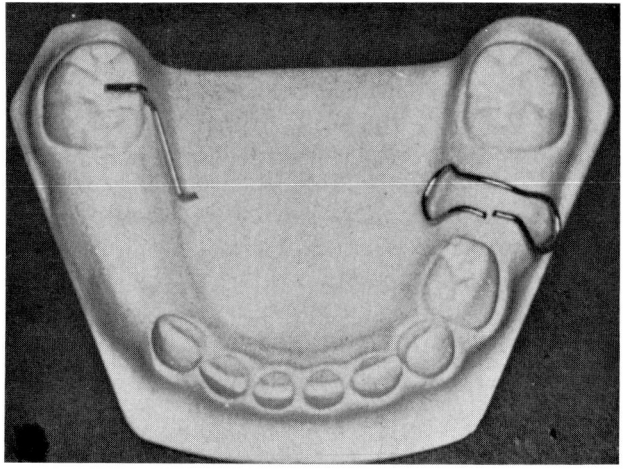

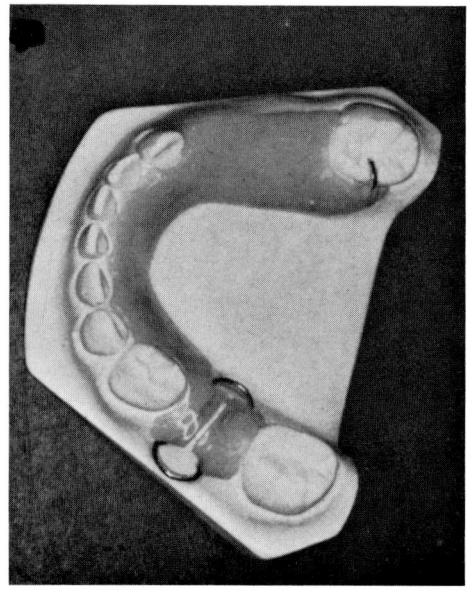

Figure 11-62 Split acrylic space regainer. The appliance is activated by opening the wire loops and inserting the appliance with slight pressure. This is done periodically until the tooth is tipped back into position. However, not more than 2 to 3 mm. of movement should be expected from this appliance. (From Norton, L. A. and Proffit, W. R.: Molar uprighting as an adjunct to fixed prostheses. J.A.D.A. 76:312-315, Feb., 1968.)

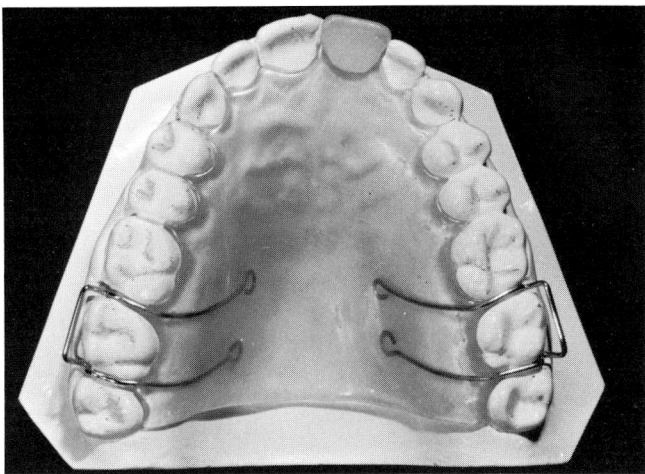

Figure 11-63 Adams clasps used to stabilize and add retention to a temporary partial denture. The Adams clasp is an effective one when used in interceptive orthodontic appliances. Note similarity between this clasp and the appliance shown in Figure 11-27. (Appliance courtesy Rocky Mountain Dental Products Co.)

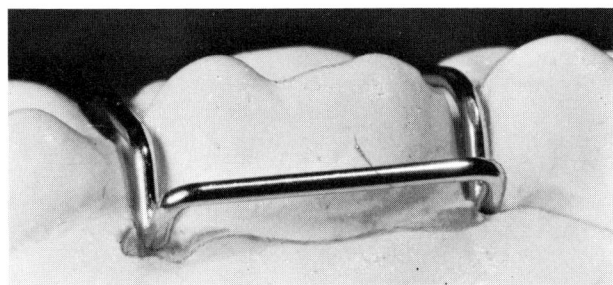

Figure 11-64. Close-up buccal view of the Adams clasp.

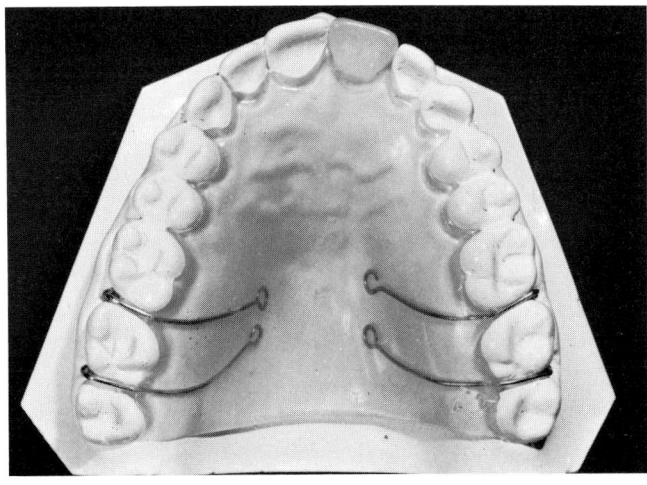

Figure 11-65 Ball clasps used to stabilize and add retention to a temporary partial denture replacing a maxillary central incisor. (Appliance courtesy Rocky Mountain Dental Products Co.)

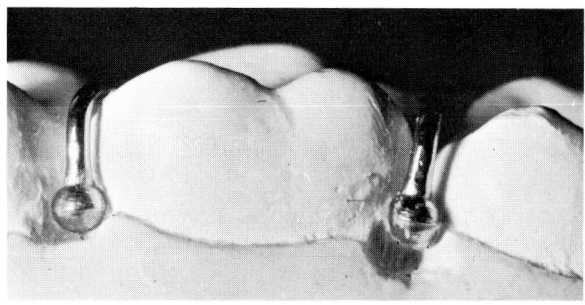

Figure 11-66 Close-up buccal view of the ball clasp.

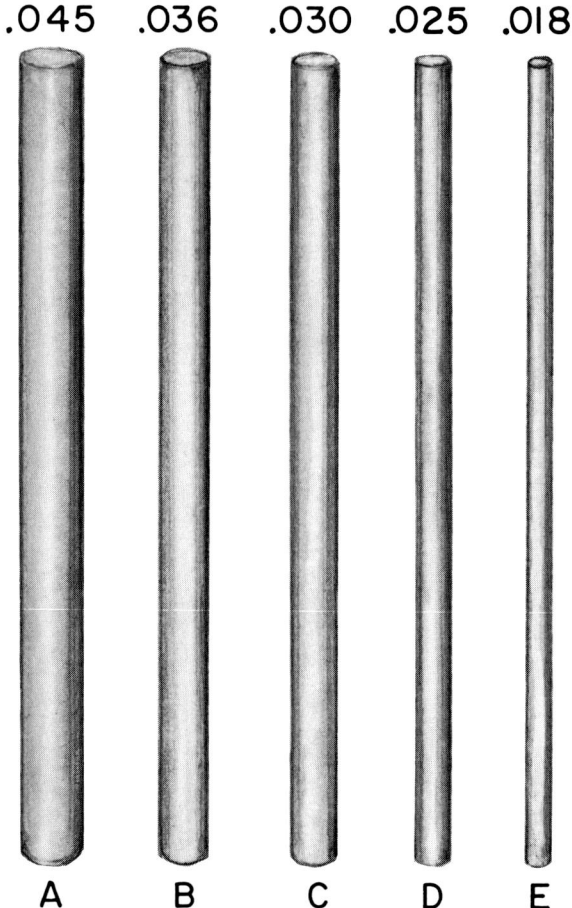

Figure 11-67 Suggested sizes of stainless steel wire to be used for space maintenance and interceptive orthodontics:
  A, 0.045 inch, used for maxillary labial arch wires in correcting bilateral posterior crossbites.
  B, 0.036 inch used for crown and loop, and band and loop unilateral space maintainers and also lingual arch wires.
  C, 0.030 inch, used for Hawley labial arch wires and molar clasps.
  D, 0.025 inch, used for cuspid clasps and auxiliary springs.
  E, 0.018 inch, used as auxiliary wire soldered onto heavier wire.

SPACE MAINTENANCE AND INTERCEPTIVE ORTHODONTICS 245

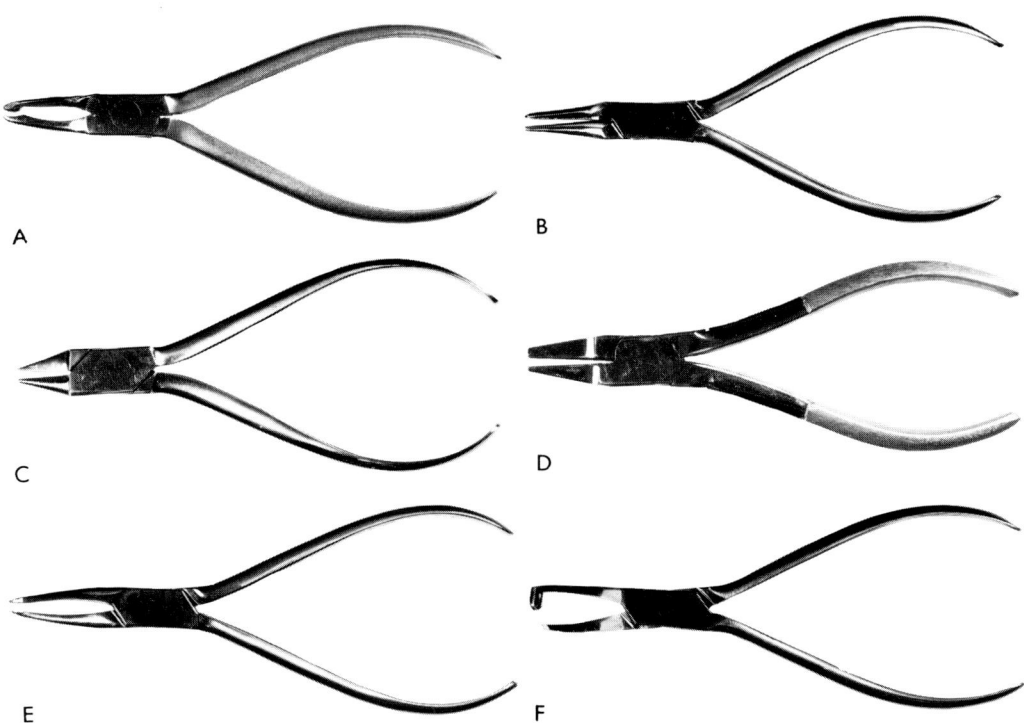

Figure 11-68 Suggested pliers for space maintenance and interceptive orthodontics:
A, No. 114 contouring plier, used to contour stainless steel crowns and bands.
B, No. 53 wire bending plier, excellent for bending the loop contacting the adjacent tooth on unilateral crown and loop, and band and loop spacers.
C, No. 139 wire bending plier, excellent for general use in bending wire.
D, No. 82 optical plier, excellent for contouring lingual or labial arch wires.
E, No. 110 How plier (straight) good for inserting and removing lingual arch wires.
F, Band remover (posterior).

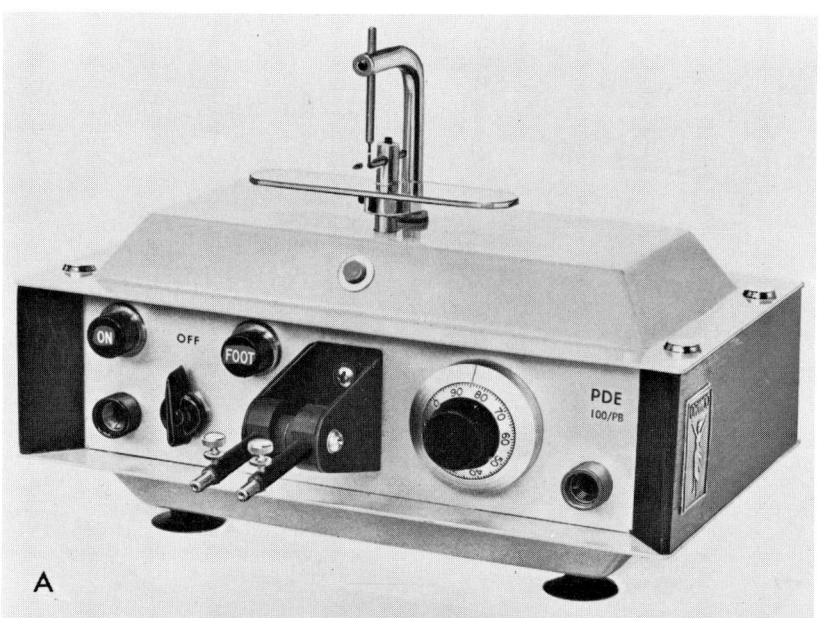

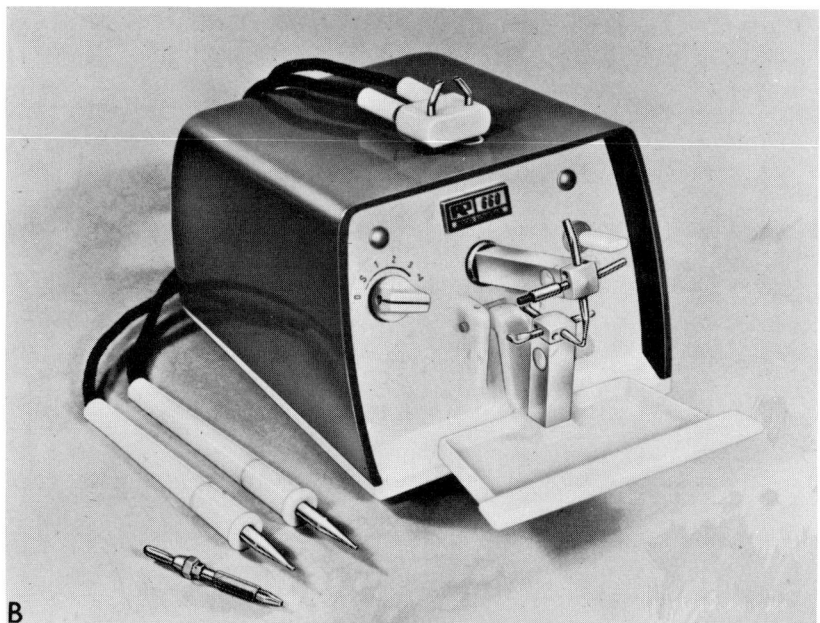

Figure 11-69 Spot welding and soldering units which may be used to make spacers and interceptive orthodontic appliances.
- A, P.D.E. welding and soldering unit. (Courtesy Ormco Corp.)
- B, No. 660 welding and soldering unit. (Courtesy Rocky Mountain Dental Products Co.)
- C, No. 506 Dial-A-Weld, welding and soldering unit. (Courtesy Rocky Mountain Dental Products Co.)
- D, No. 1082 welding and soldering unit. (Courtesy Unitek Corp.)

SPACE MAINTENANCE AND INTERCEPTIVE ORTHODONTICS 247

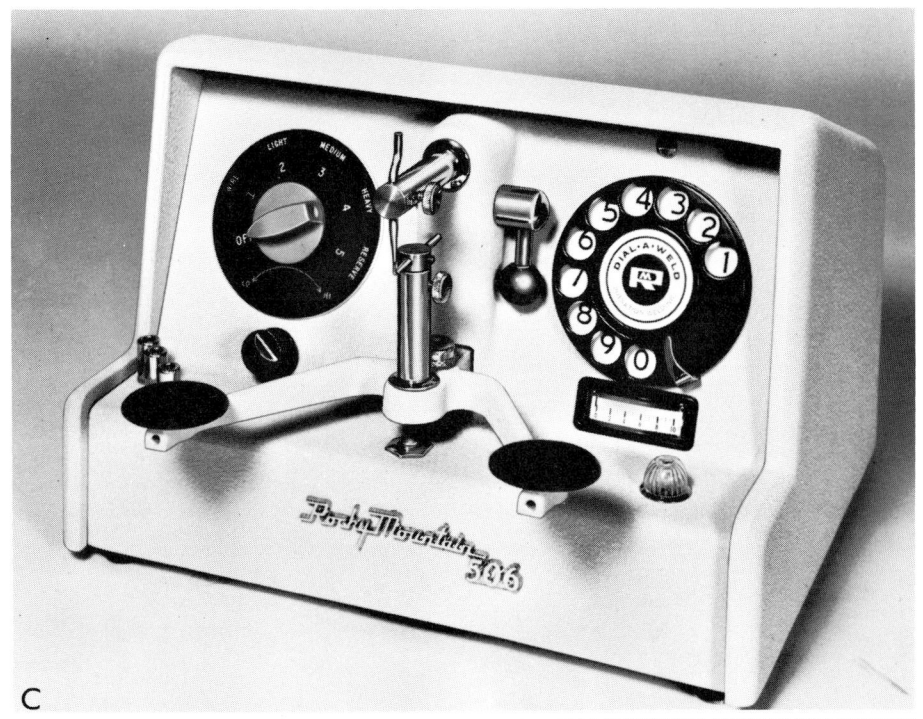

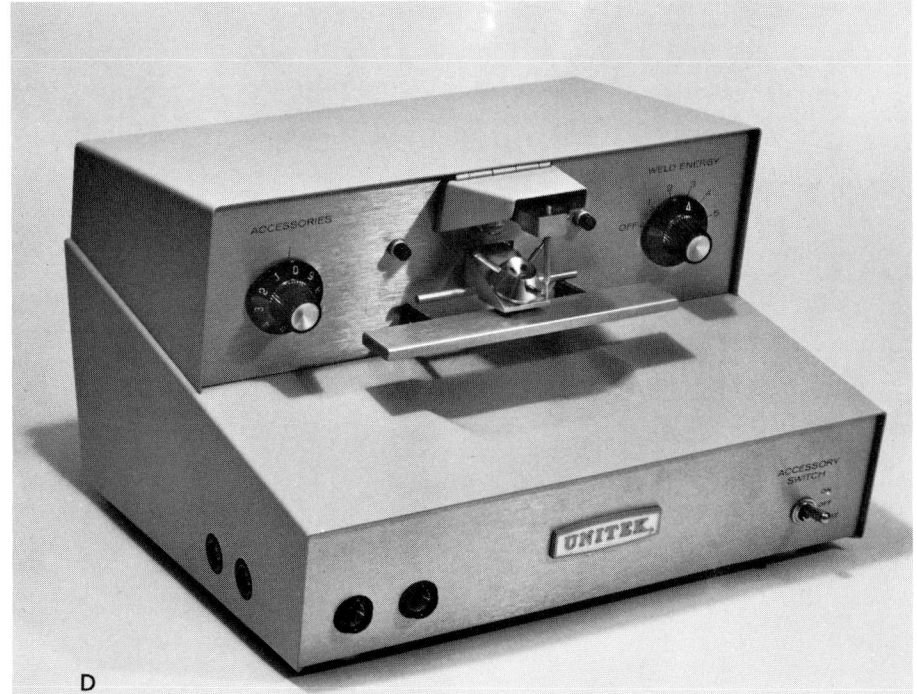

Figure 11-69 *Continued*

Chapter 12
PROSTHODONTICS

Prosthodontics for the child patient is differentiated from space maintenance and minor orthodontic procedures in order to simplify organization of the material. Full and partial dentures are the chief topics of discussion in this chapter.

Complete dentures are occasionally required to provide esthetics and function for a preschool child. There may be anodontia as a result of hereditary ectodermal dysplasia, or multiple extraction of teeth may have been performed because of rampant caries. In general, small children tolerate dentures very well. Their tissues are healthy and resistant, and their mental attitude is one of lack of concern over small irritations. They usually start eating immediately upon being fitted with dentures and seldom complain afterward. No inhibition of growth will be caused be dentures. In time, as changes occur, the dentures will simply no longer fit properly and it will be obvious that alterations or a complete remake is required. The same procedures that are employed in preparing dentures for the adult should be followed in treating the child. In general, it is inadvisable to attempt to make complete dentures for a child under the age of 4 years because of his lack of comprehension and understanding at this young age.

The chief problems with complete dentures in children arise during the period of the eruption of the maxillary and mandibular incisors. The dentures must be cut away and relieved to allow room for the new teeth. This in turn destroys the seal of the denture flange, and poor retention results. Even if the child continues to wear the denture there is usually the problem of cleanliness and food retention around the cut-away areas.

Partial dentures are quite successful with children of all ages and are usually well tolerated. If at all possible, partial dentures should be constructed rather than complete dentures. Frequently, in planning treatment for a badly broken down mouth in a preschool child, a few teeth can be saved by heroic measures. It is worth crowning two cuspids and perhaps a primary molar if they can be retained and used as abutments for a removable denture. During the transition period of the anterior teeth the partial denture can be successfully retained, whereas full dentures offer many problems.

In most clinical cases the choice of partial denture material will be acrylic resin. However, in cases that involve long-term use of the appliance, such as complete loss of permanent anteriors at an early age, the use of cast chrome-cobalt alloy partial dentures should be considered.

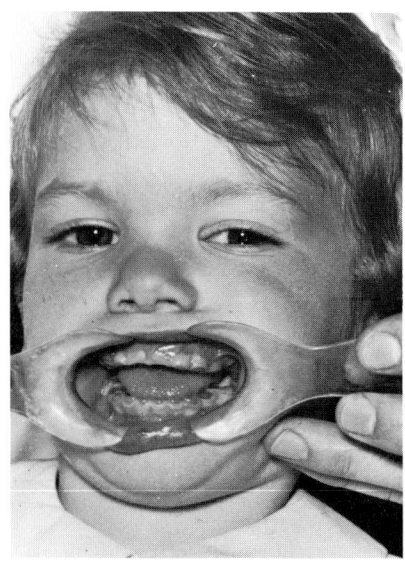

Figure 12-1 Patient J. B., a 3½ year old girl with hereditary dentinogenesis imperfecta. Rapid wearing away of enamel and dentin is common with this condition. Prostheses are necessary for both function and esthetics. Management of this case will be illustrated through age 15 (Figure 12-1 through 12-20).

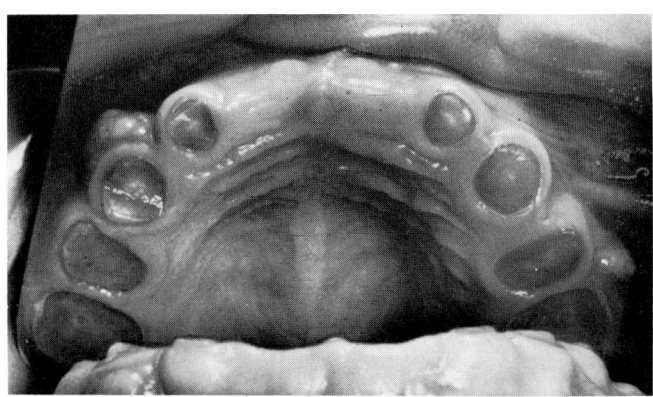

Figure 12-2 Maxillary arch. Note abrasion of teeth and chronic abscess over right primary molar. Pulpal exposures may occur in these cases because of the wearing away of enamel and dentin, and extractions become necessary.

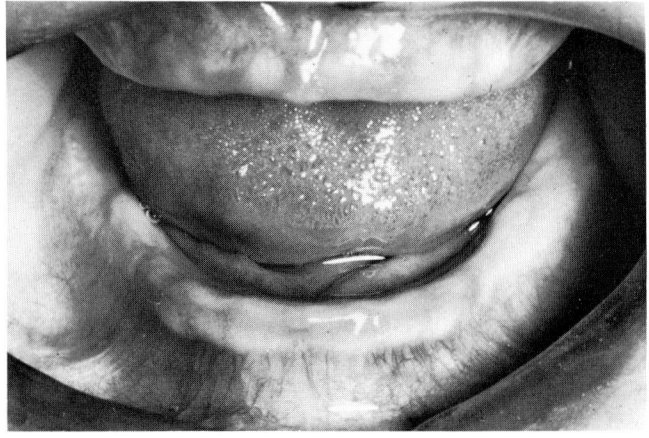

Figure 12-3 Age 4 years. All primary teeth have been extracted because of development of pulpal abscesses. Full dentures are now indicated for the health of this patient.

PROSTHODONTICS 251

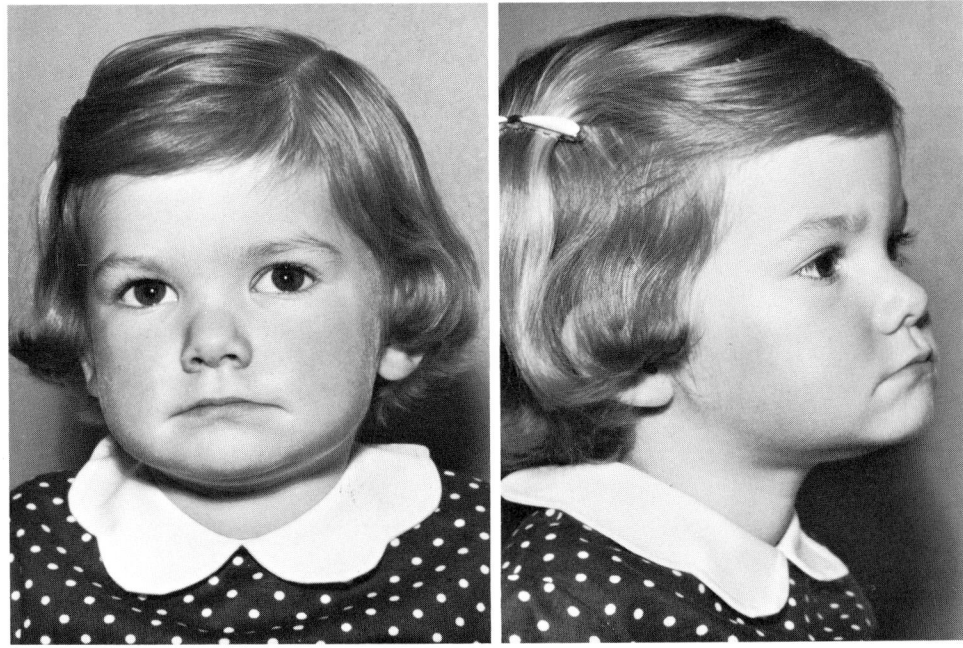

Figure 12-4 Profile and full face view. Patient is 4 years old. Extraction of all primary teeth has resulted in loss of vertical dimension.

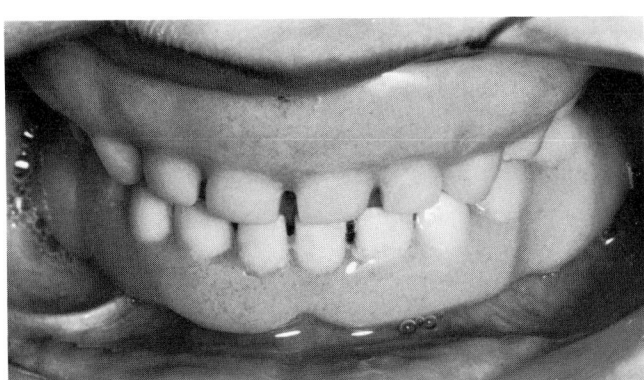

Figure 12-5 Full dentures in place. Note shape, size, color, and spacing of the denture teeth to resemble those of natural primary teeth. The same steps in fabrication of full dentures for adults should be used in the child patient.

Figure 12-6 Full face view. Note the improvement in appearance and personality. Small children adapt very quickly to prosthetic appliances and very few adjustments are usually necessary.

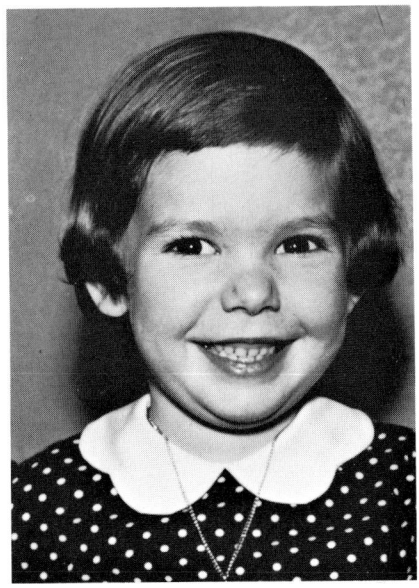

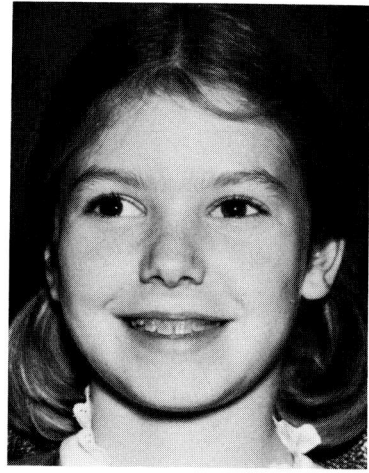

Figure 12-7 Patient is now 11 years of age. Permanent teeth have typical brown-opalescent color and are beginning to show abrasion and wear.

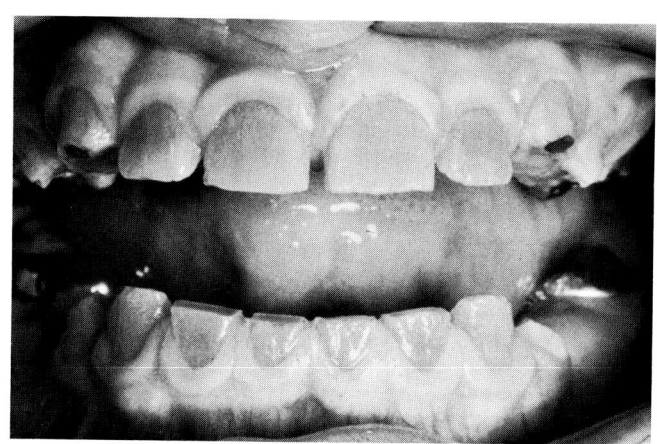

Figure 12-8 Anterior view. Mandibular incisors appear more worn than maxillary.

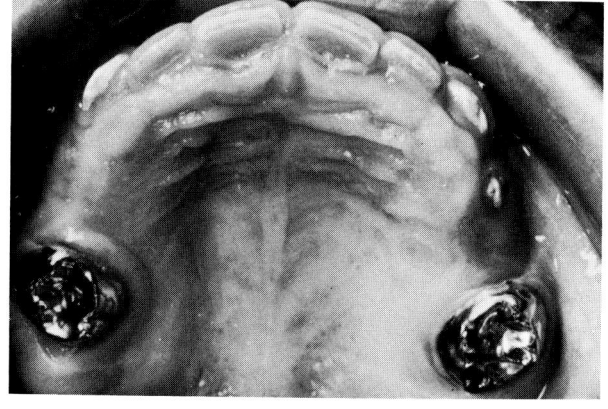

Figure 12-9 Maxillary arch. First permanent molars have been protected with stainless steel crowns. A simple acrylic palatal space maintainer was used as a temporary space holding appliance during this age period.

Figure 12-10 Mandibular arch. Permanent molars protected with stainless steel crowns. A simple acrylic space maintainer was also constructed for this arch.

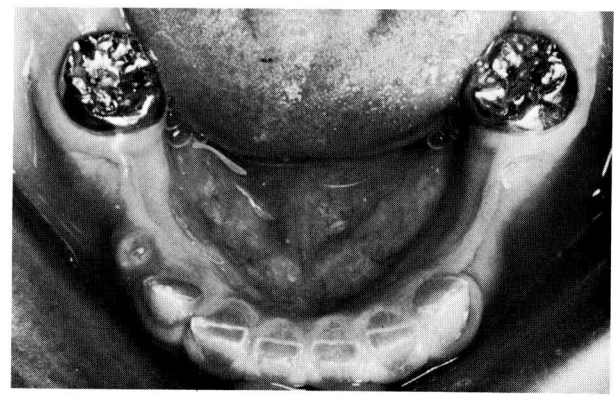

PROSTHODONTICS 253

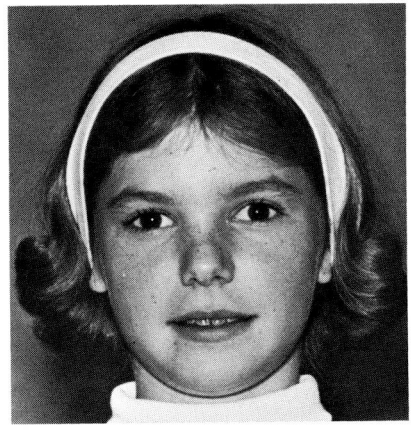

Figure 12-11 Age 13 years. The problem of esthetics is increasingly important during these years.

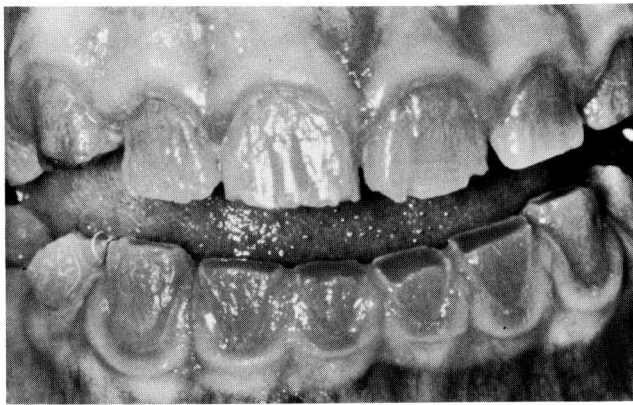

Figure 12-12 Anterior view. Chipping and abrasion are evident on the incisors.

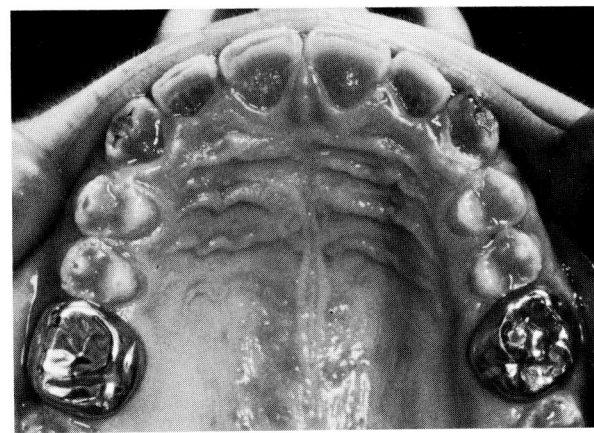

Figure 12-13 Maxillary arch. Patient is 13 years old.

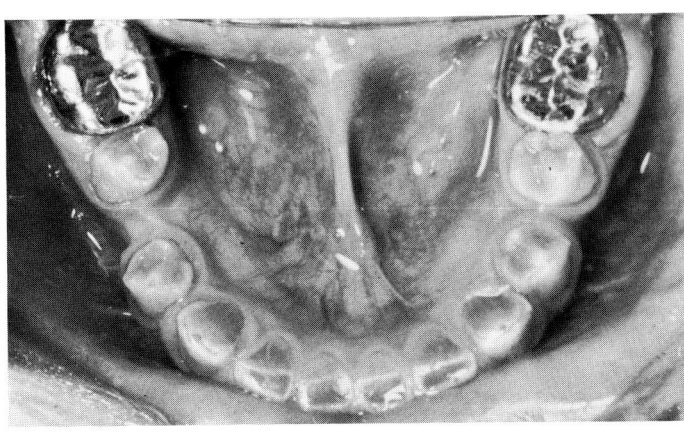

Figure 12-14 Mandibular arch. Patient is 13 years old. A decision as to further treatment must be made before significant loss of tooth structure occurs.

254 PROSTHODONTICS

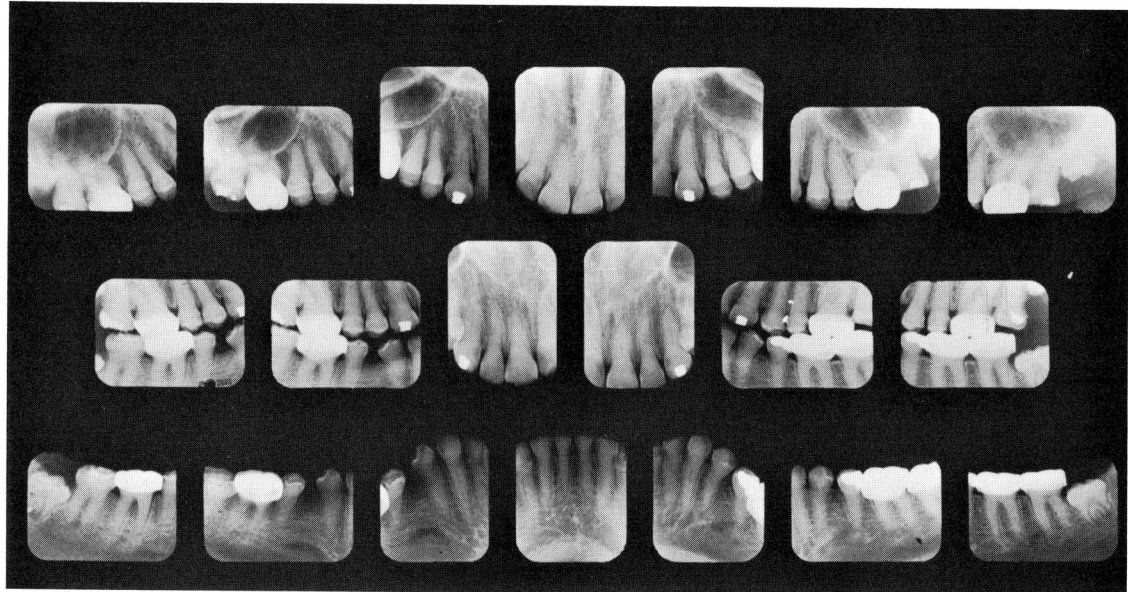

Figure 12-15 Radiographs of patient J. B. at age 14, just prior to complete tooth coverage. Note typical appearance of dentinogenesis imperfecta with obliteration of pulp canals.

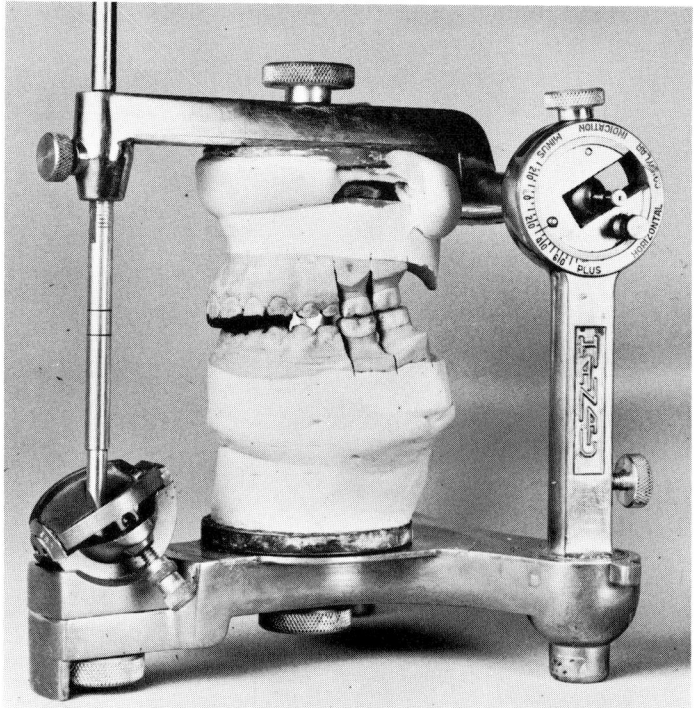

Figure 12-16 Articulator with stone models and posterior crowns showing the increase in vertical dimension.

Figure 12-17 Age 15, following full mouth reconstruction.

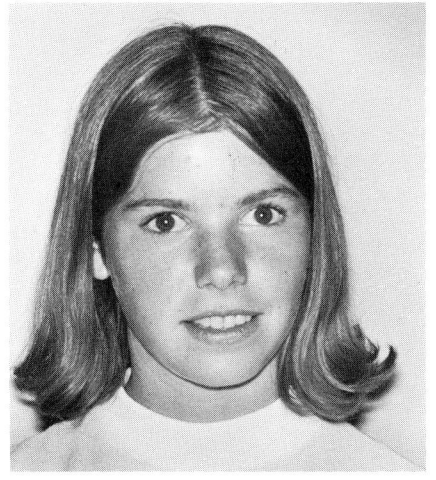

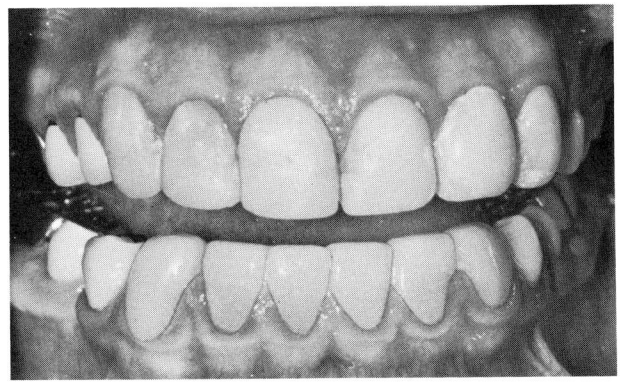

Figure 12-18 Anterior view following reconstruction. Porcelain bonded to gold crowns were constructed for all maxillary and mandibular permanent incisors.

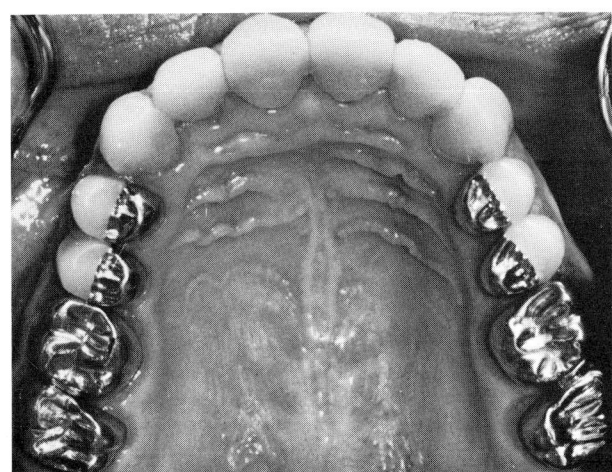

Figure 12-19 Maxillary view. Note complete coverage of all bicuspids and molars.

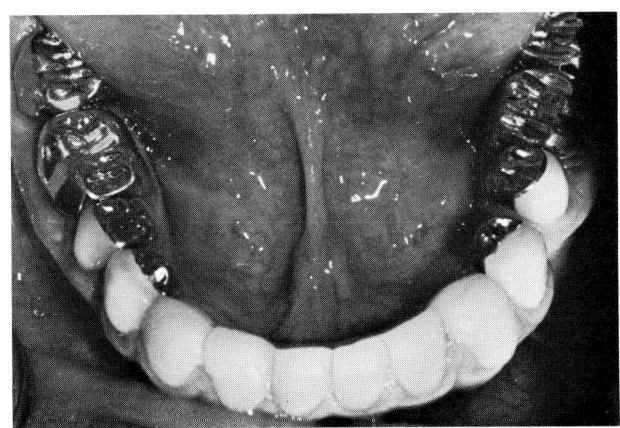

Figure 12-20 Mandibular arch. Note porcelain bonded crowns in bicuspid region and full cast gold crowns on molars.

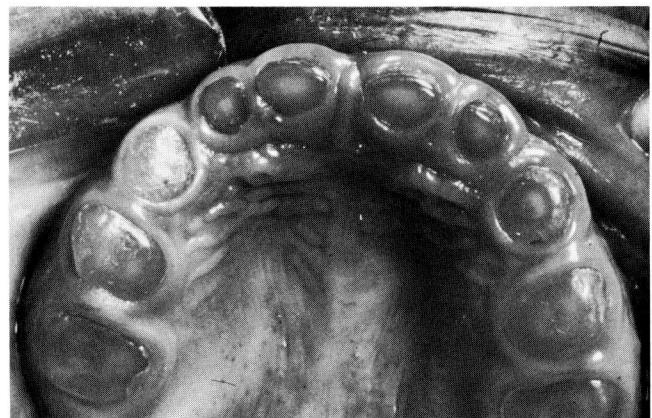

Figure 12-21 Maxillary arch of a 5-year-old girl, D. C., with dentinogenesis imperfecta. No tendency to develop pulpal abscesses was observed and it was decided to retain the teeth and construct the maxillary denture over them. Figures 12-21 through 12-26 illustrate this case.

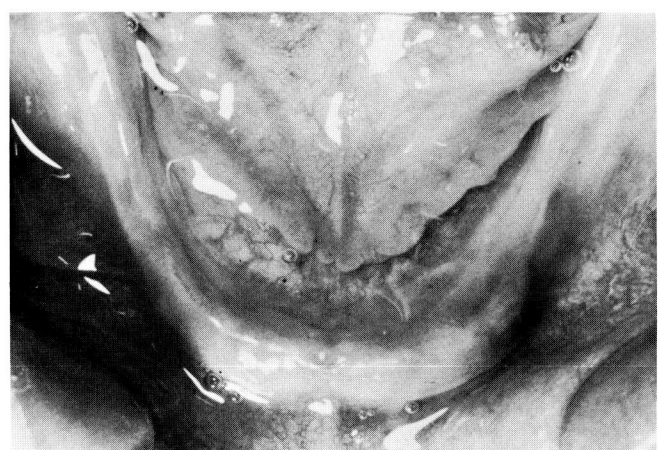

Figure 12-22 Mandibular arch. Teeth had previously been extracted when patient was first seen by authors.

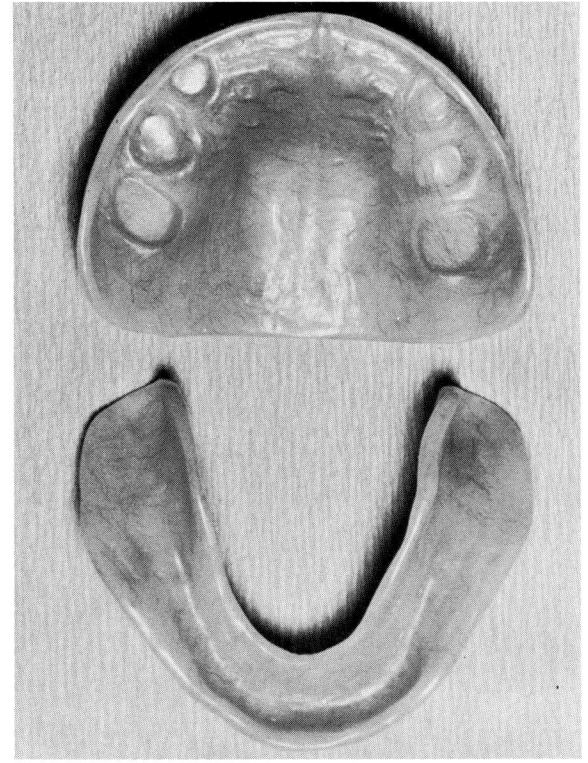

Figure 12-23 Tissue side of maxillary and mandibular dentures. Note impressions of maxillary crowns in the upper denture.

PROSTHODONTICS 257

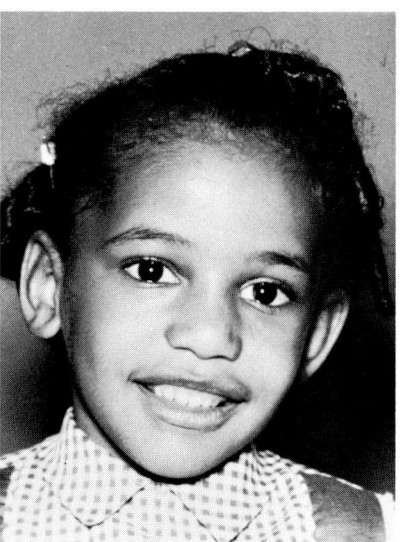

Figure 12-24 Dentures in place. No problem was encountered in retention of the maxillary denture.

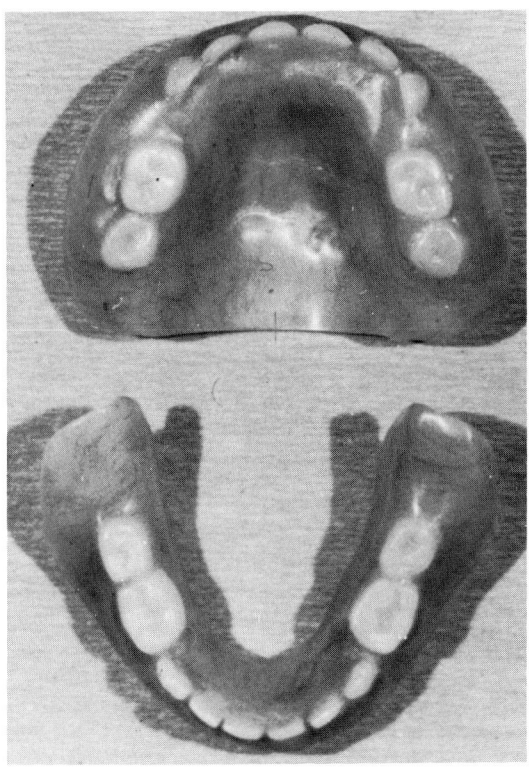

Figure 12-25 Occlusal view of dentures.

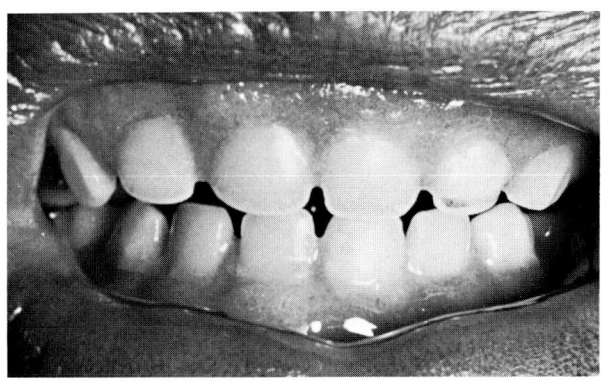

Figure 12-26 Anterior view, showing properly spaced and shaped denture teeth for a preschool child.

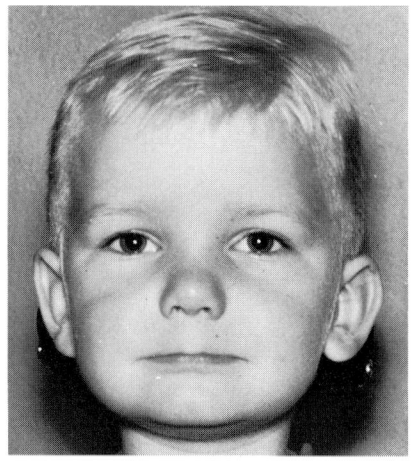

Figure 12-27 A 4-year-old boy in whom all primary teeth were extracted because of pulpal abscesses resulting from dentinogenesis imperfecta. Facial appearance is typical of overclosure in these cases.

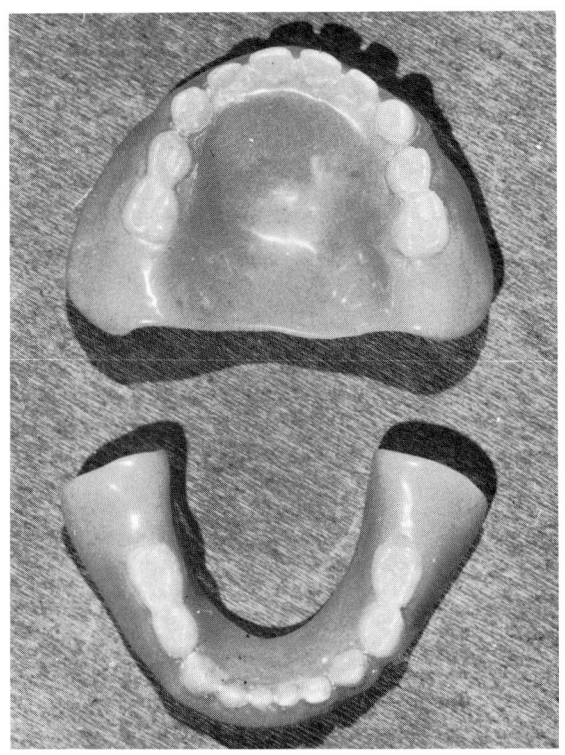

Figure 12-28 Maxillary and mandibular dentures fabricated for boy shown in Figure 12-27. Note distal extensions of denture to gain maximum stability.

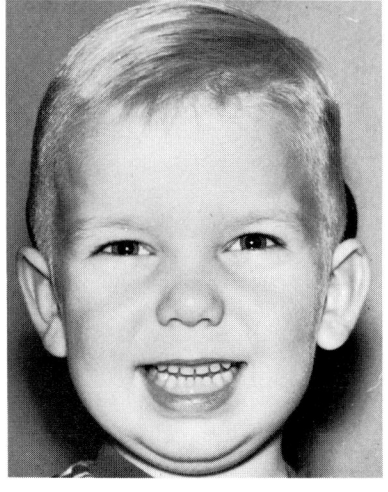

Figure 12-29 Same boy as seen in Figure 12-27 with maxillary and mandibular dentures in place. Note improved appearance. The spacing of denture teeth is important when making dentures for children.

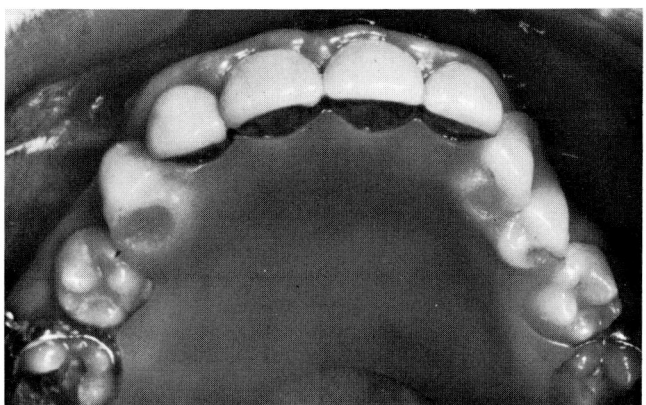

Figure 12-30 Maxillary acrylic partial denture constructed for a child with ectodermal dysplasia. Anterior teeth were conical and were restored with porcelain bonded to gold crowns.

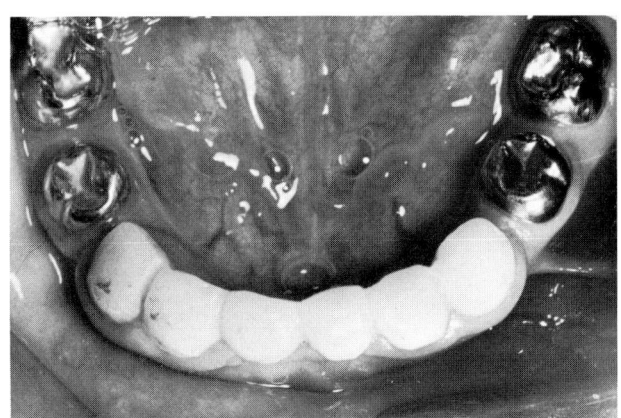

Figure 12-31 A mandibular acrylic bridge constructed for a child with missing mandibular incisors.

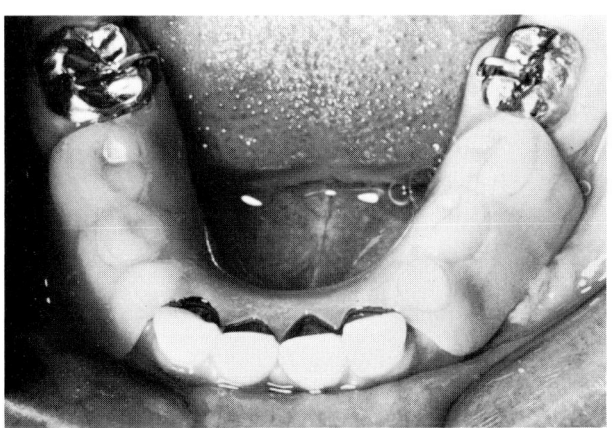

Figure 12-32 Mandibular acrylic partial denture for a child with ectodermal dysplasia. Conical incisors have been restored with porcelain bonded to gold crowns.

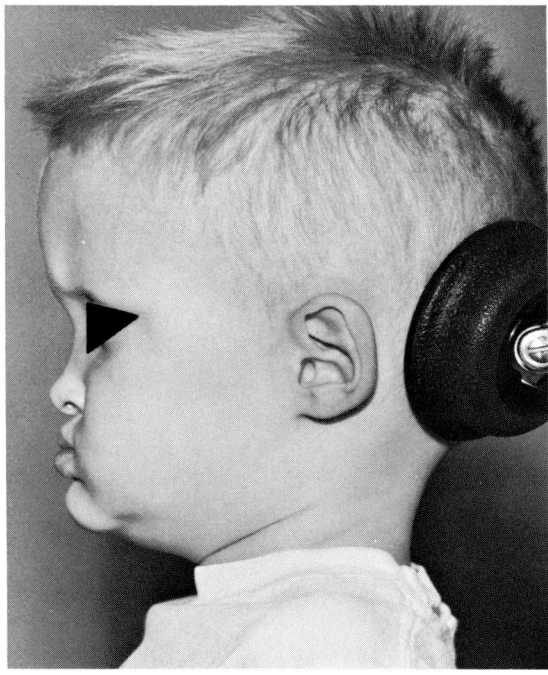
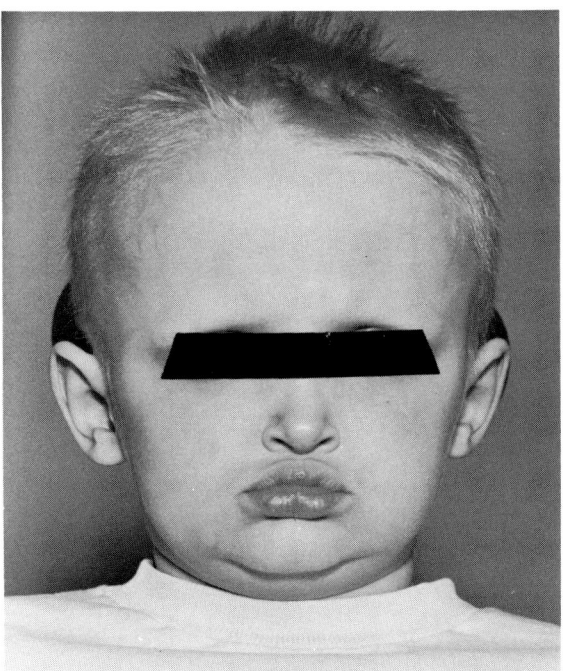

Figure 12-33   Figure 12-34

Figure 12-33   Profile of J. W., 4½-year-old boy with hereditary ectodermal dysplasia. Note typical appearance of saddle nose, everted lips, and absence of eyebrows. Lack of teeth causes overclosure. (From Bolender, C. L., Law, D. B., and Austin, L. B.: Prosthodontic treatment of ectodermal dysplasia. J. Pros. Dent. *14*(2):317-325, March-April, 1964.) Figures 12-33 to 12-43 illustrate this case.

Figure 12-34   Anterior view. These patients require full or partial dentures to restore function as well as esthetics.

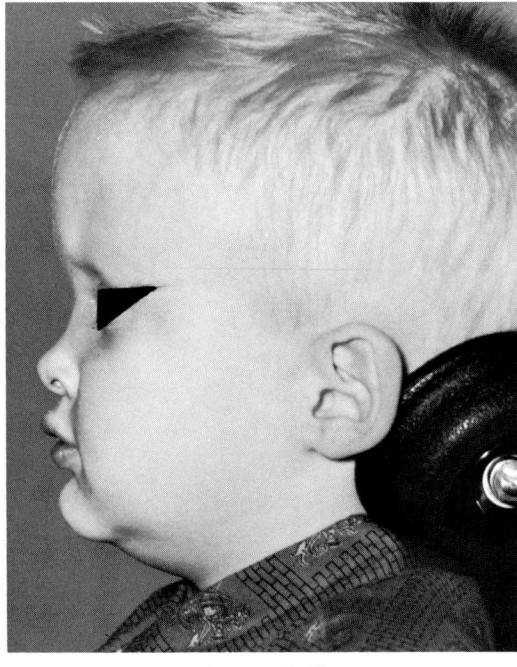
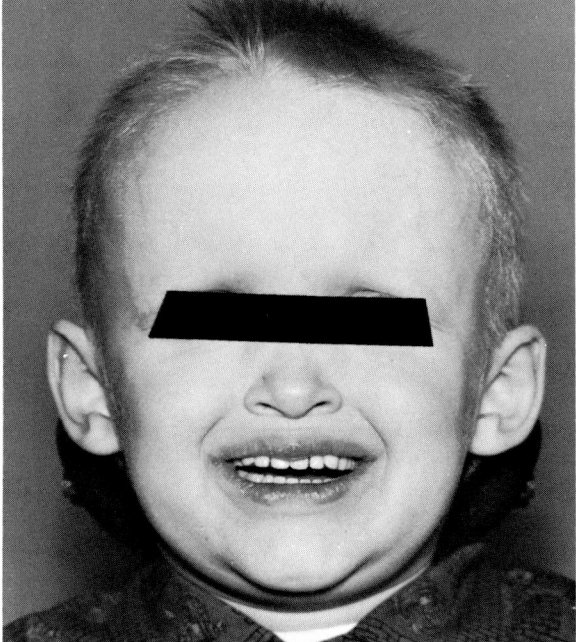

Figure 12-35   Figure 12-36

Figure 12-35   Complete prosthetic rehabilitation. Note improved profile.

Figure 12-36   Anterior view, showing natural appearance after treatment has been completed.

PROSTHODONTICS 261

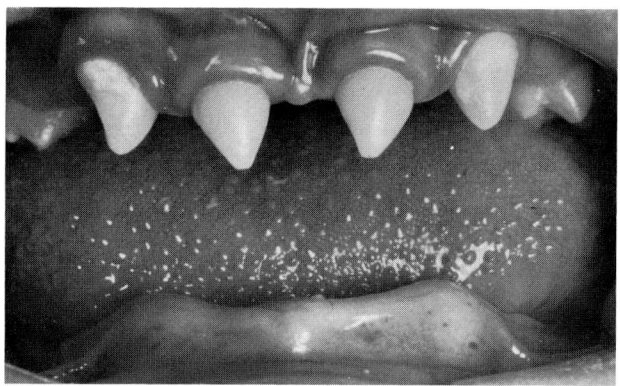

Figure 12-37 Intraoral view, before treatment. There is complete absence of erupted teeth in the mandibular arch. The maxillary arch has two erupted molars and four anteriors.

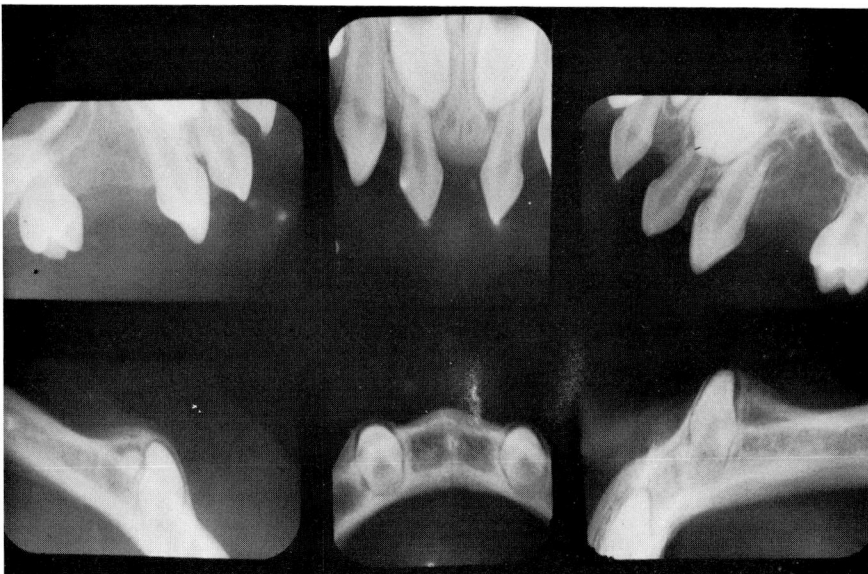

Figure 12-38 Radiographs demonstrate unerupted teeth. There is noticeable lack of alveolar bone because of the absence of teeth.

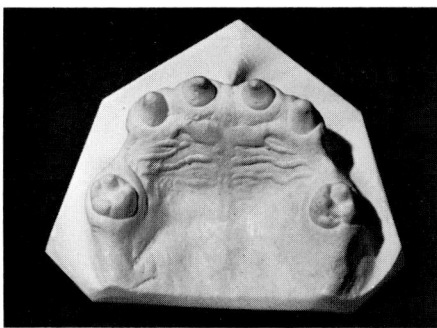

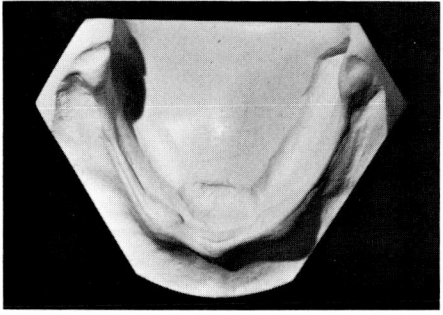

Figure 12-39 Study models. Note lack of ridge development in the mandibular arch.

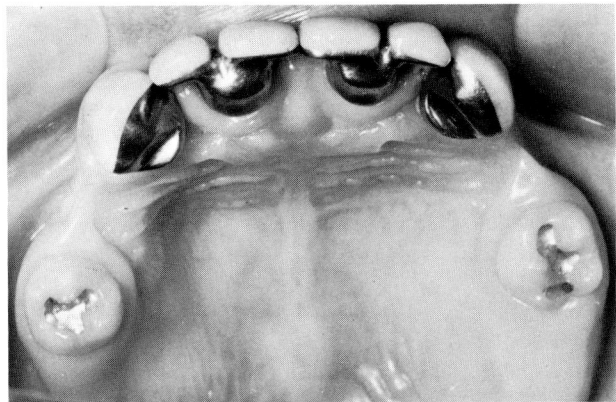

Figure 12-40 Cantilevered crowns (porcelain bonded to gold) on two maxillary conical incisors. This was done to render the typical appearance of four primary incisors. The conical cuspids were also crowned. Note lingual rest areas on these crowns for support of the partial denture.

Figure 12-41 Cast cobalt-chromium alloy partial seated in maxillary arch. The wide flat teeth were necessary because of the discrepancy in width between the two arches.

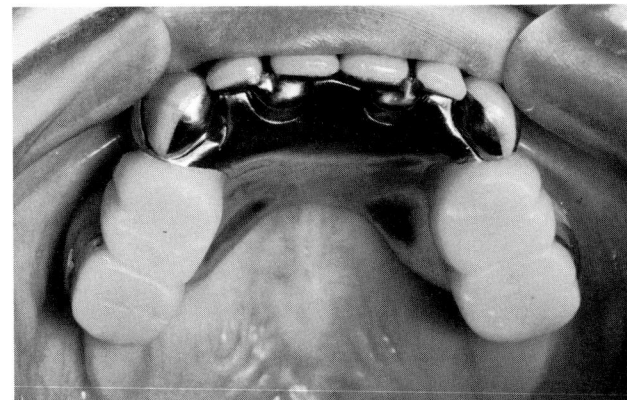

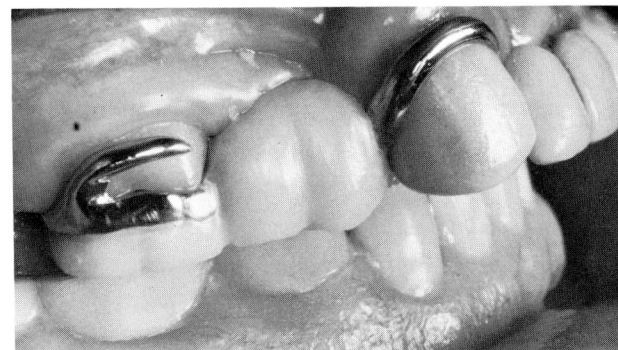

Figure 12-42 Lateral view showing the clasps on the primary cuspid and molar. The molar is covered by the partial in order to build up adequate vertical dimension.

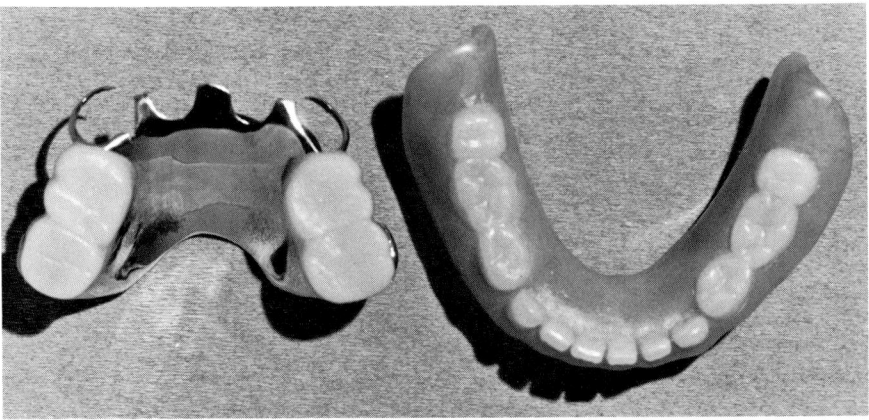

Figure 12-43 Upper partial and lower full denture. Note distal extension of mandibular denture flanges to gain stability.

PROSTHODONTICS

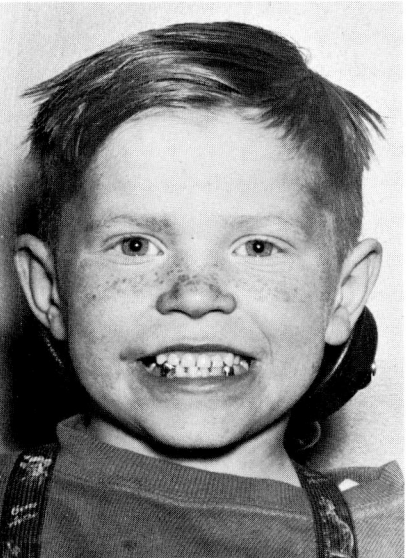

Figure 12-44 A 5-year-old boy with a full maxillary denture and mandibular partial. Teeth were extracted because of rampant caries.

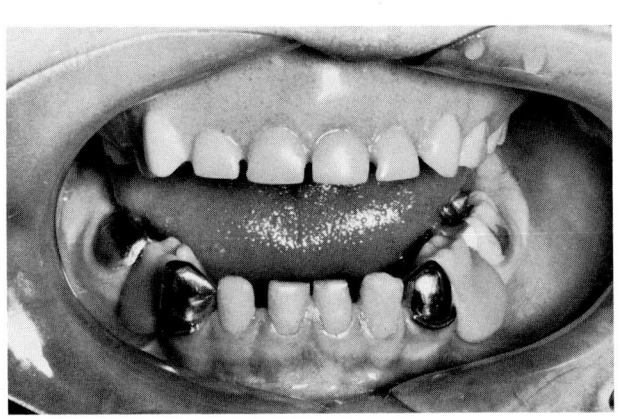

Figure 12-45 Same boy as seen in Figure 12-44. Solder was flowed on the gingival area of the steel crowns on the cuspids. This was done to provide better retention for the wire clasps.

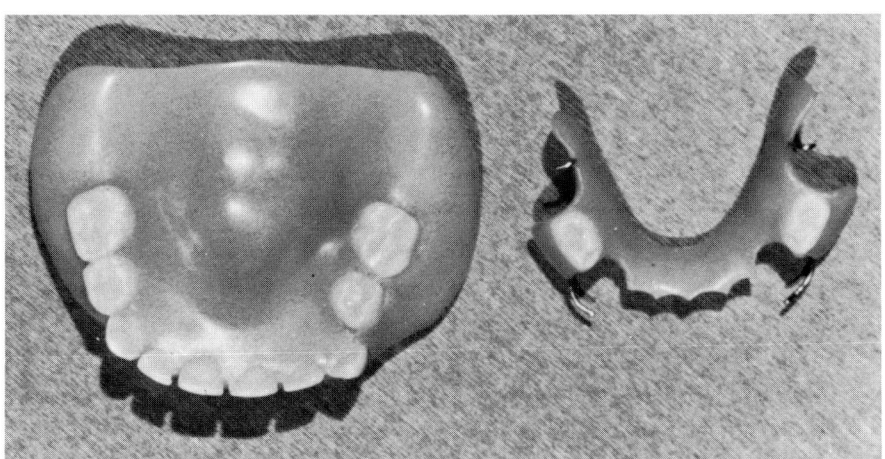

Figure 12-46 View of maxillary denture and mandibular partial of patient shown in Figure 12-45. Note extension of maxillary denture. Mandibular partial has rests on the second primary molars.

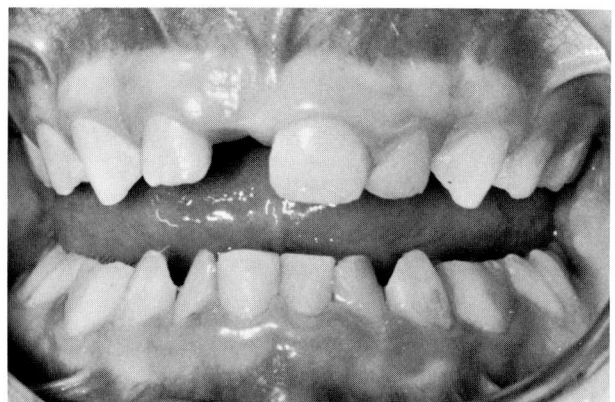

Figure 12-47 This case illustrates the construction of a fixed bridge for a 4-year-old girl who lost a maxillary primary central incisor in a fall from a swing. Although replacement of primary incisors is not usually considered necessary for space maintenance, parents may request such replacement for esthetic reasons. (See Figures 12-48 through 12-58.) (See Figures 13-20 through 13-23 for treatment of a similar case with a removable partial denture.)

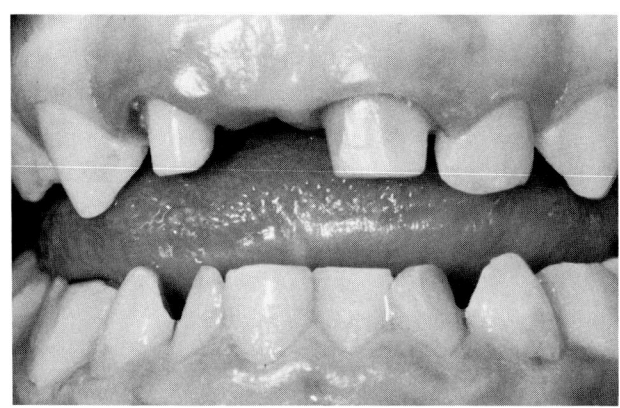

Figure 12-48 Intraoral view showing reduction of primary lateral and central for porcelain bonded to gold abutments.

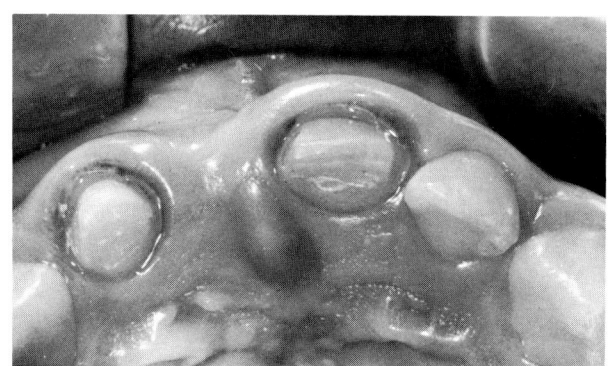

Figure 12-49 Incisal view of preparations showing shoulder of minimal width, on proximal and labial surfaces only.

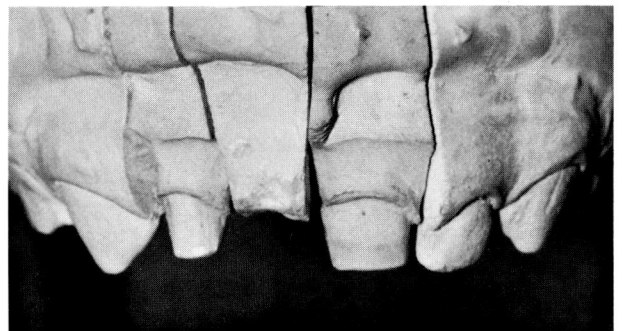

Figure 12-50 View of stone dies on articulator.

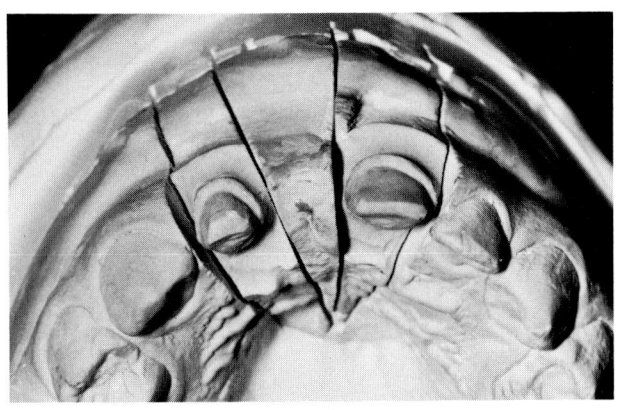

Figure 12-51 Incisal view of stone dies. Detail of the shoulder preparation can be seen.

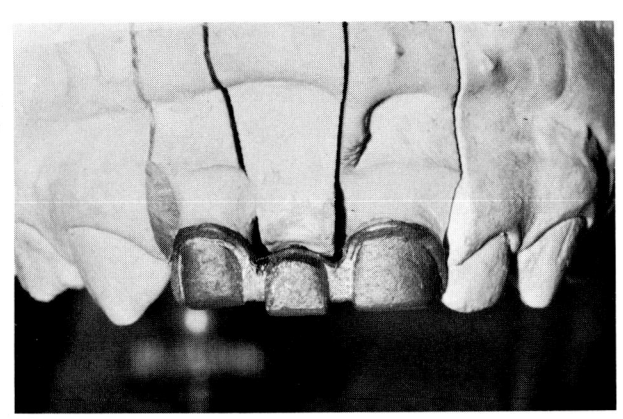

Figure 12-52 Anterior view of gold casting for bridge in place on dies.

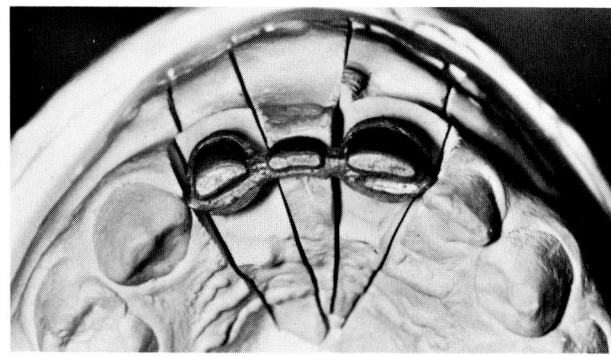

Figure 12-53 Incisal view of gold casting for bridge.

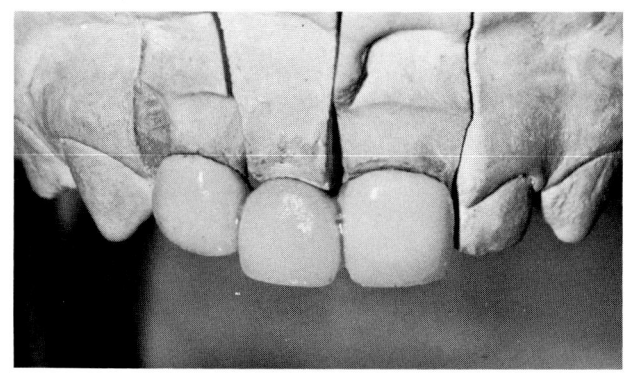

Figure 12-54 Labial view of completed bridge on stone model.

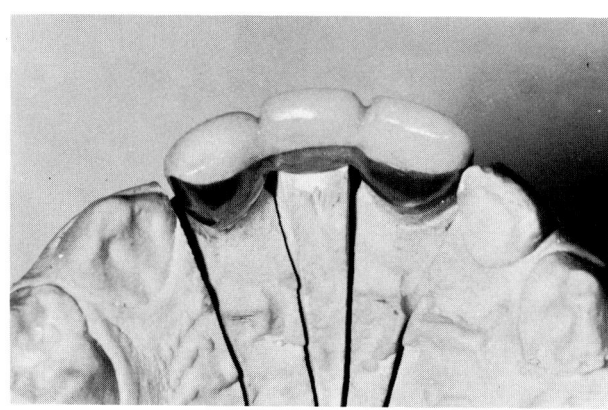

Figure 12-55 Lingual view of completed bridge on model.

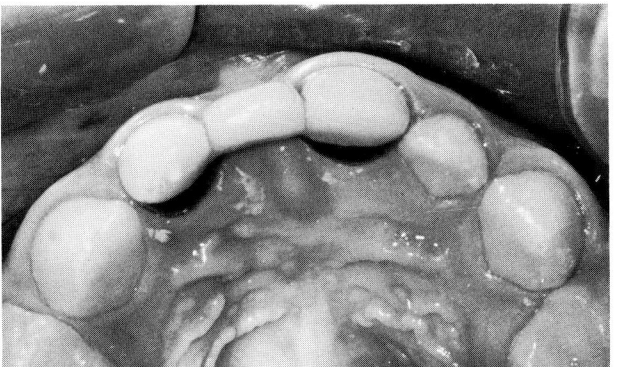

Figure 12-56 Incisal view of completed bridge in the mouth.

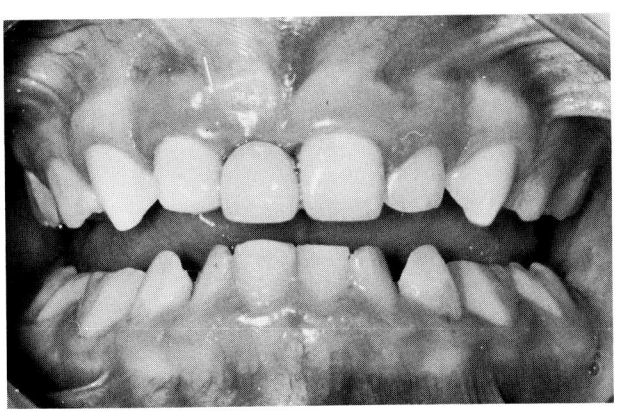

Figure 12-57 Anterior view of completed bridge in place in the mouth.

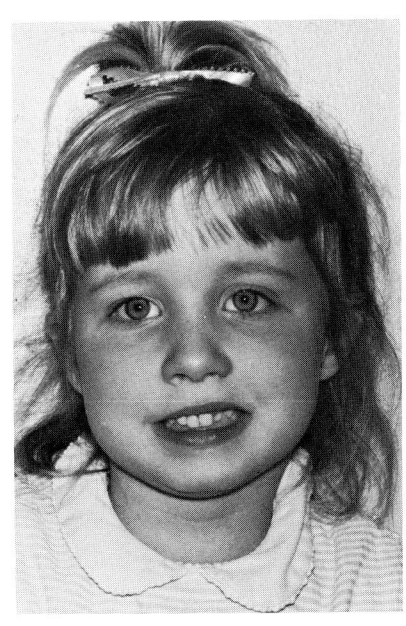

Figure 12-58 Porcelain bonded to gold bridge replaces maxillary right primary central incisor.

TRAUMA TO THE PRIMARY DENTITION

Chapter 13

Accidents to the primary dentition are extremely common; however, many accident cases are never seen by the dentist since they are of a very minor nature. In a clinical study[1] of 500 5-year old children, it was found that 28 per cent evidenced some kind of injury to their anterior teeth. The most common type of trauma was caused by a fall and resulted in small enamel and dentin fractures of the incisors. These accidents accounted for 82 per cent of the total injuries observed. Of the entire group of children, only 4 per cent had experienced complete avulsion or displacement of teeth—a surprisingly low percentage. This probably accounts for the low incidence of observed hypoplasia on permanent incisors, since this is the type of injury which is most likely to damage underlying permanent teeth. Schrieber[2] followed 42 cases of intrusion or displacement of primary teeth and found that over 20 per cent of these children later evidenced hypoplastic areas on the permanent incisors. He also found that the most common age at which injuries occur to primary teeth is between 1½ and 2½ years. This is the stage of learning to walk, when the small child is relatively uncoordinated.

If the dentist is called in for any emergency involving traumatic injuries to small children, he should make every effort to see the patient as soon as possible. It is never advisable to rely on the parent's assessment of the extent of damage. Frequently the child is not very cooperative at this age level, and it may be necessary to postpone radiographic examination and definitive treatment until soft tissue bruises have healed and the child has calmed down. It is very important to carefully examine the dentition for loose or cracked fragments of teeth, for trauma to opposing teeth, and for pulpal exposure. Displaced teeth can be repositioned and even splinted if necessary. Intrusions are usually left alone, and the teeth allowed to re-erupt. In all such cases, periodic recalls with radiographic evaluation are absolutely necessary. Radiographic coverage must be adequate, and should include the areas adjacent to the traumatized tooth and also the opposing teeth. Discolored and traumatized primary teeth are always a potential hazard since infection can develop and involve the underlying permanent teeth. If there is any question concerning pathology around a suspected nonvital incisor, the tooth should be observed closely or else extracted. The parent's concern is an important consideration whenever a young child damages his primary teeth. In most instances, if the injury is limited to enamel and dentin fracture, it can be predicted that there will be no effect on the permanent successor. However, if there is intrusion or displacement, especially at ages 1½ to 2½, there is the distinct possibility that there will be hypoplastic defects on the underlying tooth when it erupts. This must be considered when questions of medicolegal liability are involved.

In any severe traumatic injury to the primary teeth, jaw fracture should be considered as a possibility. A blow to the chin for example, may result in fracture of the condyle. It also should be pointed out that whenever soft tissues are bruised and teeth damaged in injuries occurring out of doors, the child should be referred to his physician for possible tetanus booster injections.

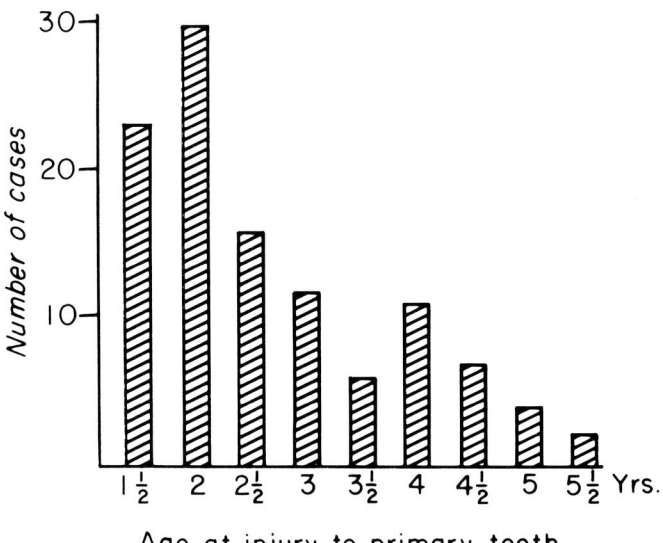

Figure 13-1 Accidents to primary teeth are most common at 1½ to 2½ years of age. This is the stage of learning to walk and is a period of underdeveloped motor coordination. (From Schreiber, C. K.: The effect of trauma on the anterior deciduous teeth. Brit. Dent. J. *106*:340-343, May, 1959.)

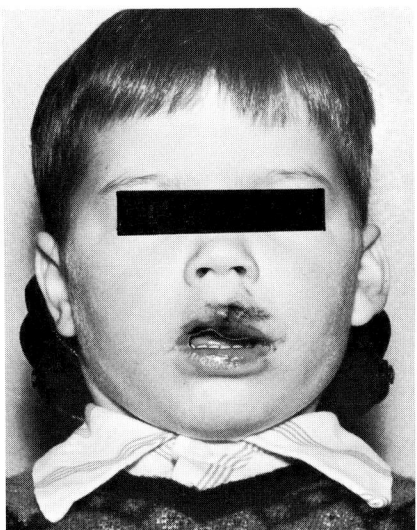

Figure 13-2 Typical appearance of a preschool child following an injury to the lips and teeth. In many of these cases the physician is consulted first. If possible, elective treatment should be deferred until the soft tissue bruising has subsided.

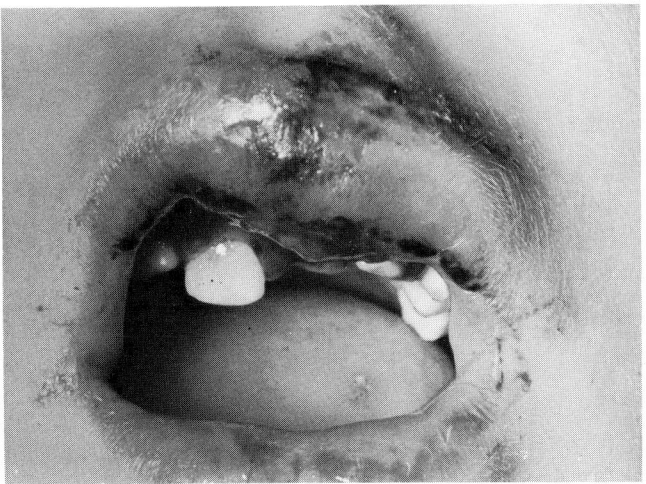

Figure 13-3 Close-up view of the case illustrated in Figure 13-2. One incisor has been avulsed or intruded, the other is quite mobile. Treatment consists of carefully removing loose fragments, taking radiographs to ascertain root condition, and closely observing the dentition over a 6-month period. The opposing arch should always be checked for possible damage. No positive statement can be made at this time concerning possible effects on the underlying permanent teeth.

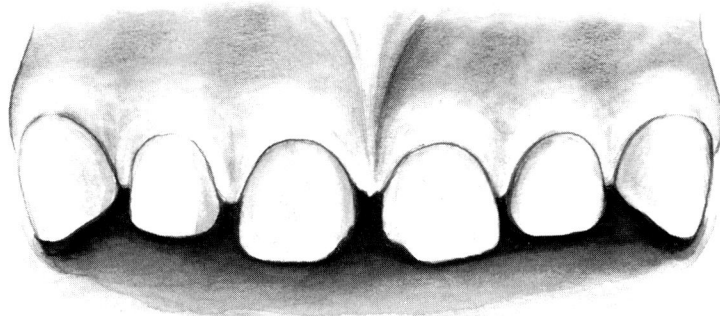

Figure 13-4 Enamel fracture of a maxillary primary incisor.
Treatment
1. Take radiographs to determine the full extent of the injury. Save films for future reference.
2. Smooth the fractured enamel if there are any sharp edges.
3. Schedule periodic checkups at 6-month intervals.
4. Tooth may become necrotic at a later date and require endodontic therapy or extraction.
5. Tooth may undergo internal resorption and necessitate extraction.

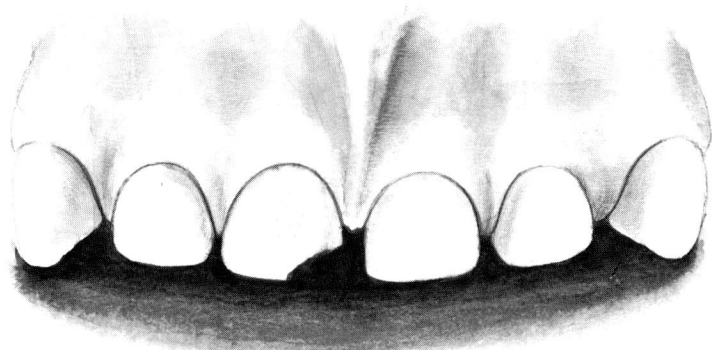

Figure 13-5 Dentin fracture of a maxillary primary incisor.
Treatment
1. Take radiographs to determine the full extent of the injury and save for reference for future examination.
2. Depending on the extent of the exposed dentin, the fractured area may be smoothed over with discs, or if necessary, a protective base of calcium hydroxide may be placed and the tooth covered with a stainless steel crown.
3. Schedule periodic checkups at 6-month intervals. If tooth becomes necrotic, extraction or endodontic therapy will be required.

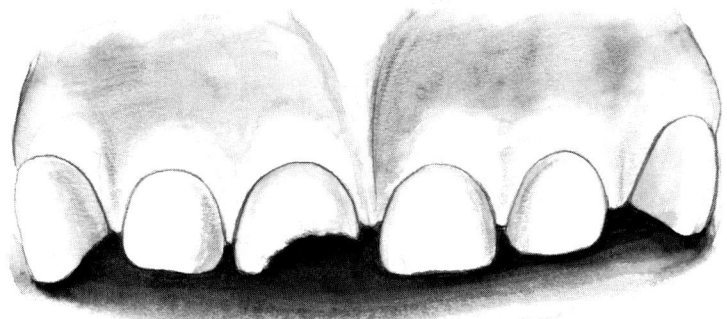

Figure 13-6 Fracture involving the pulp in a maxillary primary incisor.

Treatment

1. Take radiographs and save for reference for future examinations.
2. If pulpal exposure is very small and patient is seen immediately after the accident, cap the pulp with calcium hydroxide and place a protective steel crown.
3. If pulpal exposure is large, perform a pulpotomy utilizing formocresol, and place a steel crown.
4. Schedule periodic checkups at 6-month intervals. If tooth becomes necrotic, extraction or endodontic therapy will be required.

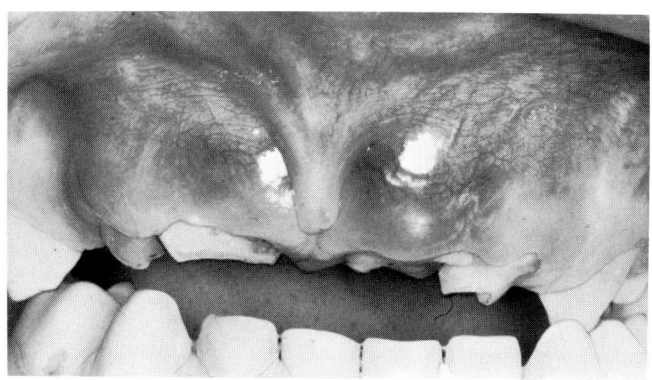

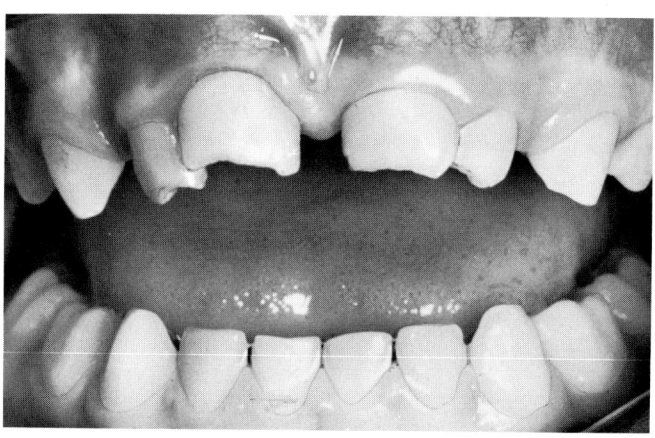

Figure 13-7 Severe intrusion of all four maxillary primary incisors. Careful clinical examination for pulpal exposure is always indicated. Radiographs must be taken to ascertain root damage. Usually these cases should be left alone and the teeth allowed to re-erupt. Careful follow-up observation is necessary, since the teeth frequently are devitalized by the injury. When this occurs, they should be either treated endodontically or extracted to prevent abcess formation around the developing permanent teeth.

Figure 13-8 Same case as illustrated in Figure 13-7, after 5 months. Note the re-eruption of the fractured teeth. Loss of vitality occurred in this instance and the involved incisors were eventually extracted to eliminate abscess formation around the developing permanent teeth. Intrusions of primary teeth, as contrasted to simple fractures, are more likely to cause hypoplasia of underlying permanent teeth.

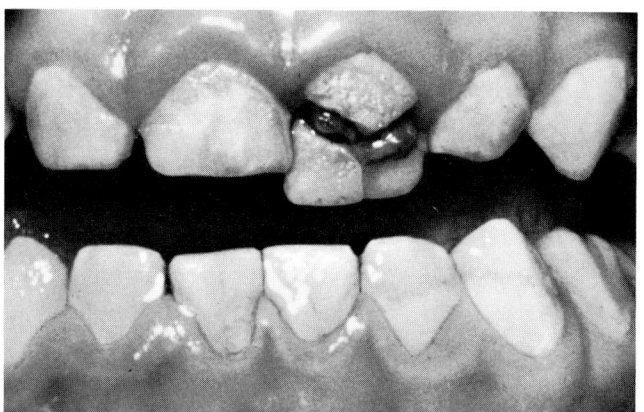

Figure 13-9 A horizontal and vertical fracture of the crown of a maxillary primary central incisor. When a primary tooth is so severely mutilated, extraction is usually the treatment of choice.

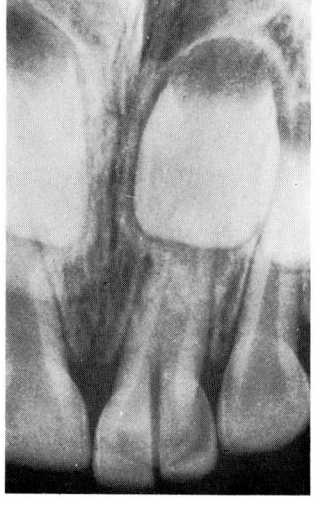

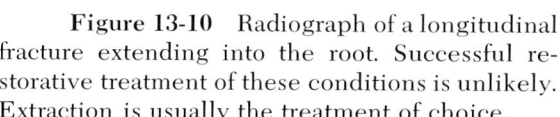

Figure 13-10 Radiograph of a longitudinal fracture extending into the root. Successful restorative treatment of these conditions is unlikely. Extraction is usually the treatment of choice.

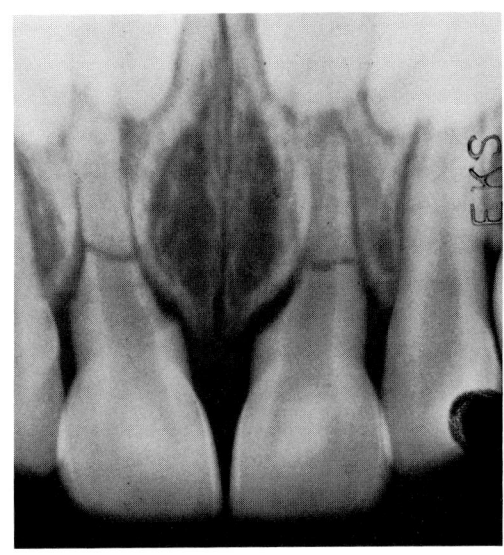

Figure 13-11 Radiograph showing fractured roots of the maxillary primary incisors following a fall. In this case stabilization of the injured teeth is not indicated and extraction is the treatment of choice.

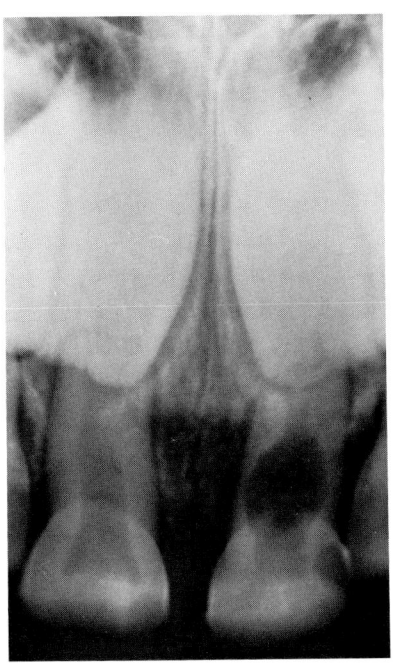

Figure 13-12 Internal resorption in a maxillary primary incisor after a traumatic injury. Note that there is no fracture of tooth structure in this case. Extraction is the treatment of choice.

Figure 13-13 Endodontic treatment of a traumatized primary incisor which became nonvital. Zinc oxide and eugenol is the filling of choice for the root canal since it can be resorbed. (Courtesy Dr. Harold D. Rosenbaum.)

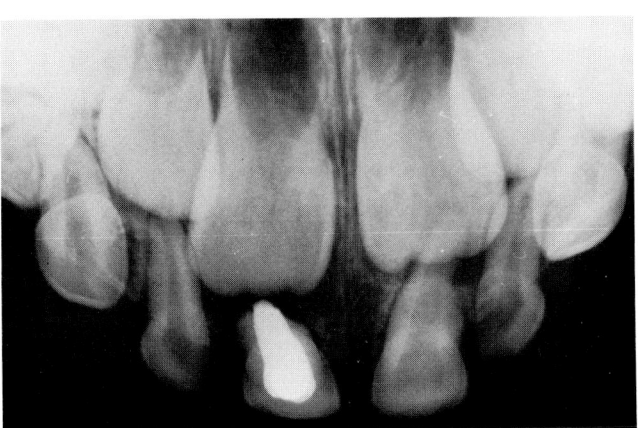

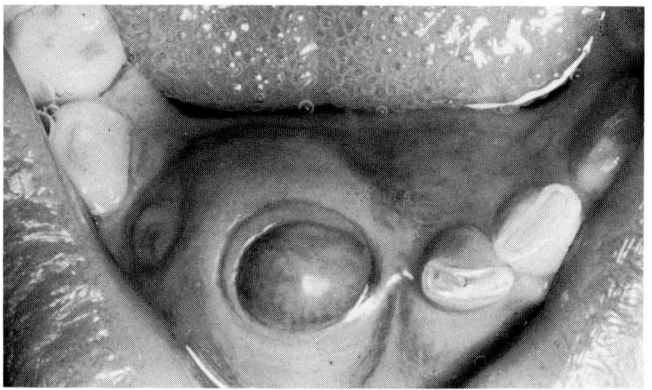

Figure 13-14 Large acute abscess occurring 1 year following a traumatic accident to the mandibular primary incisors. One discolored and nonvital incisor was allowed to remain in the arch because it was asymptomatic. The case was not observed closely and the resultant infection caused gross displacement of the underlying permanent central incisor.

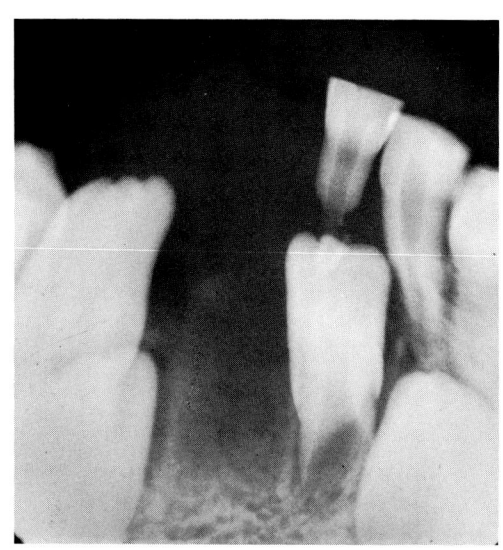

Figure 13-15 Radiograph of teeth shown in Figure 13-14. Note the extensive bone loss and the extreme malposition of the permanent central incisor. This case clearly shows the need for constant observation of traumatized primary teeth and their prompt treatment if they become nonvital and undergo periapical change.

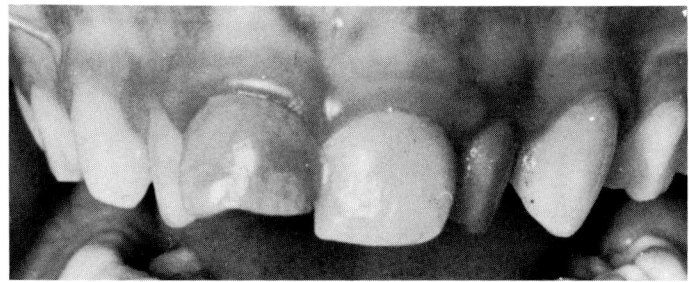

Figure 13-16 Discoloration of maxillary primary central caused by trauma. Condition occurred as the result of escape of hemosiderin pigments into dentinal tubules. Tooth may become lighter or darker. Semiannual examination should be made to check for development of periapical involvement. Tooth should be treated endodontically or extracted if pathology develops.

Figure 13-17 Mandibular primary incisor is missing; parents mistakenly considered it to have been completely "knocked out" after a fall.

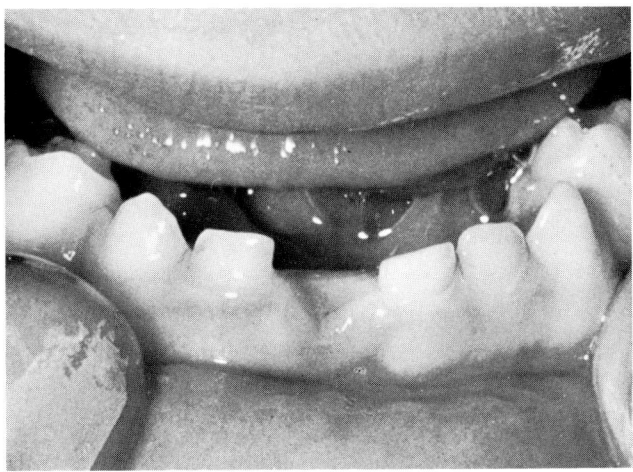

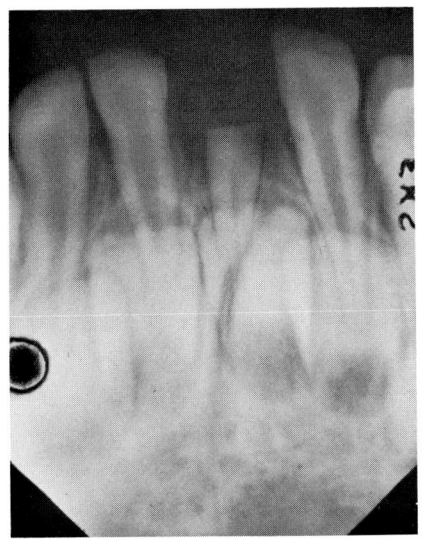

Figure 13-18 Radiograph of teeth shown in Figure 13-17. A retained root is present as a result of the traumatic accident in which only the crown was fractured off. A thorough examination by a dentist, including radiographs, is always desirable in any case of trauma.

Figure 13-19 Drifting of maxillary primary incisors following the loss of one central. When a primary incisor is lost after 3 to 3½ years of age, intercanine space usually remains the same. However, some shifting of the remaining incisors may occur. Construction of a bridge or removable appliance is ordinarily not necessary, but may be indicated in some cases when improved esthetics is desired or unusual conditions prevail, such as crowding. (See Chapter 12, Prosthodontics.)

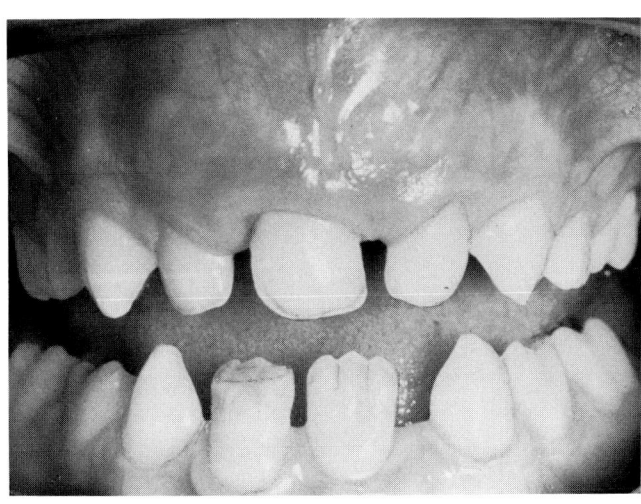

278   TRAUMA TO THE PRIMARY DENTITION

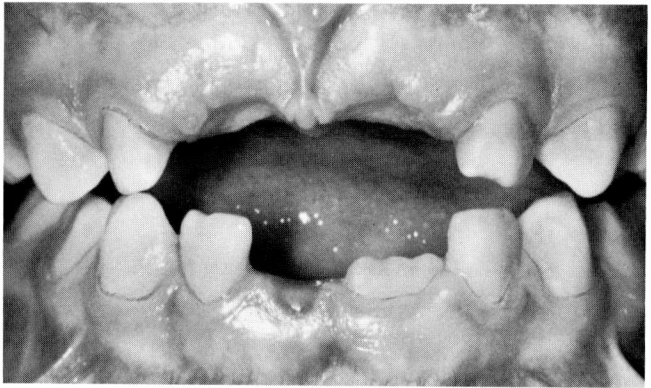

Figure 13-20 At 3½ years of age this child lost both maxillary primary central incisors in an accident. A partial denture was fabricated to restore esthetics.

Figure 13-21 Partial denture for child shown in Figure 13-20. Note that no clasps are used. Although retention in this case is excellent without clasps, the clasps should be used when problems of retention are anticipated.

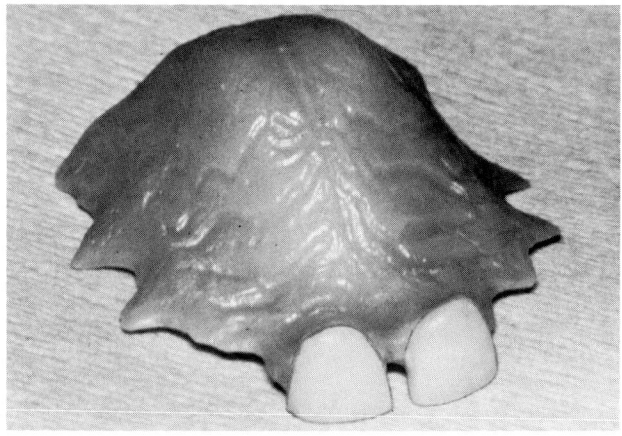

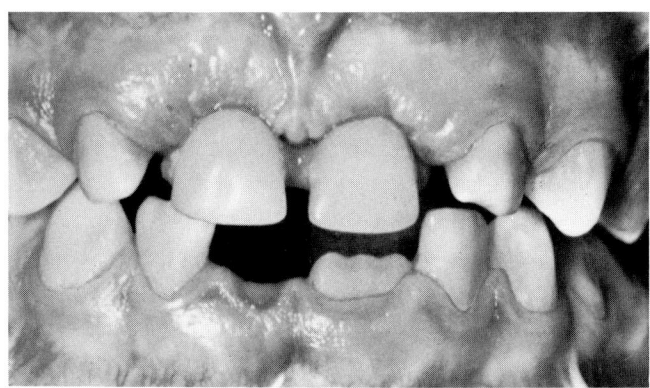

Figure 13-22 Partial denture in place. Note size and spacing of teeth to achieve natural dental appearance for a child of this age.

Figure 13-23 Full-face view of child with partial denture in place. Partial is no longer used once the permanent maxillary incisors start to erupt.

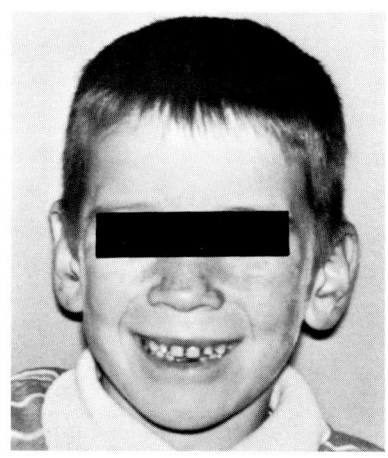

Figure 13-24 Hypoplasia of the maxillary right permanent central incisor with a history of a traumatic intrusion of the primary incisor at age 2½. These sequelae are impossible to predict with certainty at the time of the accident.

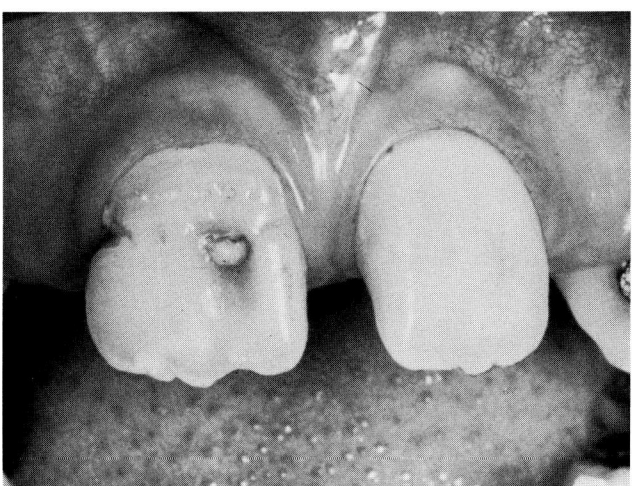

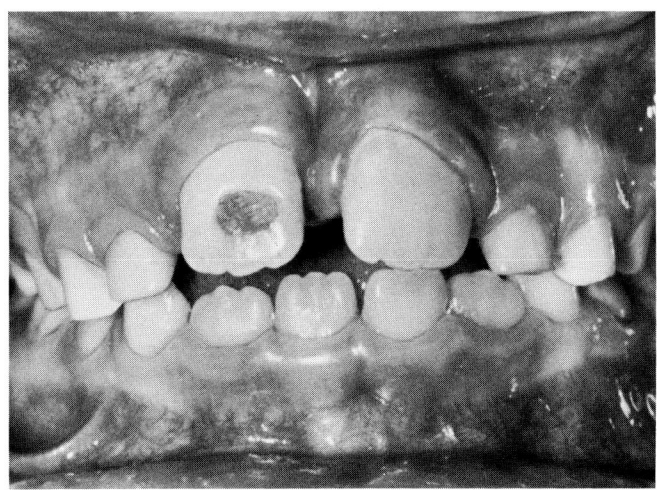

Figure 13-25 Hypoplasia of the maxillary right permanent central incisor. History of trauma similar to that of patient shown in Figure 13-24.

Figure 13-26 Circumscribed spots of Turner's hypoplasia on the mandibular permanent central incisors. Case history revealed a severe fall at age 2. Injuries to mandibular teeth are far less common than to maxillary.

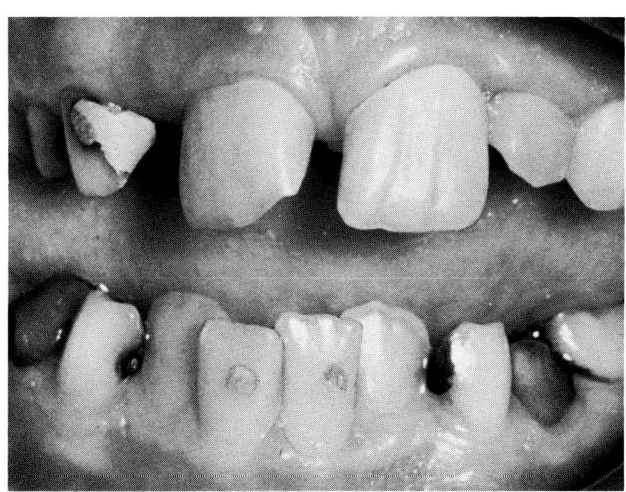

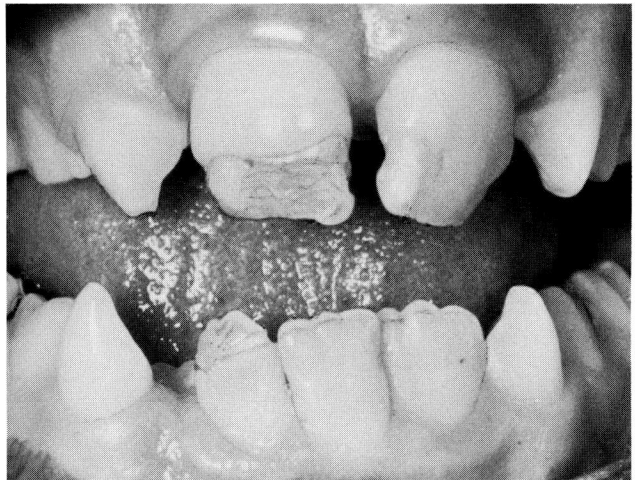

Figure 13-27 Severe hypoplastic defects in maxillary and mandibular permanent incisors. There was a history of facial injury during infancy as a result of an automobile accident. Frequently the dentist is called on to assist in insurance settlements in such cases. Consideration should always be given to the possibility of extensive coronal restorations at some future date.

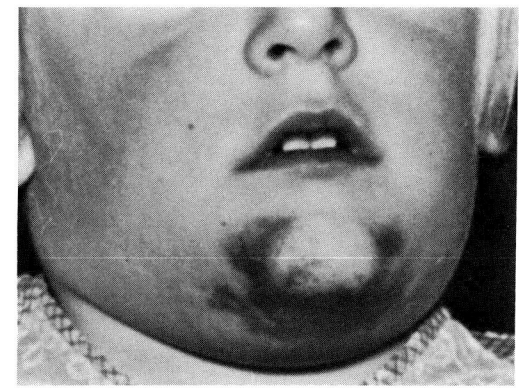

Figure 13-28 Chin of a child who fell over the handlebars of a tricycle. These injuries usually cause trauma to the posterior teeth and possibly the condyle of the mandible.

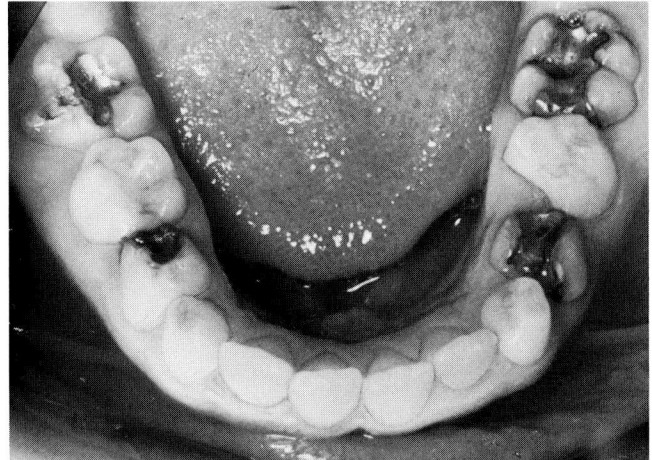

Figure 13-29 Fracture of posterior teeth as a result of a blow under the chin. There was no condylar fracture in this case. Examination of any patient after an accident should always include gross clinical inspection of all the teeth. Fractured posterior teeth should be treated and followed the same as fractured anterior teeth.

References

1. Hunton, R. T., and Lust, W. B.: Injuries as found in the anterior primary dentition. Senior thesis. University of Washington, June, 1961.
2. Schreiber, C. K.: The effect of trauma on the anterior deciduous teeth. Brit. Dent. J. *106*:340-343, May, 1959.

TRAUMA TO THE PERMANENT DENTITION

Chapter 14

Management of injuries to the newly erupted permanent anterior teeth constitutes a recurring problem to the practicing dentist. Studies of these injuries indicate that over 75 per cent occur in children between the ages of 8 and 11 years, the elementary school period. This is a period of growth and development characterized by unrestrained physical activity; the dentition is vulnerable because of the prominence of the permanent anterior teeth during the development of the facial complex. Many minor injuries to these teeth are never seen by the dentist, consequently his experience is likely to be associated with the more traumatic incidents involving gross dentin fracture, pulpal exposure, and occasionally complete avulsion. Davis[3] reported from a study of 2,237 students between 7 and 17 years of age that 22.8 per cent had experienced some type of traumatic accident to the anterior teeth. In fractures of the incisors, 74.2 per cent involved the enamel, 24.7 per cent were in the dentin, and only 1.1 per cent involved the pulp. The pulpal fractures are extremely important, however, since these cases are usually the ones that require emergency dental treatment. A report from the Eastman Institute[7] indicates that only 2 per cent of fractured incisors involve root fracture. Little or no information is available concerning the incidence of complete avulsion but it is comparatively rare.

The causative factors in dental injuries during the childhood years have been documented by Law[4] and are presented in Table 14-1. A wide variety of factors are responsible for these injuries.

Boys are reported to have twice as many injuries as girls at comparable

TABLE 14-1 CAUSES OF FRACTURES AND ENVIRONMENT IN WHICH THEY OCCURRED IN 1,643 ELEMENTARY SCHOOL CHILDREN

Fall	6	Kicked	1
Golf club	2	Door handle	1
Swimming pool	3	Ice	3
Car	6	Roller skating	1
Sidewalk	4	Bathroom	1
Eating candy	1	Telephone	1
Fall from tree	2	Push-ups	1
Beads	1	Trapeze	1
Bike	15	Go-Kart	1
Sink	2	School bus	1
Truck	1	Playground	2
Summer camp	1	Baseball	3
Fight	5	Basketball	1
Sled	4	Boxing	1
Pop bottle	3	Jump rope	1
Pole vaulting	1	Baton	1
Sling shot	1	Merry-go-round	1
Rock	1	Fire escape	1
Marble	1	Train	1

age levels, which is probably attributable to their participation in more active games and sports.

Prevention is an important consideration, and the only truly preventive measure the dentist can suggest during the elementary school years is early orthodontic correction of markedly protruding maxillary incisors. The child with pronounced labioversion of maxillary teeth is more susceptible to injury than one with a flat profile with good soft tissue coverage. Lewis[5] and Davis[3] reported a significantly higher incidence of fractured permanent incisors among children with maxillary protrusions in excess of 4 mm. Early referral to the orthodontist is particularly desirable if the child is known to be "accident prone."

The use of mouthguards is especially helpful in preventing accidents to anterior teeth during participation in organized athletics. This is most helpful during the teenage years. Cohen[2] reported excellent results in prevention of dental injuries to Philadelphia high school football players with the mandatory use of individually fitted mouthguards. Most high schools and colleges now require the wearing of these appliances in all types of contact sports.

In all cases of accidental injuries to young permanent incisors there are two considerations of prime importance to the dentist: (1) conservation of the pulp; (2) restoration of the crown. It is recognized that young incisors should be maintained in the dental arch if at all possible. Each anterior tooth aids in assuring the proper eruptive position of the neighboring tooth. If an immature anterior tooth is lost, however, the only prosthesis that can be employed is the removable appliance because it is not advisable to construct fixed bridgework at this stage of development of the dentition. Unfortunately, the appearance of the removable appliance is usually more satisfactory than its function. One way to improve the latter is through the use of chrome-cobalt alloy cast partials which will provide maximum strength, comfort, and retention.

Appropriate treatment of the fractured incisor for pulpal conservation depends on the nature and severity of the injury. As previously stated, most fractures of the immature permanent tooth do not directly involve the pulp. Many fractures do, however, involve the dentin and irritants can pass via the dentinal tubules to the pulp. Therefore, the treatment of choice is a sedative dressing held in place by a strong support. Such a treatment consists of a zinc oxide type of dressing sealed in with an unmodified stainless steel crown. Esthetics are admittedly poor, but for the 6 to 12 months needed to give the pulp an opportunity to recover, this is the preferred treatment.

If there is actual exposure of the pulp, immediate treatment is indicated consisting of pulpotomy with calcium hydroxide, or if conditions warrant, endodontic treatment.

Complete avulsion of one or more permanent incisors is not a common accident, but when it occurs it necessitates immediate, definitive treatment. Studies by Andreasen and Hjorting-Hansen[1] indicate that the length of time the avulsed tooth is out of the mouth before replantation determines the likelihood of success of the treatment. They studied 110 replanted teeth, and found that when the extraoral period did not exceed 30 minutes, replantation was successful in 90 per cent of the cases based on absence of root resorption or other pathology. When the extraoral period was 30 to 90 minutes, replantation was successful in 43 per cent of the cases. When teeth were replanted after a 90-minute extraoral period, success was achieved in only 7 per cent of the cases. It would seem advisable in most instances to wash the root of the avulsed tooth and immediately replant and splint, postponing the endodontic treatment for several weeks.

Coverage of the crown subsequent to traumatic injury will depend on the extent of damage, age of the patient, and development of the dentition. Usually a permanent crown can be fabricated within 6 to 12 months following injury to the permanent tooth. Significant psychological effects can be anticipated if mutilated anterior teeth are not adequately restored, particularly in the younger teenager.

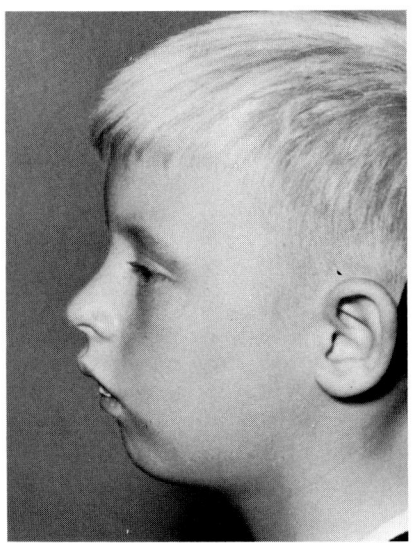

Figure 14-1 Profile of a 10-year-old boy with protruding maxillary central incisors. Children with this type of malocclusion are more susceptible to dental injuries. To help reduce this high rate of dental accidents, children with protruding anterior teeth should receive some orthodontic correction as soon as possible.

Figure 14-2 Same child as shown in Figure 14-1, exhibiting fractured wrist. The "accident prone" child frequently experiences trauma to the teeth. Note the protruding and elongated central incisors with very little lip coverage.

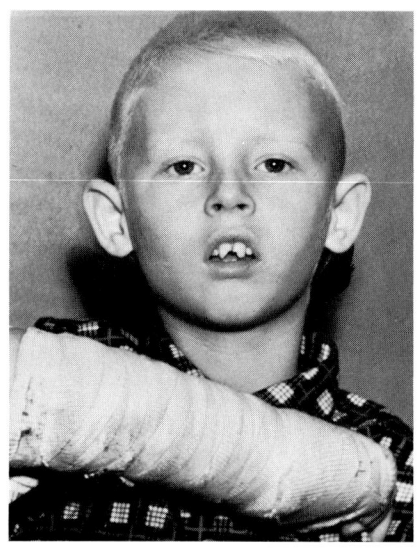

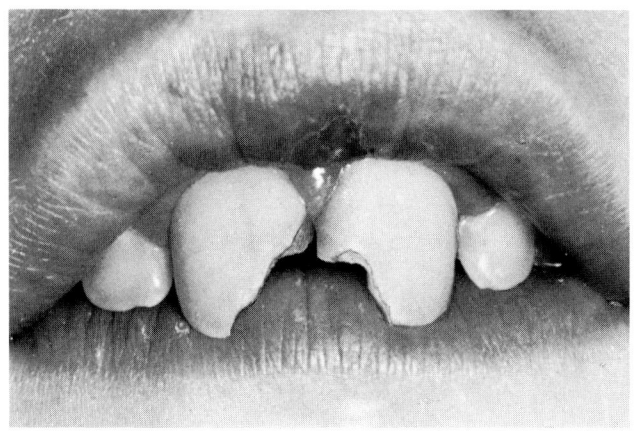

Figure 14-3 Close-up from Figure 14-2, showing diagonal fractures of the enamel and dentin with slight lip involvement. Any fracture involving the dentin requires immediate treatment and should be covered with a temporary crown and a palliative cement in order to preserve the vitality of the tooth.

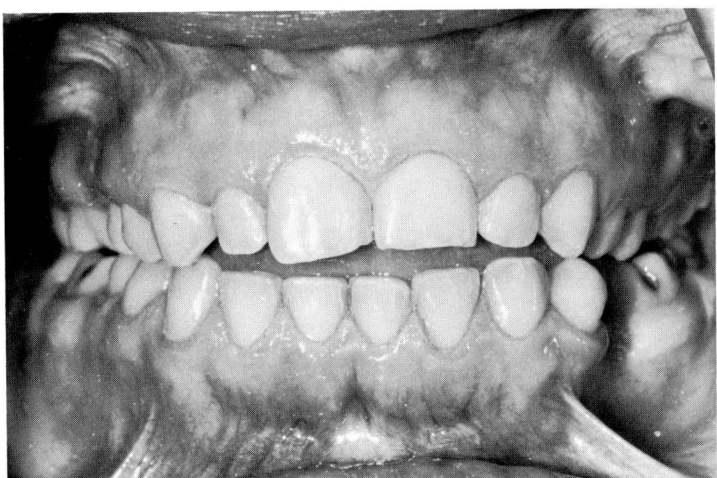

Figure 14-4 Enamel fractures of the maxillary permanent central incisors. The following treatment is recommended:
1. Obtain a history of the accident.
2. Do a thorough oral examination to determine the extent of the injury including any tooth mobility.
3. Take three periapical radiographs of the involved area, one central and both lateral incisor views, and at least one occlusal view of the opposing arch.
4. Gently smooth the rough edges of fractured enamel.
5. It is wise to check the teeth 3 and 6 months following the accident. The teeth may have sustained a severe blow and yet only have slight enamel fractures. In this case, the effect of the concussion may have been great enough to cause loss of vitality of the involved teeth. Therefore, a vitality test should be made. A vitality test taken less than a month following the accident may be unreliable because the pulp may be in a temporary state of shock.
6. These teeth may be reshaped within 3 to 6 months to make them more esthetically acceptable, if desired.

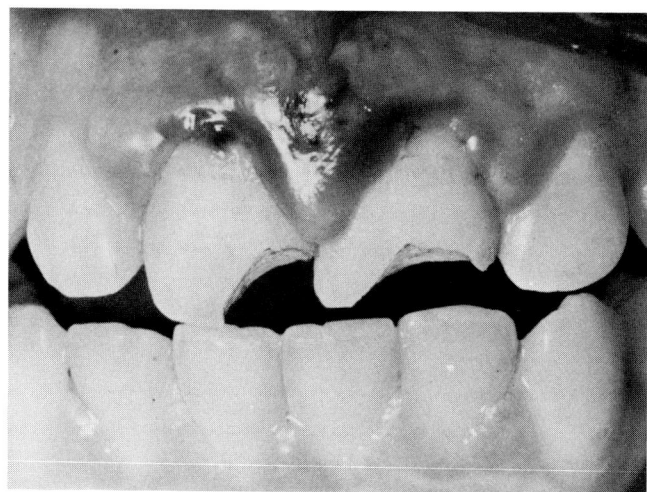

Figure 14-5 Dentin fractures of the maxillary permanent central incisors. The following treatment is recommended:
1. Obtain a history of the accident.
2. Do a thorough oral examination to determine the extent of the injury including mobility.
3. Take three periapical radiographs of the involved area, one central and both lateral incisor views and at least one occlusal view of the opposing arch.
4. Place a paste of calcium hydroxide or zinc oxide and eugenol over the exposed dentinal tubules. Cement a temporary crown, preferably stainless steel, over the fractured tooth and leave in place for a minimum of 3 to 6 months. (For examples of temporary crowns see Figure 14-14.) Try to avoid tooth reduction and unnecessary manipulation during the visit for emergency treatment.
5. The patient should be checked at 3-month and 6-month intervals at which time a vitality test can be taken.
6. Once the fractured teeth have sufficiently erupted and the pulp has receded so that a crown preparation can be made without involving the pulp, then permanent restorations may be placed.

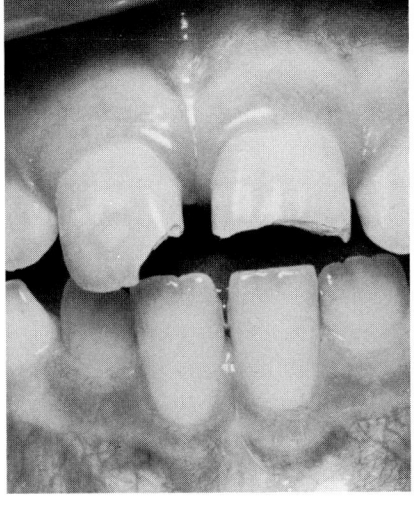

Figure 14-6 A mesial diagonal dentin fracture of the maxillary right central incisor and a horizontal dentin fracture of the maxillary left central incisor.

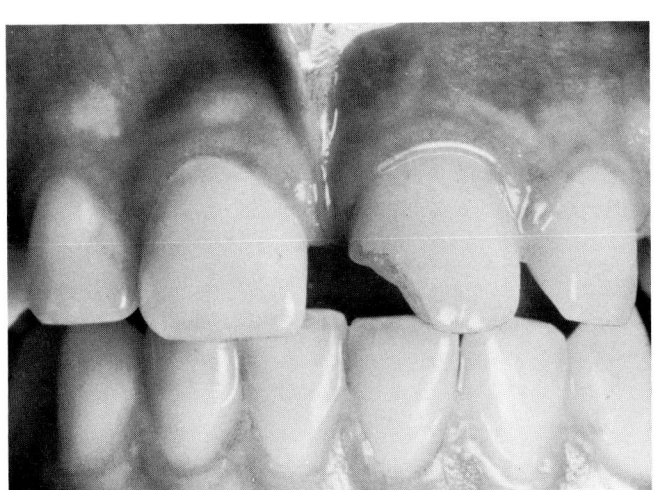

Figure 14-7 A mesial diagonal dentin fracture of the maxillary left central incisor. Rarely is the pulp exposed in this type of injury.

Figure 14-8 A horizontal dentin fracture of the maxillary left central incisor. Note the wide spaces and lack of support to injured teeth in all of the aforementioned cases.

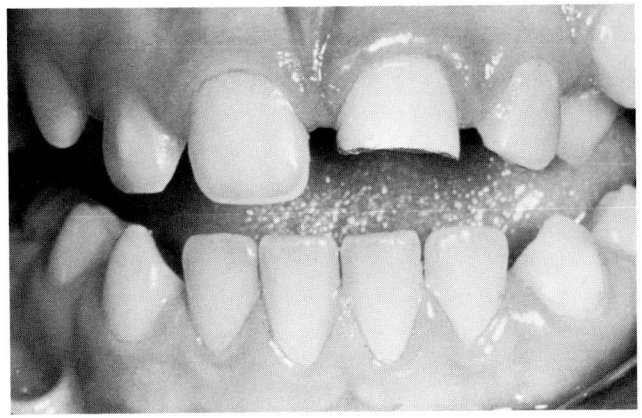

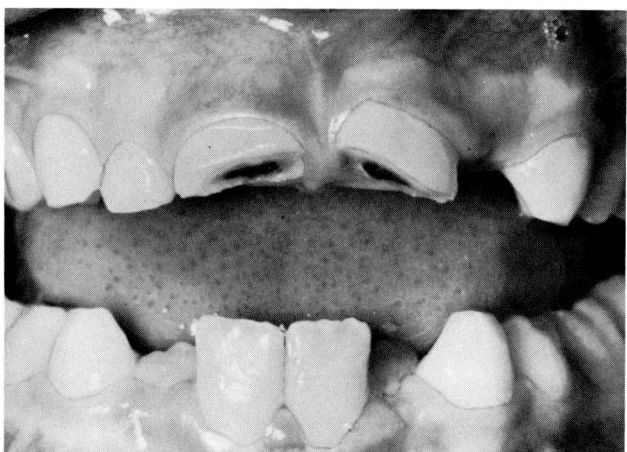

Figure 14-9 Fractures of the maxillary permanent central incisors exposing the pulp. The following treatment is recommended:
1. Obtain a history of the accident.
2. Do a thorough oral examination to determine the extent of the injury including any tooth mobility.
3. Take three periapical radiographs of the involved area, one central and both lateral incisor views and at least one occlusal view of the opposing arch.
4. A pulpotomy should be done if the following conditions exist:
   a. The dental pulp is exposed.
   b. The pulp is vital and shows moderate hemorrhage.
   c. The apex of the root is not fully developed.
5. Pulpotomy technique is as follows:
   a. Isolate the tooth with a rubber dam.
   b. Amputate the coronal pulp.
   c. Place a paste of calcium hydroxide over the amputated pulp (approximately 1 mm. thick).
   d. Fill the chamber with zinc oxide and eugenol or zinc phosphate cement.
   e. Cement a temporary crown, preferably stainless steel, over the fractured tooth.
   f. In 2 to 3 months there should be a bridging of dentin over the amputation site, and in 3 to 6 months a permanent restoration may be placed.
6. If a pulpotomy is not indicated, then endodontic treatment should be initiated to save the tooth.

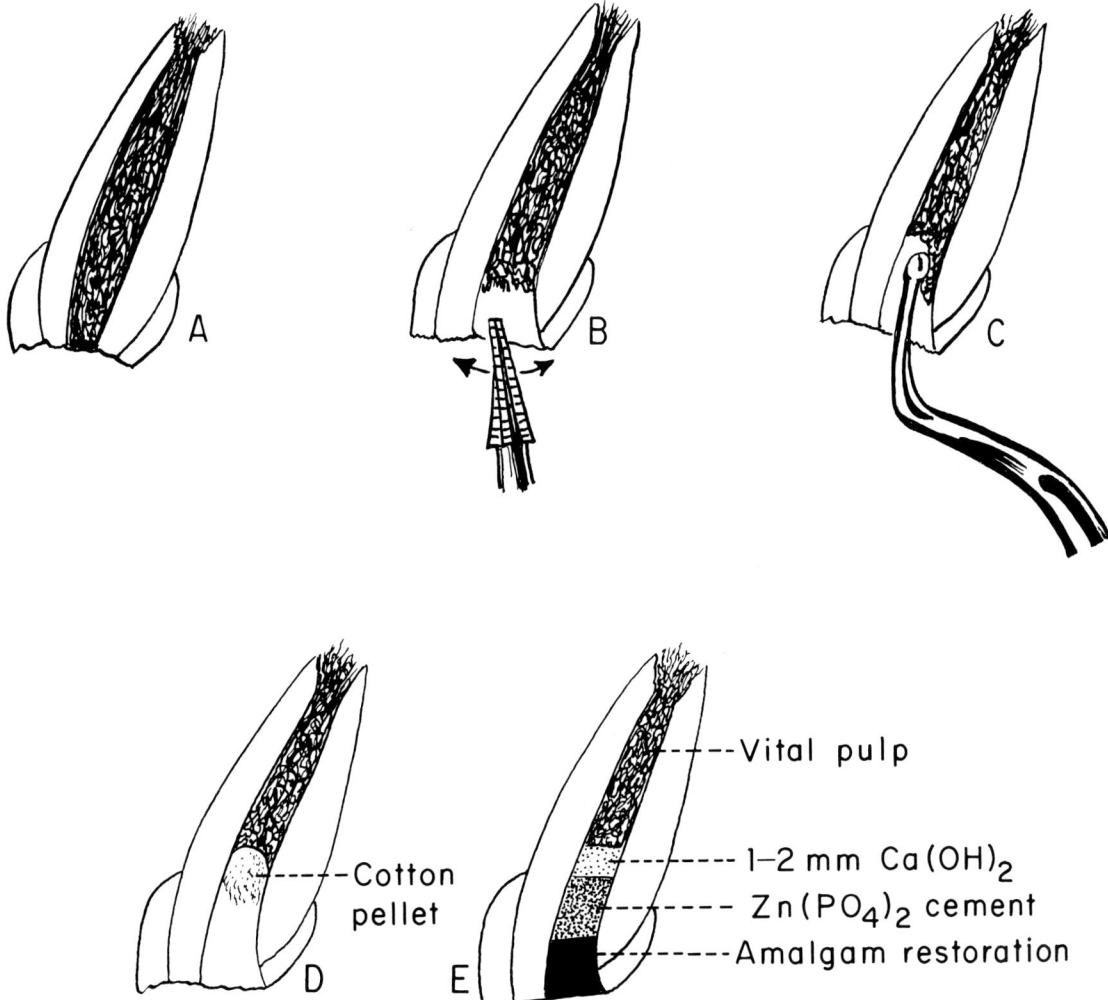

Figure 14-10 Procedure for pulpotomy on young permanent incisor:
A, Pulp exposure caused by traumatic injury in a young permanent incisor with incomplete apical development.
B, Access is gained with a tapered fissure bur.
C, Pulp is amputated at cementoenamel junction with sharp spoon excavator.
D, A sterile cotton pellet is used to control hemorrhage.
E, A layer of calcium hydroxide (approximately 1-2 mm. thick) is placed against the amputated pulp followed by a base and amalgam restoration or temporary crown. An esthetic permanent crown may be placed at a later date.

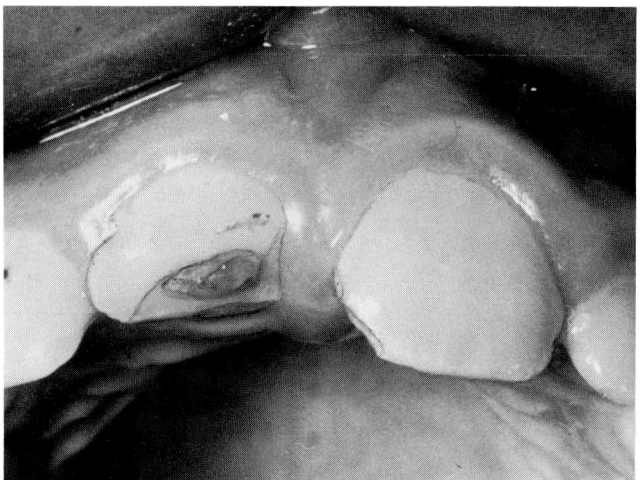

Figure 14-11 Pulpal fracture of the maxillary right central incisor. A pulpotomy with calcium hydroxide was the treatment of choice for this tooth. Note dentin fracture of the maxillary left central incisor.

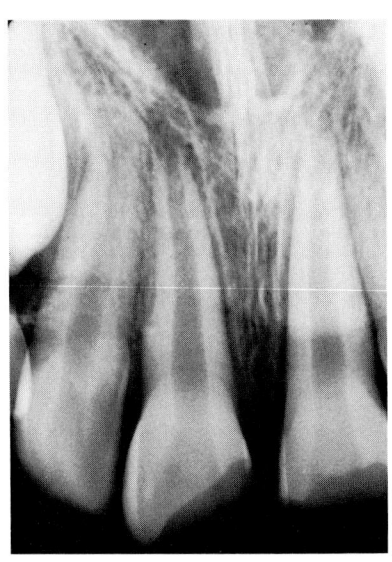

Figure 14-12 Preoperative radiograph showing two severely damaged central incisors. The pulp was exposed on the right central incisor and a pulpotomy performed. Note incomplete apical development.

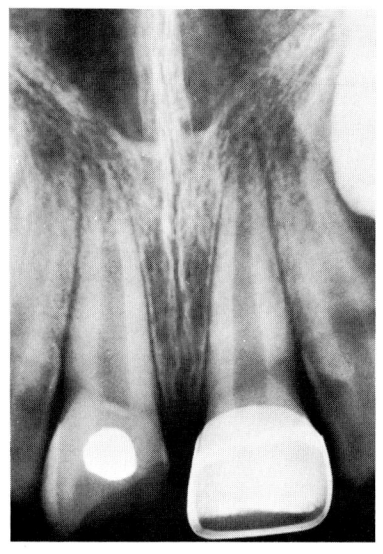

Figure 14-13 Same patient as shown in Figure 14-12, 6 months postoperatively. A dentin bridge has formed at the site of the pulpal amputation on the maxillary right central incisor. This is a good indication of a successful pulpotomy. Note continued root development on both central incisors which suggests that the pulps have remained vital.

TRAUMA TO THE PERMANENT DENTITION 291

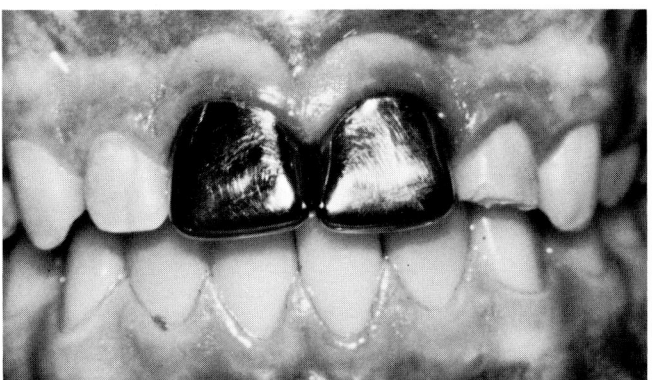

Figure 14-14 Unaltered stainless steel crowns. Although these restorations are not esthetic, they provide maximum protection to the dental pulp. Such crowns are the treatment of choice for emergency treatment of dentin or pulpal fractures.

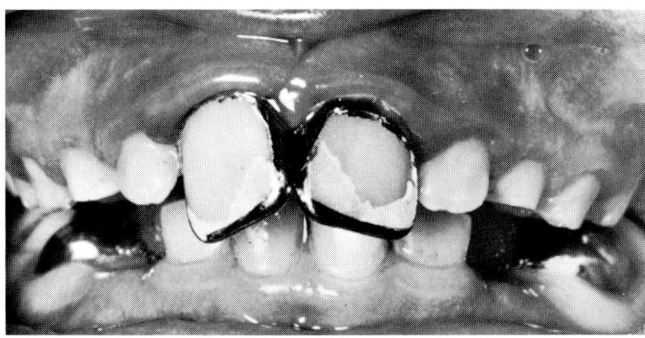

Figure 14-15 Stainless steel crowns with labial window removed to improve esthetics. Alteration of crowns makes them more susceptible to becoming loosened which defeats the purpose of protecting the dental pulp.

Figure 14-16 Mutilated crown. Lack of sufficient coronal tooth structure and extension of the fracture below the gingival margin complicates treatment of this tooth.

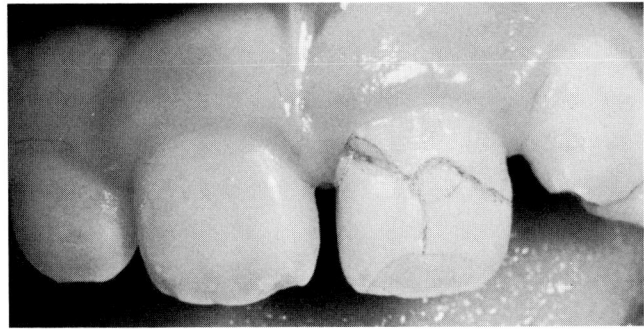

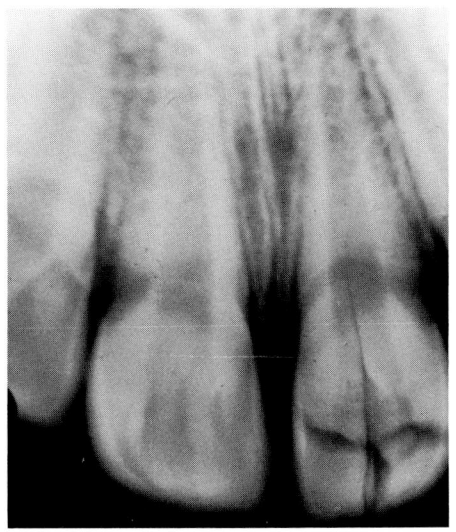

Figure 14-17 Radiograph of the tooth shown in Figure 14-16. Note the longitudinal fracture which penetrates the root. Successful endodontic treatment of this case would be questionable. Extraction may be necessary.

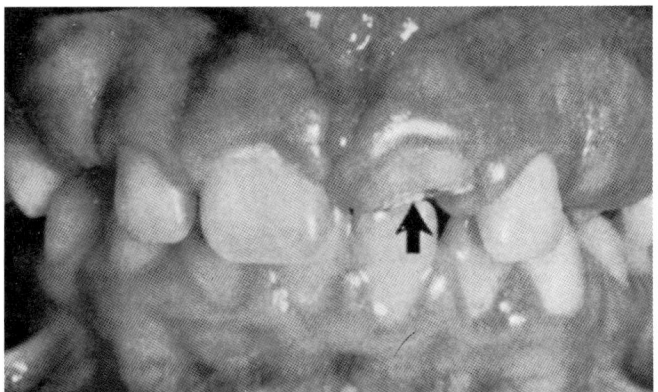

Figure 14-18 Coronal fracture of maxillary left central incisor involving the dental pulp in a 9-year-old child. (Courtesy Dr. Myron Warnick, from Ingle, J. I.: *Endodontics.* 1st ed., Lea & Febiger, Philadelphia, 1965, p. 574.)

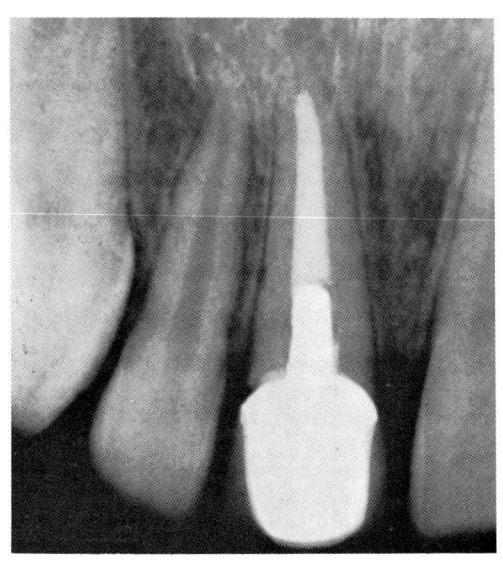

Figure 14-19 Radiograph following completion of root canal therapy. Dowel and bonded porcelain crown in place. (Courtesy Dr. Myron Warnick, from Ingle, J. I.: *Endodontics.* 1st ed., Lea & Febiger, Philadelphia, 1965, p. 574.)

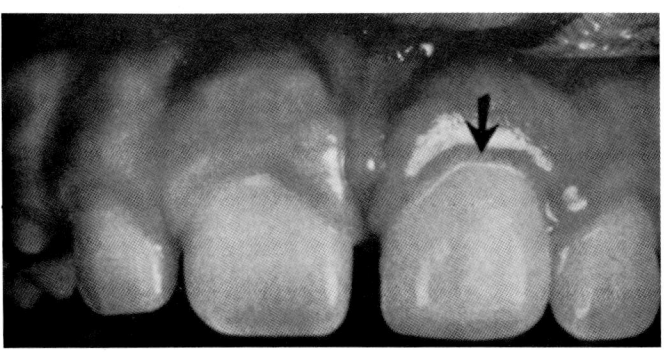

Figure 14-20 Clinical view showing highly esthetic restoration. (Courtesy Dr. Myron Warnick, from Ingle, J. I.: *Endodontics.* 1st ed., Lea & Febiger, Philadelphia, 1965, p. 574.)

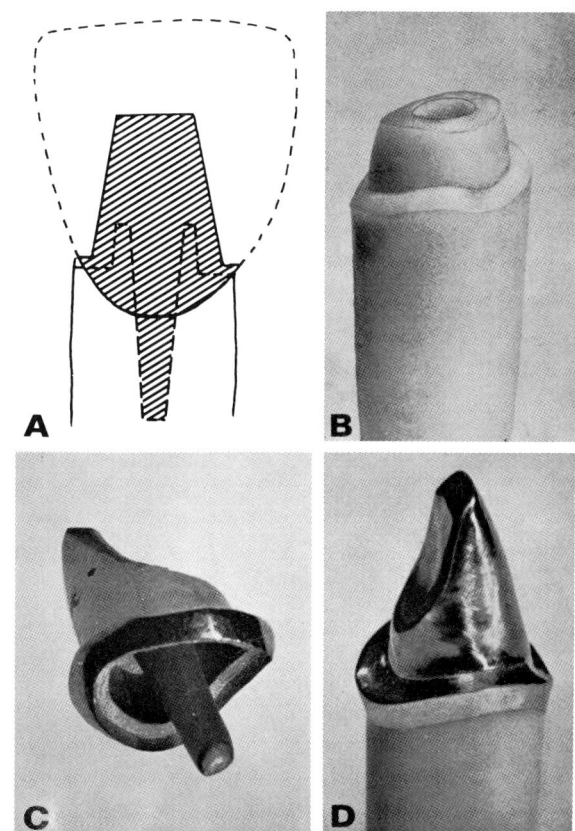

Figure 14-21 Full coping with collar and dowel. Preparation for restoration with a jacket crown. (From Ingle, J. I.: *Endodontics*. 1st ed., Lea & Febiger, Philadelphia, 1965, p. 621.)

A, Schematic drawing of the preparation and casting.
B, Preparation which emphasizes subgingival shoulder.
C, Internal surface of the casting. Note the shoulder and collar and the bulk and length of dowel.
D, Casting cemented in place. Restoration with a jacket crown will complete the case.

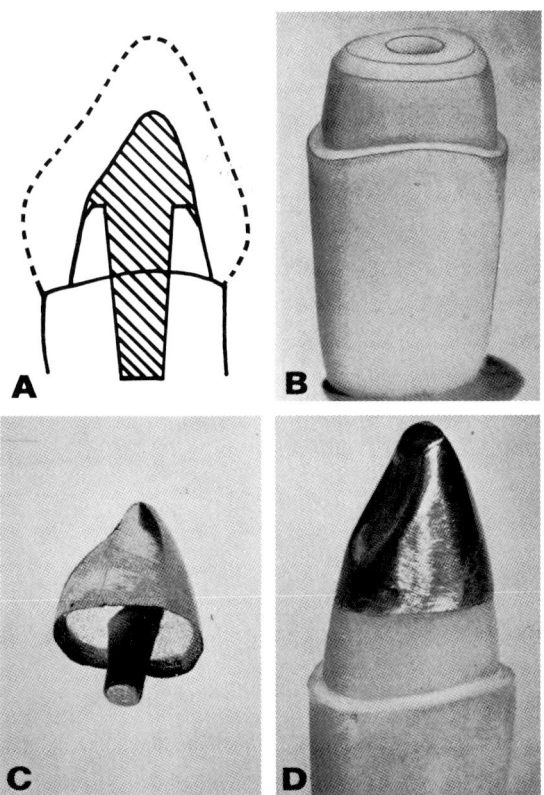

Figure 14-22 Dowel and extension for increasing the length of preparation of a fractured crown. (From Ingle, J. I.: *Endodontics*. 1st ed., Lea & Febiger, Philadelphia, 1965, p. 623.)

A, Schematic drawing.
B, Preparation for coping to extend length of remaining tooth.
C, Internal surface of the casting. Note the collar and the bulk and length of the dowel.
D, Casting cemented in place ready for impression for jacket coverage.

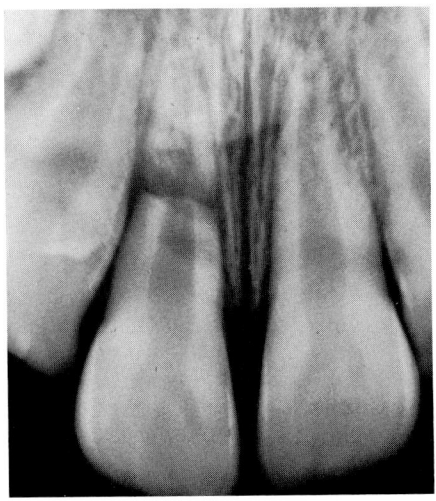

Figure 14-23 Root fracture of a maxillary right central incisor. The following treatment is suggested:
1. Stabilize the tooth with a splint, leaving it on for 6 to 8 weeks.
2. Eliminate trauma to the occlusion.
3. Allow the root to heal. (See Figures 14-24 and 14-25.)
4. If the pulp becomes devitalized, endodontic treatment should be initiated. (See Figure 14-27.)

Figure 14-24 Root fracture following a traumatic injury. Tooth was stabilized with an acrylic splint for 6 weeks. (Courtesy Dr. David C. Dilts.)

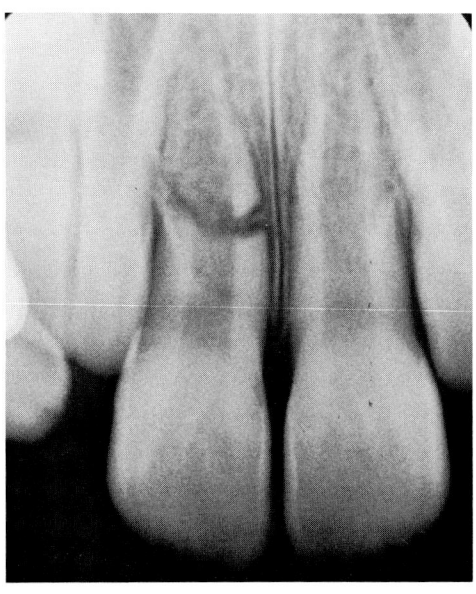

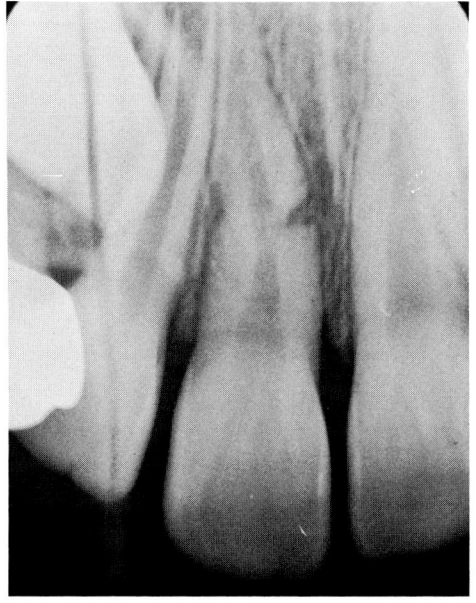

Figure 14-25 Same tooth as shown in Figure 14-24, after 1 year. Note extensive repair. The pulp of the tooth is vital. (Courtesy Dr. David C. Dilts.)

TRAUMA TO THE PERMANENT DENTITION

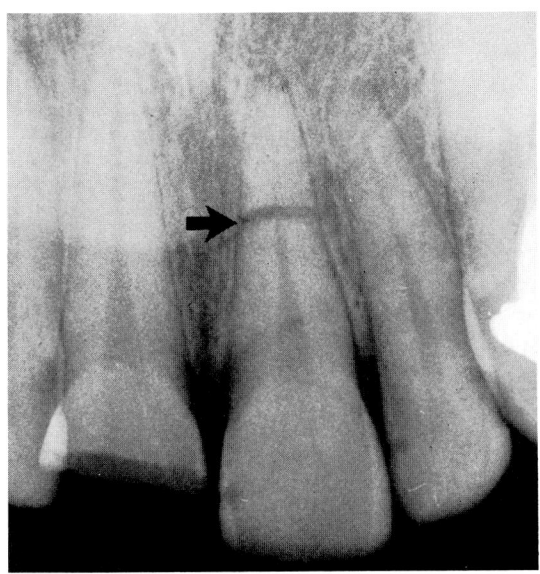

Figure 14-26 Fracture of the root of a central incisor. The pulp has been devitalized. (From Ingle, J. I.: *Endodontics*. 1st ed., Lea & Febiger, Philadelphia, 1965, p. 586.)

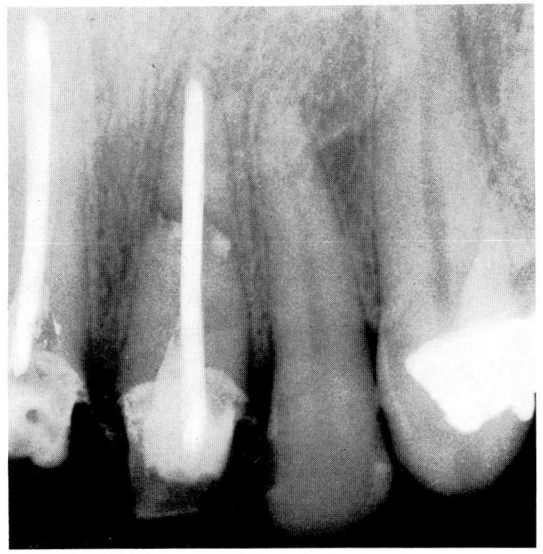

Figure 14-27 Radiograph in patient shown in Figure 14-26, 5 years postoperatively. A silver filling point has been used, and the crown has been restored with a porcelain jacket crown. Note how the silver point has stabilized the two root segments. (From Ingle, J. I.: *Endodontics*. Lea & Febiger, 1st ed., Philadelphia, 1965, p. 586.)

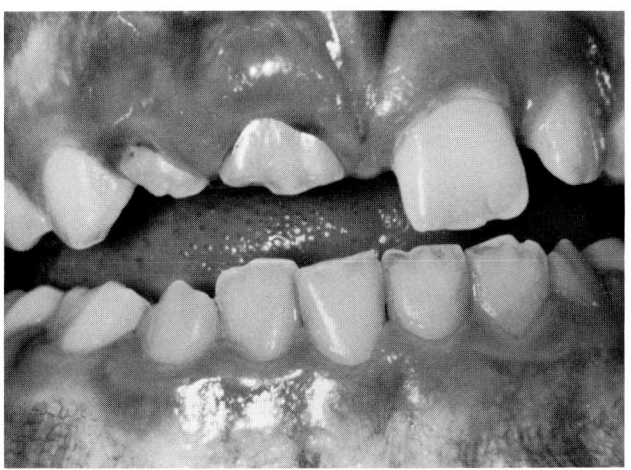

Figure 14-28 Intruded maxillary right central and lateral incisors. Treatment of choice is as follows:
1. When the roots of intruded teeth are not completely developed, the intruded teeth should be left in the intruded position to re-erupt.
2. When the roots of intruded teeth are completely developed, the intruded teeth should be repositioned and a splint placed to stabilize them.

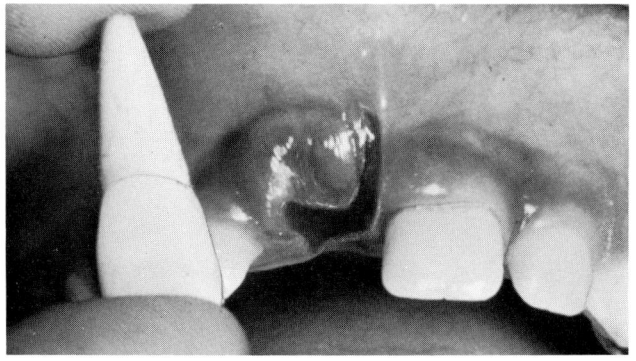

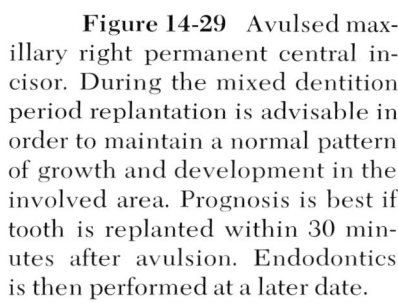

Figure 14-29 Avulsed maxillary right permanent central incisor. During the mixed dentition period replantation is advisable in order to maintain a normal pattern of growth and development in the involved area. Prognosis is best if tooth is replanted within 30 minutes after avulsion. Endodontics is then performed at a later date.

Figure 14-30 Avulsed maxillary left incisor. Root canal filling with gutta percha points. Filling material is sealed with hot spatula. The lingual opening into the pulp chamber is filled with a silicate restoration. The tooth should be held in a piece of moist gauze while out of the mouth and during all manipulative procedures. The root should be kept moist, but should not be scraped. Extra oral root canal filling is usually performed when a period of 60 minutes or more has elapsed after avulsion.

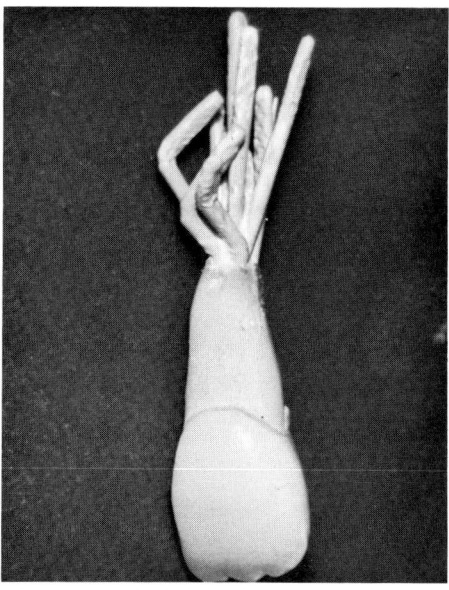

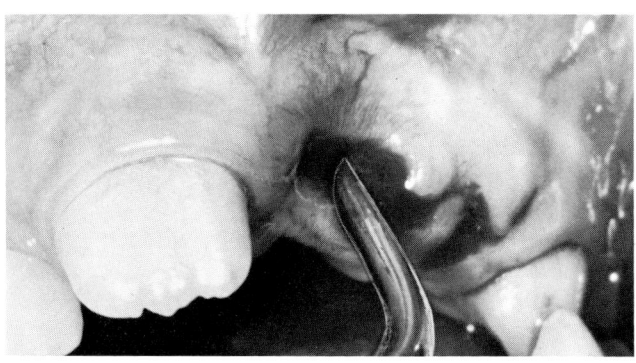

Figure 14-31 Curette used to stimulate hemorrhage in tooth socket. Note incision and opening into apical area of alveolus. This vent will allow escape of fluids and permit complete seating of tooth. The prognosis for replantation in cases involving alveolar fracture is poor.

Figure 14-32 Replanted tooth held in position with acrylic splint for from 2 to 4 weeks.

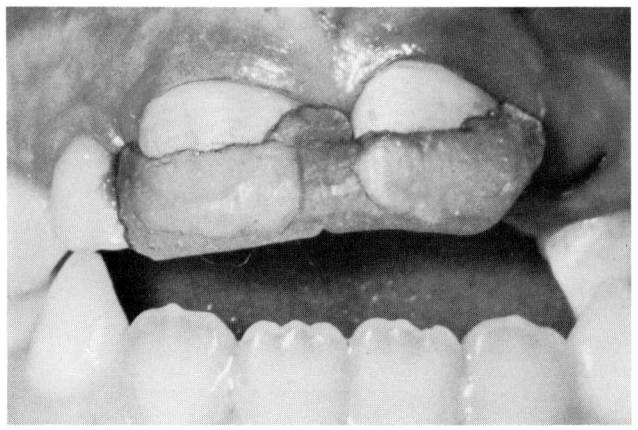

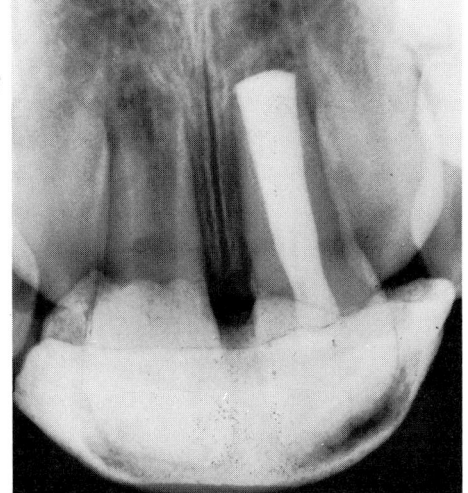

Figure 14-33 Radiograph of replanted tooth. Note well-sealed blunderbuss canal.

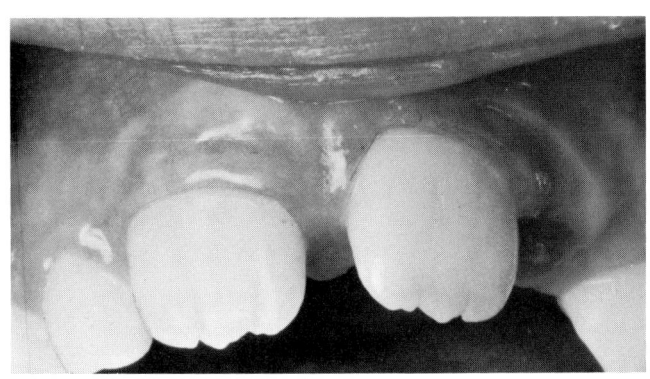

Figure 14-34 Tooth in position 1 month after replantation. Ankylosis, followed by resorption of the root, often occurs in these cases. However, if the tooth remains in position until all the permanent teeth have erupted, the replantation should be considered a success.

Figure 14-35 Ankylosis of a maxillary left central incisor after replantation. The adjacent teeth continued to erupt, leaving the replanted incisor at the former incisal level. When this occurs the replanted tooth may be restored to the new incisal level with a full crown or porcelain jacket. (From Ingle, J. I.: *Endodontics.* 1st ed., Lea & Febiger, Philadelphia, 1965, p. 601.)

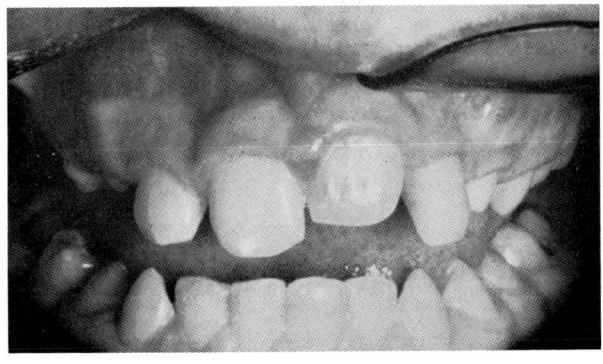

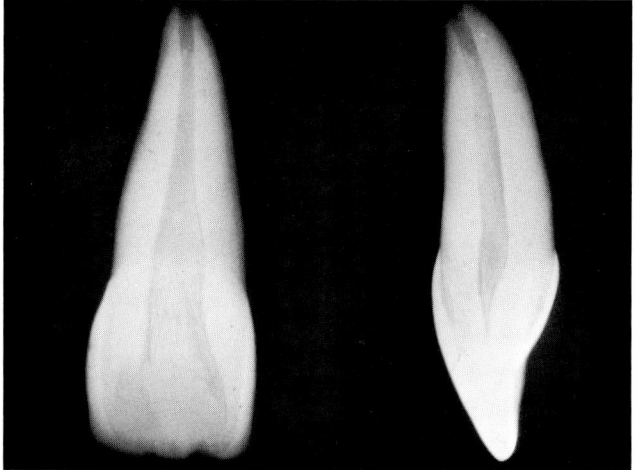

Figure 14-36 Radiograph of immature permanent incisor. Labial view shows wide extension of pulp chamber mesiodistally. Mesial view shows ample dentin on labial and lingual to permit tooth reduction or placement of a cingulum pin.

Figure 14-37 Lingual view of preparation of a young permanent tooth to receive a gold three-quarter crown with acrylic window. Note mesial and distal grooves and cingulum pin hole. Reduction of enamel is at the expense of the lingual to preserve esthetics. Advantages of this restoration are simplicity, durability, and the fact that the labialgingival is not involved.

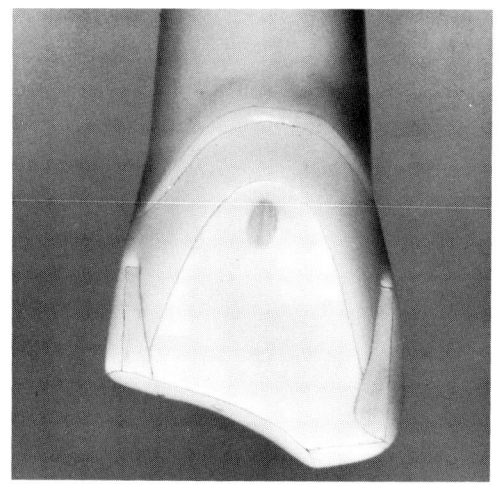

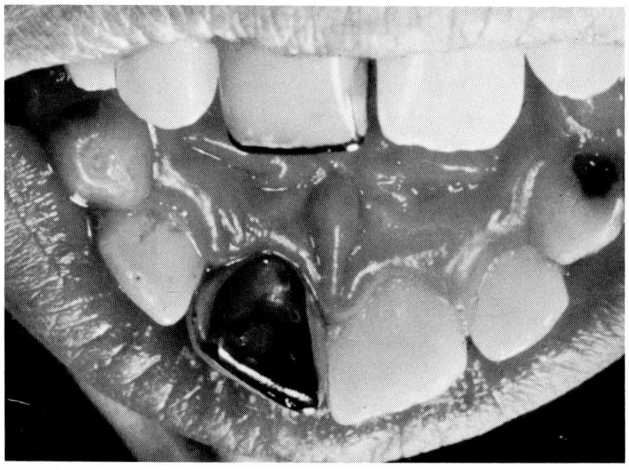

Figure 14-38 Labial and lingual view of completed three-quarter crown with acrylic window. The original mesiodistal, and lingual dimensions of the tooth should not be exceeded. Disadvantages of this restoration include extension of gold on incisal edge and difficulty in obtaining good esthetics in area of fracture.

TRAUMA TO THE PERMANENT DENTITION 299

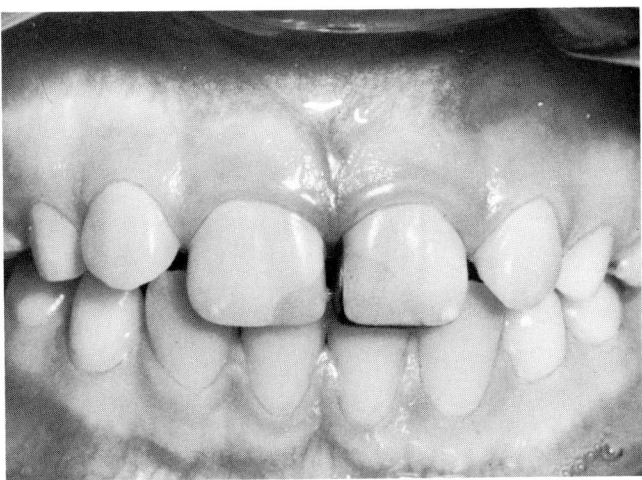

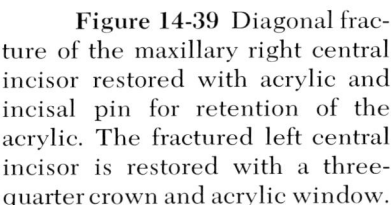

Figure 14-39 Diagonal fracture of the maxillary right central incisor restored with acrylic and incisal pin for retention of the acrylic. The fractured left central incisor is restored with a three-quarter crown and acrylic window.

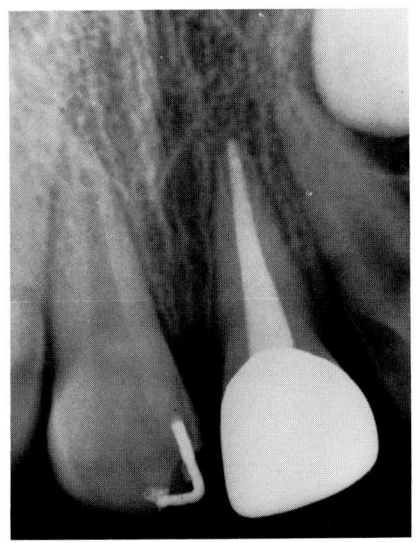

Figure 14-40 Radiograph of restorations shown in Figure 14-39. Note the pin for retention of acrylic in the maxillary right central incisor. A straight pin will usually provide adequate retention. Endodontic treatment was performed on the left central incisor.

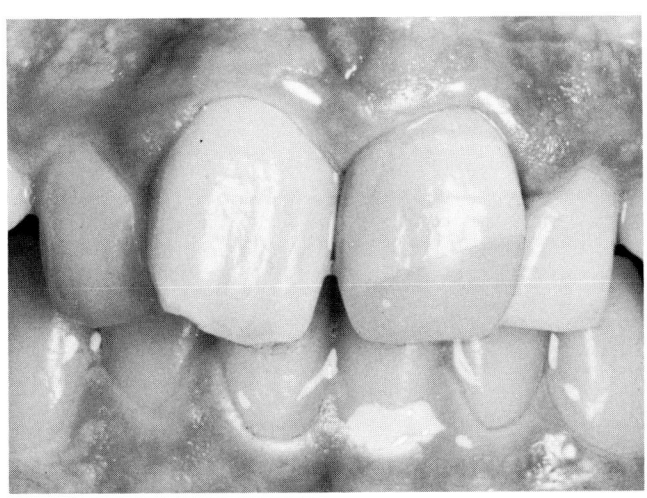

Figure 14-41 A large coronal fracture restored with acrylic. The acrylic restoration was anchored in the pulp chamber after endodontic treatment was completed. The difficulty of trying to match natural and artificial colors on the same tooth is apparent in this view.

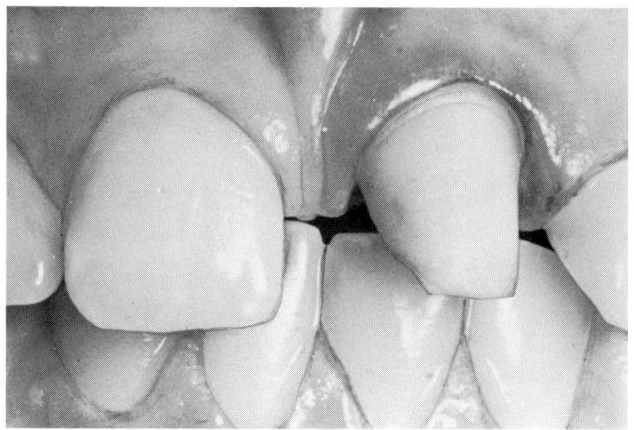

Figure 14-42 Preparation of fractured young permanent central incisor for a porcelain fused-to-gold crown. Strength and esthetics are advantages of these restorations.

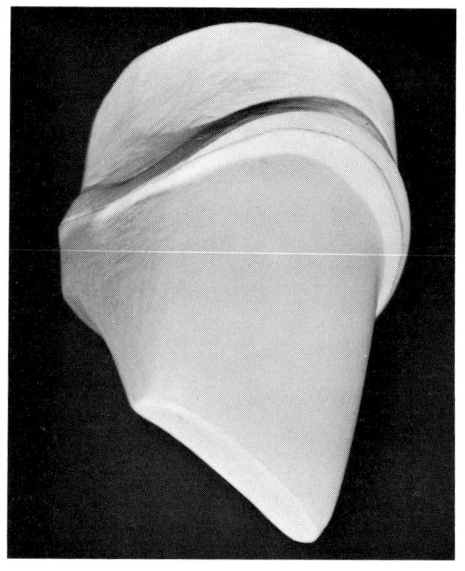

Figure 14-43 Detail of preparation for porcelain fused-to-gold crowns. Note the chamfer on the labial and the minimal reduction on the proximal to avoid exposure of the pulp. (See Figure 14-36 for illustration of lateral extension of pulp chamber in a young permanent central incisor.)

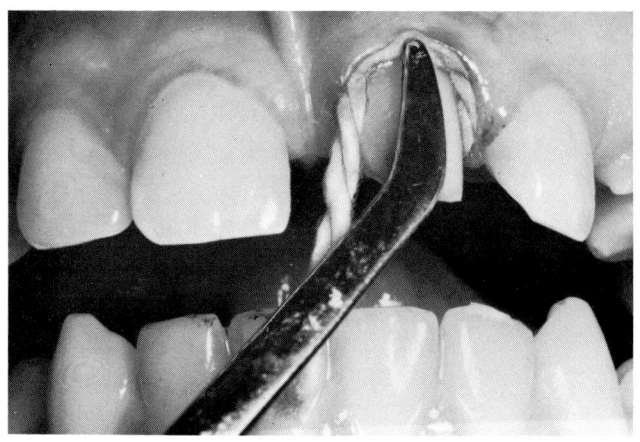

Figure 14-44 Retraction of gingival tissue around crown preparation prior to taking impression.

TRAUMA TO THE PERMANENT DENTITION 301

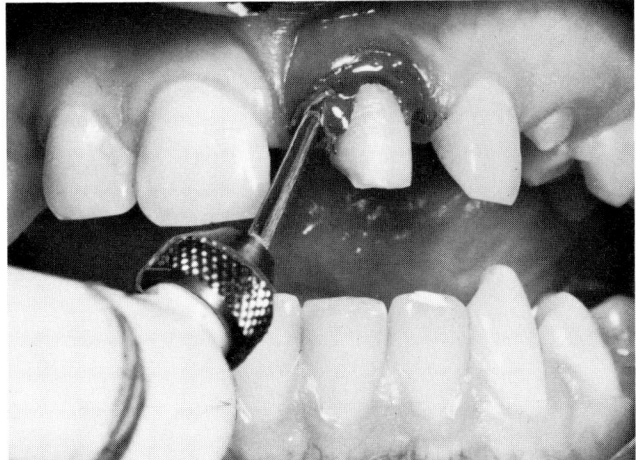

Figure 14-45 Securing impression with rubber base material.

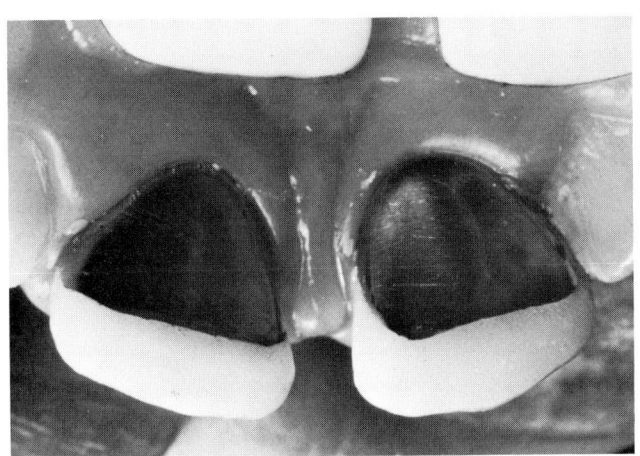

Figure 14-46 Lingual view of porcelain fused-to-gold restorations. Note extension of porcelain over incisal edge to improve esthetics.

Figure 14-47 Labial view of completed porcelain fused-to-gold crown. Mesiodistal and labiolingual dimensions of original tooth should not be exceeded.

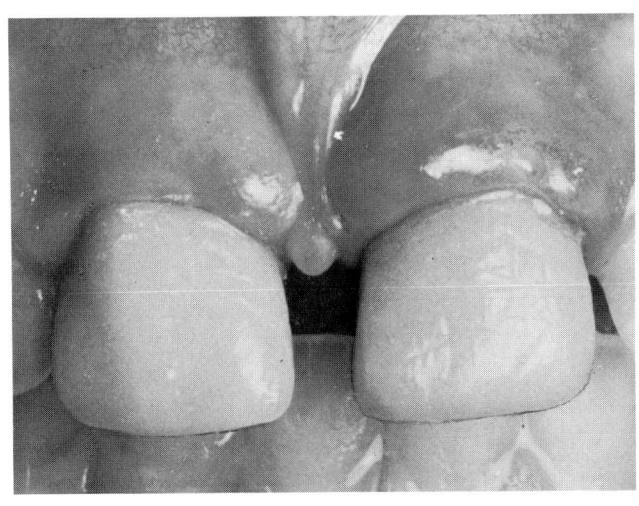

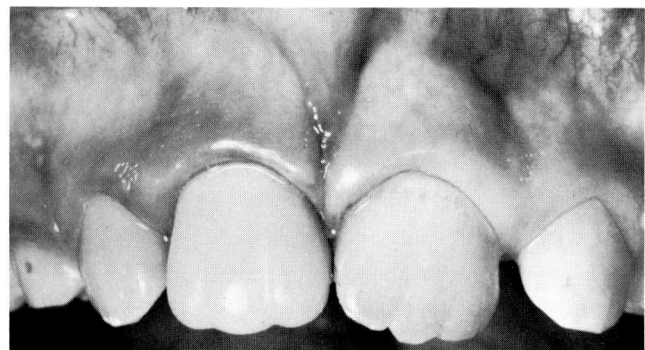

Figure 14-48 Porcelain fused-to-gold restoration of the maxillary right permanent central incisor. Note the mamelons.

Figure 14-49 An esthetic crown (porcelain fused-to-gold) on a maxillary left central incisor.

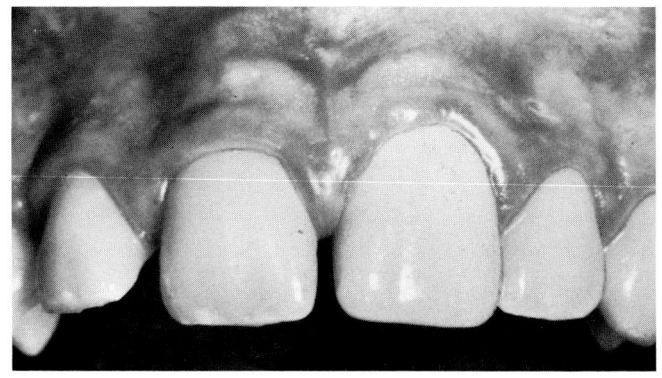

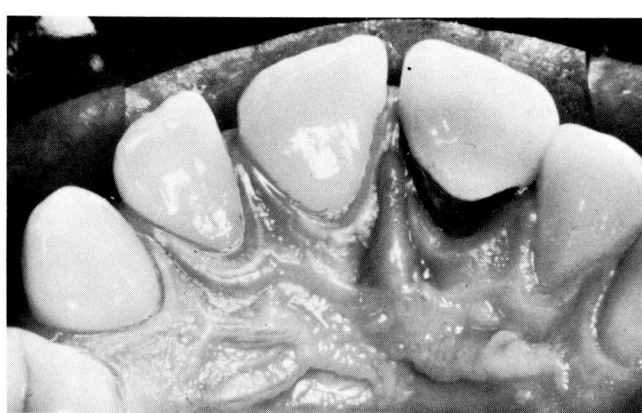

Figure 14-50 Lingual view of the crown shown in Figure 14-49.

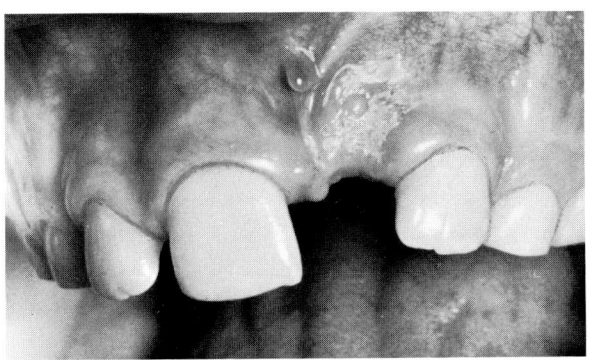

Figure 14-51 A case demonstrating mesial drifting of adjacent teeth after the maxillary permanent left central incisor was traumatically avulsed. There will invariably be a loss of space if an anterior tooth is lost during the mixed dentition period unless a prosthetic appliance is used.

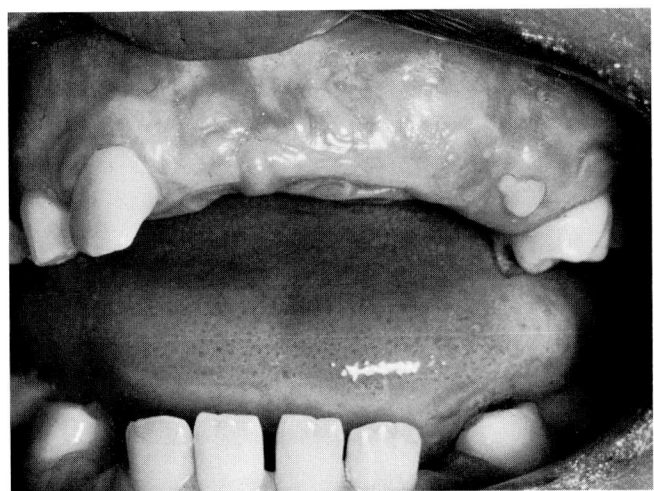

Figure 14-52 A 10-year-old girl lost the maxillary permanent right and left central incisors, left lateral incisor, and the primary left cuspid in an automobile accident. A temporary partial denture was made to restore esthetics and function in the area as well as to prevent mesial drifting of the teeth into the edentulous area. (See Figures 14-53 through 14-56.)

Figure 14-53 Acrylic temporary partial denture with stainless steel wire clasps, in case illustrated in Figure 14-52. Note the slight diastema between the central incisors to make the partial appear more realistic for the age of the patient.

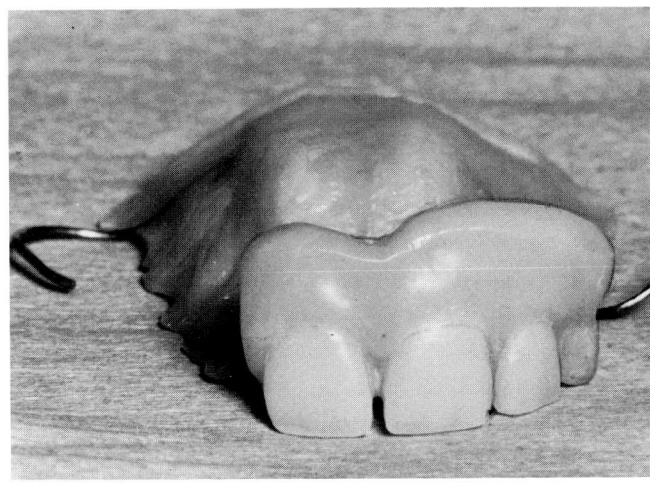

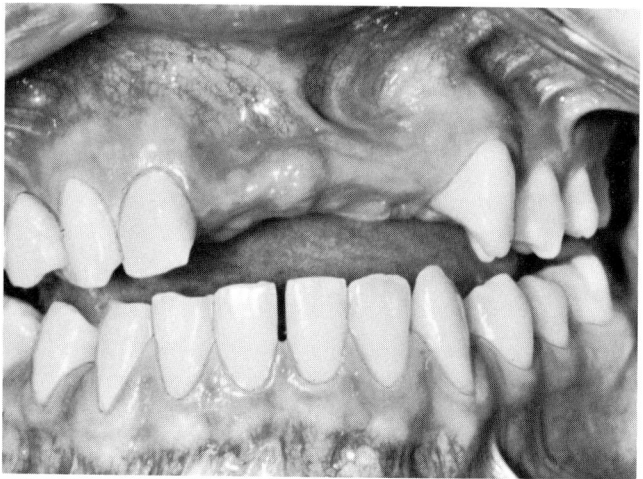

Figure 14-54 Edentulous area following eruption of the permanent cuspid. (Patient from Figure 14-52.)

Figure 14-55 Chrome cobalt partial denture made for the patient described in Figures 14-52 through 14-54, following complete eruption of the permanent teeth. A fixed bridge may be constructed when teeth have reached full maturity.

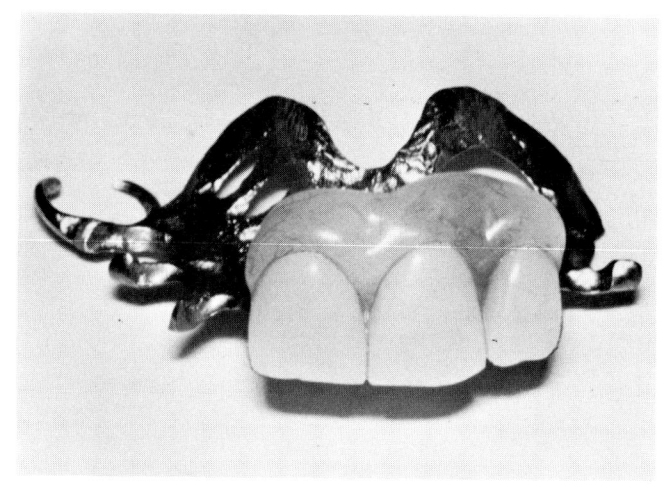

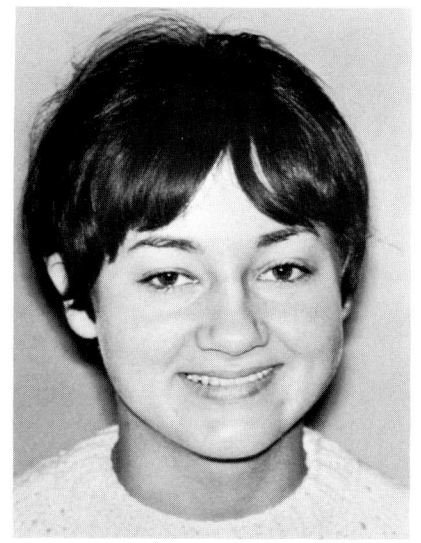

Figure 14-56 Full-face view of patient with partial denture in place.

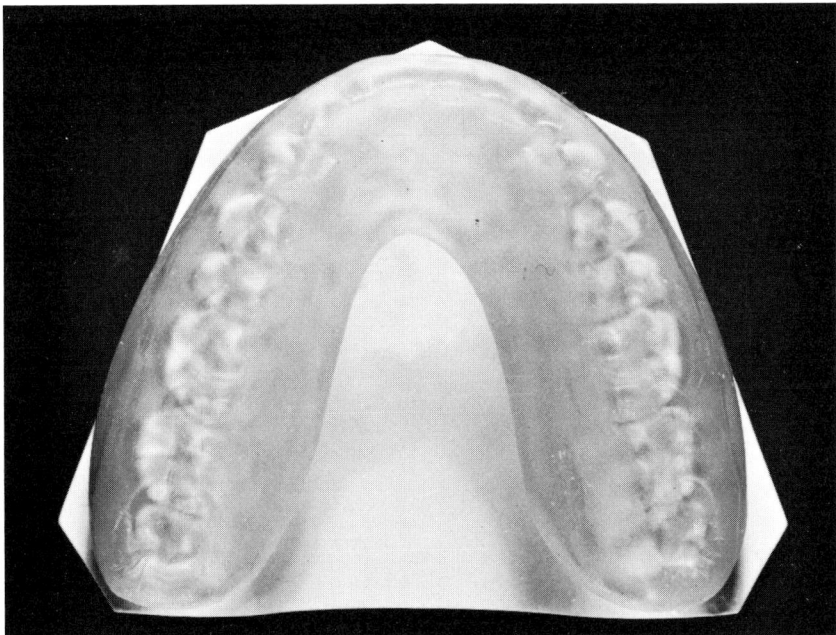

Figure 14-57 Mouth protector on model. Mouth protectors should be worn by all individuals participating in contact sports to prevent or decrease the severity of dental accidents. According to Stevens[6] the custom-made variety (fabricated from impressions and models by dentists using a durable firm material such as vinyl plastic or resilient acrylic) is the superior protector, and athletes should secure this type whenever possible. The studies of Stevens also indicate that mouth protectors should have an even occlusal imprint of the teeth from the opposing arch, or at least be graduated in thickness on the occlusal surface (thinner in the molar areas and thicker in the incisor areas). The imprints of the mandibular teeth in the protector serve to prevent posterior displacement of the mandible when impact is received.

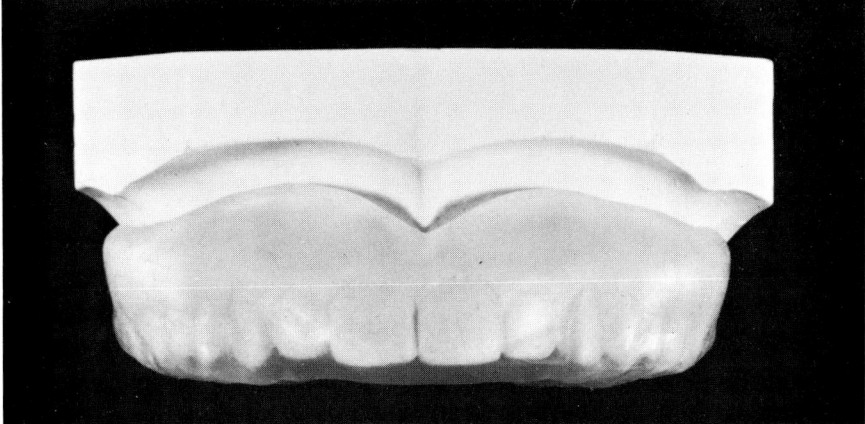

Figure 14-58 Anterior view of mouth protector. The mouth protector must not impinge on the frenum areas.

References

1. Andreasen, J. O., and Hjorting-Hansen, E.: Replantation of teeth. I. Radiographic and clinical study of 110 human teeth replanted after accidental loss. Acta Odont. Scand. 24:263-286, Nov., 1966.
2. Cohen, A.: Improvements in mouthguards. Dental Digest 71:68-70, Feb., 1965.
3. Davis, J. M.: The relationship of overjet to the incidence of subjects with fractured young permanent anterior teeth. Master's thesis, University of Washington, June, 1967.
4. Law, D. B.: Prevention and treatment of traumatized anterior teeth. Dent. Clin. North Amer., Nov. 1961, pp. 616.
5. Lewis, T. E.: Incidence of fractured anterior teeth as related to their protrusion. Angle Orthodont. 29:128-131, April, 1959.
6. Stevens, O. O.: Mouth protectors: evaluation of twelve types—second year. J. Dent. Child. 32:137-143, 1965.
7. Sundvall-Hagland, I.: Olycksfallsskador paa Tänder och Parodontium under Barna-aaren. Chapter 11, III, 1, in Nord. Klin. Odont., Vol. II, 1960.

THE HANDICAPPED CHILD

Chapter 15

In the average community the dentist who includes the handicapped child among his patients will be well rewarded far beyond monetary considerations. The total number of handicapped children is relatively small, and even those persons limiting their practices to children are called upon to treat relatively few. The handicapped do, however, require extra time, energy, preparation and thought as compared to normal children. Fortunately, there is increased emphasis today on the need for adequate dental service for this segment of the population.

The words "handicapped child" denote an exceedingly wide range of conditions. It should be recognized that the handicapped condition can be physical, mental, or social. The actual dental problems associated with these children are usually the same as those affecting normal children. They are often more severe however, because of neglect, and almost always more difficult to correct, especially from a management standpoint.

Except in institutions where the children's total health is supervised by administrative personnel, the dental care of the handicapped is frequently neglected. Causative factors in this neglect seem to be ignorance of the dental problems that can and will develop, and an aversion on the part of the parents to subject their child to additional treatment procedures not related to the main problem. In many cases the family, feeling sorry for the child, attempts to overcompensate by giving him cookies, candies, and other cariogenic foods. In addition, oral hygiene is frequently very difficult to carry out and may be totally neglected. The end-result, as might be expected, is a child who is in the most desperate need of help. To compound all of this, the family with a handicapped child oftentimes will have other associated problems, such as insurmountable medical expenses, emotional problems with other children as a result of overattention to the affected child, and even dissension between parents as to the proper care of the affected child.

Paramount to good dental care for the handicapped is the dentist's attitude toward these children and their parents. The operator must learn to accept the unusual sights, sounds, and actions which he observes and hears upon meeting these children. Some of them cannot control their physical actions (as in cerebral palsy); consequently, treatment can be very frustrating. Others who need the careful intimate attention of the dentist may not be esthetically pleasing patients. Some, such as the mentally retarded, make sounds and movements that may be quite different from those of the usual child patient. On the other hand, the hemophiliac may appear perfectly normal, but his tissue response is exaggerated and requires special consideration. The child with cystic fibrosis may have paroxysms of coughing in the middle of treatment. The dentist, therefore, must develop an attitude of concern for treating the dental problems and avoid being affected by the child's physical condition.

Whether treatment is performed in the dental office or in the hospital under general anesthesia it is wise to consult with the family physician and obtain as much information as possible concerning the nature of the condition and precautions which should be observed. The goal in treating the handicapped child is to render him the same dental care as that afforded his more normal contemporary.

THE HANDICAPPED CHILD 309

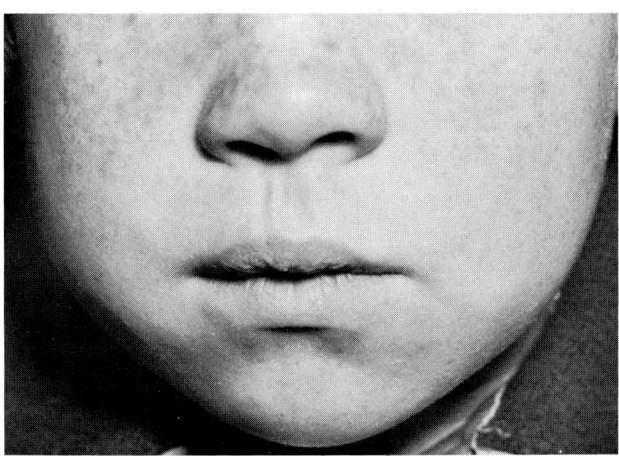

Figure 15-1 Minimal cleft lip. Note slight deformity of maxillary lip and dipping of right ala of nose.

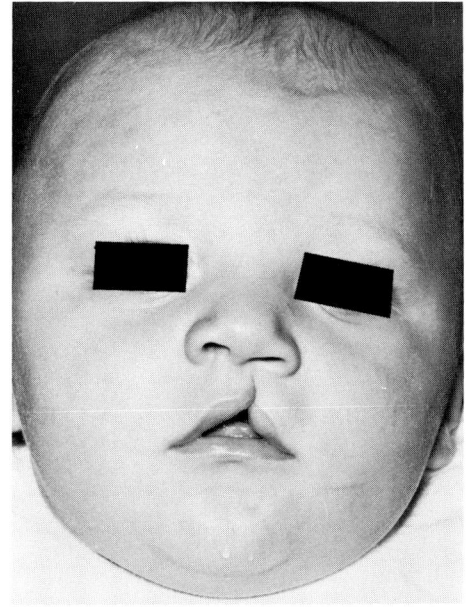

Figure 15-2 Unilateral cleft in baby boy. Most clefts occur on the left side. One in 700 children is born with a cleft lip and/or cleft palate.

Figure 15-3 Esthetic result, several years following surgery for a cleft lip.

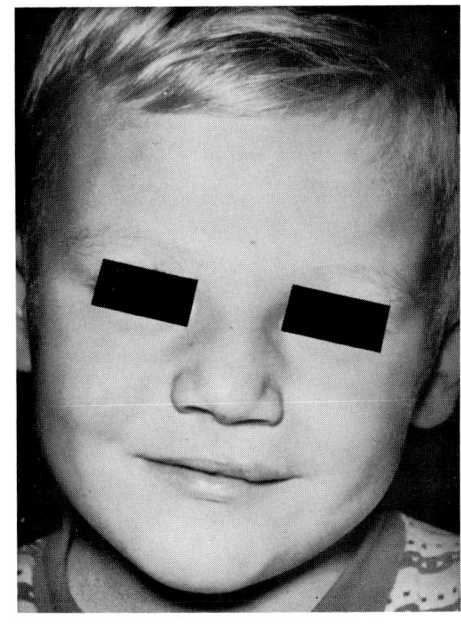

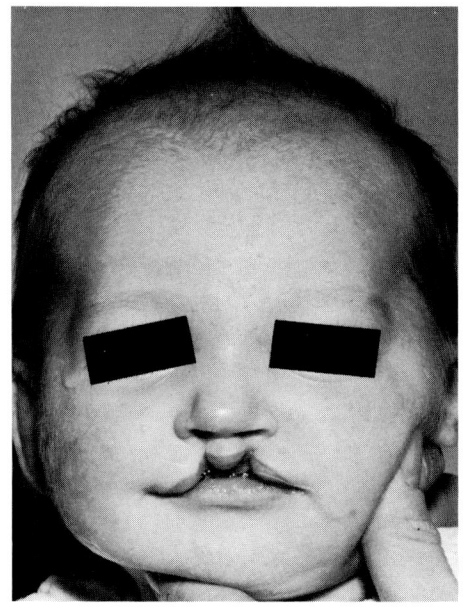

Figure 15-4 Young girl with bilateral cleft lip. This problem can be successfully treated surgically early in life.

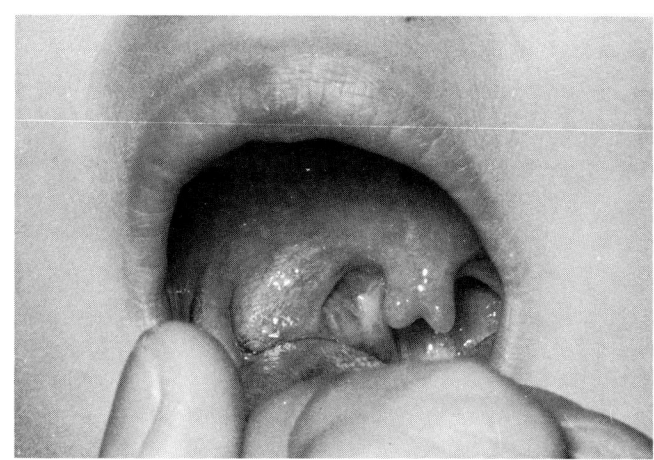

Figure 15-5 Foreshortened soft palate. A child with this condition may require surgery in addition to speech therapy, depending upon his ability to accommodate for the lack of tissue in this area. Note minimal cleft of uvula.

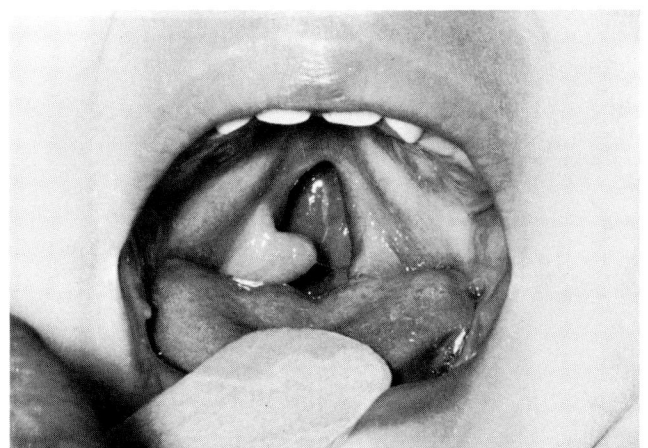

Figure 15-6 Cleft of soft palate only. Situations of this nature will require coordinated consultations among various specialists, such as the oral surgeon, plastic surgeon, prosthodontist, and speech therapist.

THE HANDICAPPED CHILD 311

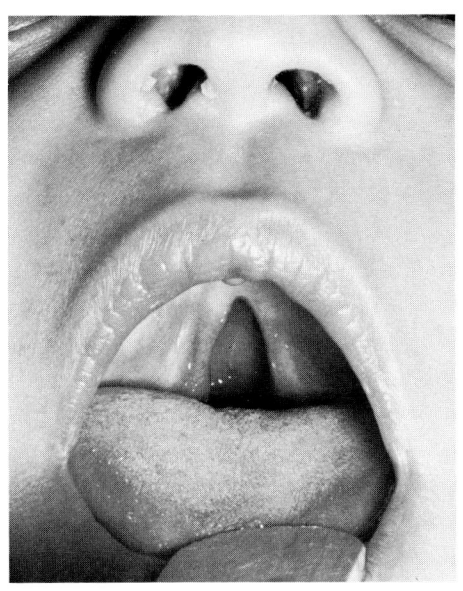

Figure 15-7 Cleft of hard and soft palate. Preventive and restorative dentistry should be administered routinely. Management of the cleft is best handled by the team approach as suggested in Figure 15-8.

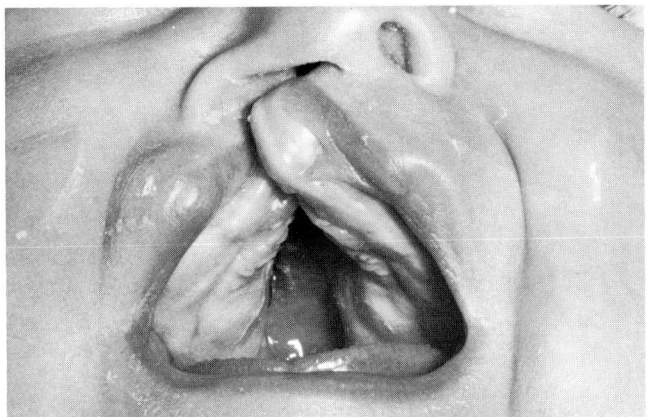

Figure 15-8 Severe unilateral cleft of lip, alveolar ridge, and palatal bone. Clefts of this nature require the joint consultation and services of the pediatrician, oral and/or plastic surgeon, prosthodontist, orthodontist, speech pathologist, otolaryngologist, and psychologist.

Figure 15-9 Bilateral cleft of hard and soft tissue of maxillary arch with premaxilla distorted superiorly. These clefts are the most difficult to treat because of the amount of tissue destruction. The modern team approach, as mentioned in Figure 15-8, can be most successful. Parents of these children, like those of all children with facial deformity, should be given great support and hope. The pedodontist or family dentist should play a decisive role in providing service and coordinating activities through the years of these children's growth and development.

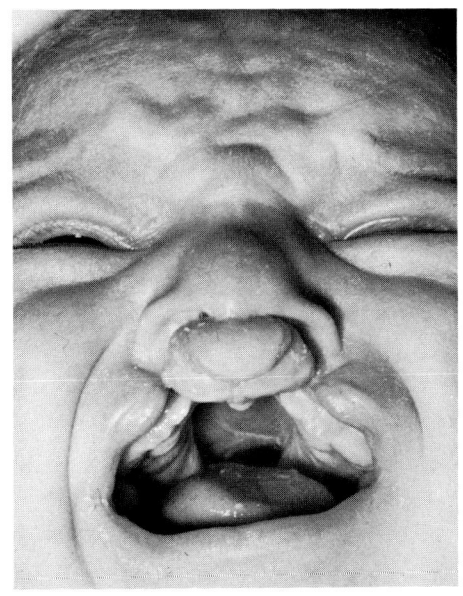

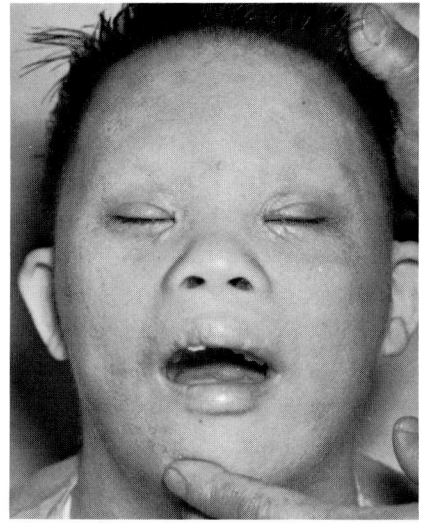

Figure 15-10 Blindness in a child requires that the dentist be careful to explain all procedures in great detail, particularly those involving noises, e.g., suction and drill. Constant physical contact is important. Patience, firmness, and kindness are key prerequisites for the successful treatment of these children.

Figure 15-11 The deaf child also requires extra attention, for demonstration of the treatment which will be carried out. Time spent at this will be repaid in a more cooperative patient. It is most important to reduce apprehension in handicapped children to the minimum.

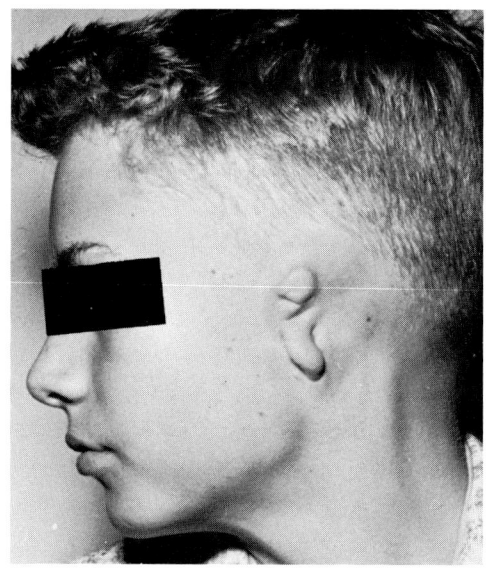

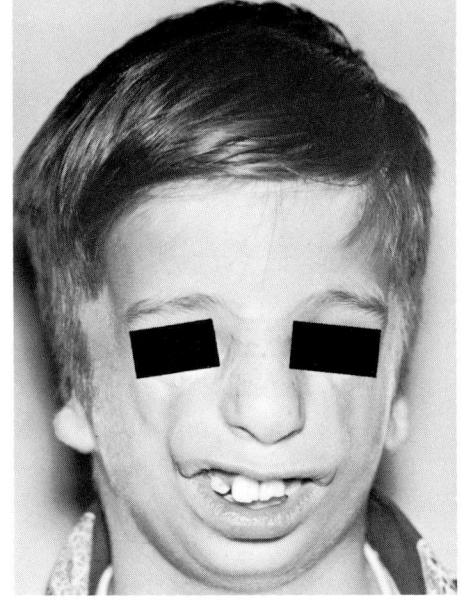

Figure 15-12 Some children may have multiple deformities. For example, this child has Treacher-Collins syndrome, which affects his eyes, facial configuration, and hearing as well as his mouth. Early, sympathetic dental care is needed for these children. The dentition must not be neglected or compromised because of these abnormalities.

THE HANDICAPPED CHILD 313

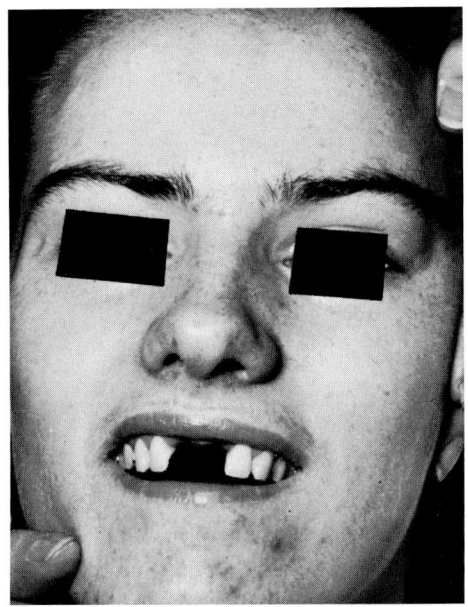

Figure 15-13 Cerebral palsy presents the special problem of maintaining good esthetics. Frequent falls and uncontrolled blows to the front of the mouth take their toll on teeth and make replacements difficult.

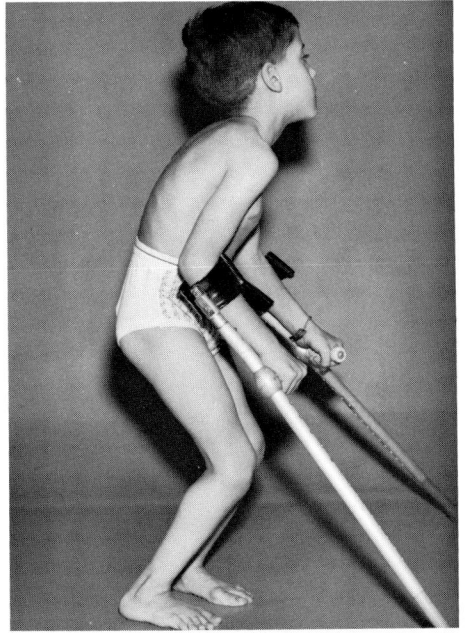

Figure 15-14 The positions assumed by cerebral palsied patients will often test the ingenuity of the dentist. Modern one-piece dental chairs help make positioning easier. Restraints, applied gently, and drugs used as relaxants are frequently helpful in making it possible for the dentist to perform his treatment.

Figure 15-15 Oral cleanliness of children with motor nerve disorders is always a problem. The electric toothbrush may be useful. Although most cerebral palsied patients have been found to be cooperative enough to be treated under local anesthesia, frequently general anesthesia is preferable when extensive care is indicated and the child cannot control his movements.

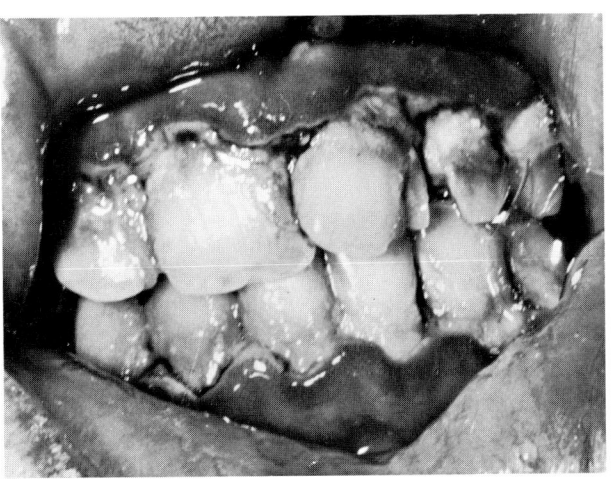

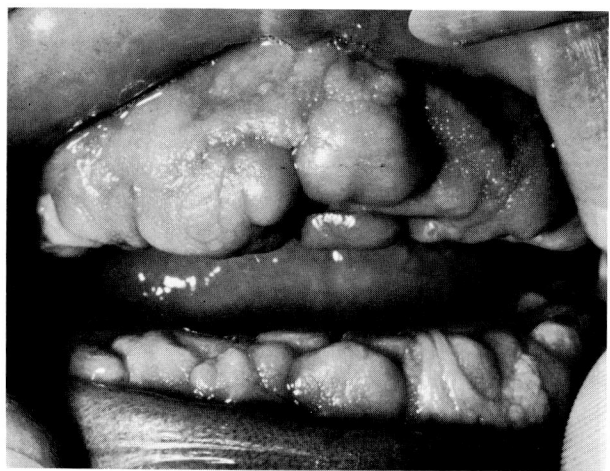

Figure 15-16 Gingival hyperplasia occurs in a large number of patients receiving Sodium Dilantin for prevention of convulsions. Surgical intervention is indicated long before this stage is reached. Although scrupulous dental care is a necessity, the tissue will regenerate as long as the drug is administered. Consultation with the pediatrician or neurologist concerning reduction in the dose of the drug, or use of a substitute, is helpful.

Figure 15-17 The teeth of many children with cystic fibrosis are stained by drugs. Paroxysmal coughing in children with cystic fibrosis or any other disease that causes lung congestion should not interfere with routine care. Short appointments following mucolytic therapy are advisable.

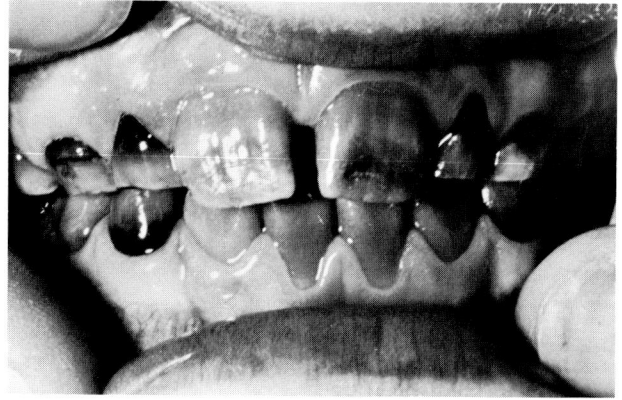

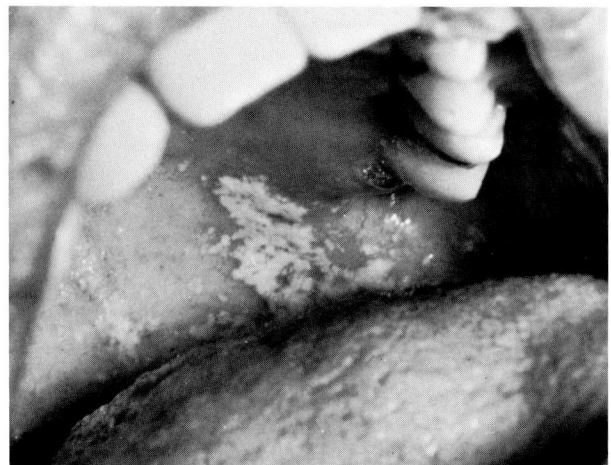

Figure 15-18 Moniliasis is often seen in sickly children. Debilitating diseases such as lupus erythematosus and reactions to certain drugs are causative factors. The dentist should be alert to the presence of these secondary problems.

THE HANDICAPPED CHILD

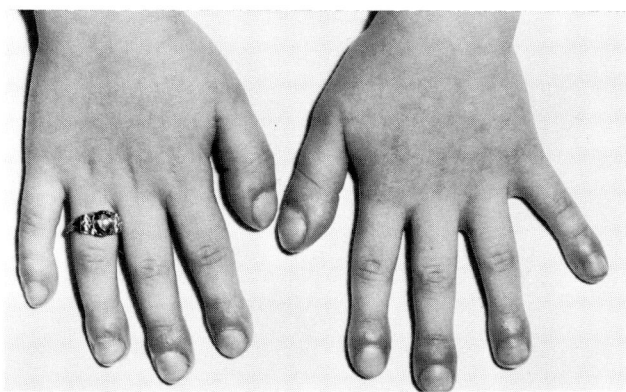

Figure 15-19 Teenage girl with inoperable congenital heart defect. Clubbing of fingers is characteristic of this condition. (See Figures 15-20 through 15-22.)

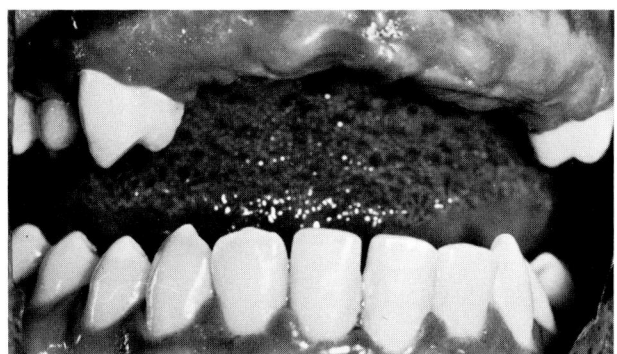

Figure 15-20 Extensive oral surgery has been performed. Severe cardiac disease should not prohibit dental care. Early preventive care is desirable.

Figure 15-21 Adequate antibiotic coverage is a prerequisite for all cardiac patients requiring dental treatment. Treatment may include scaling and polishing of teeth. Multiple extractions and major reconstruction as in this fixed anterior bridge can be successfully performed.

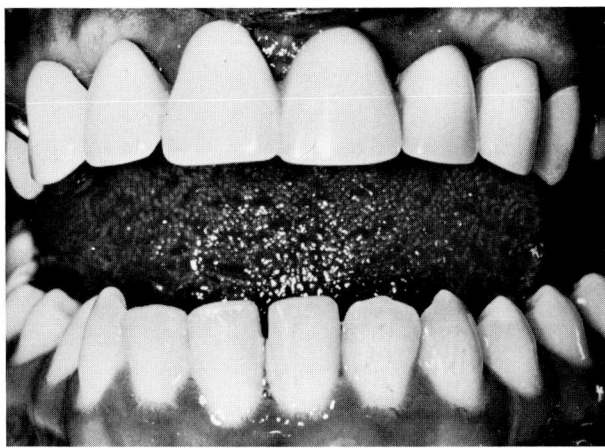

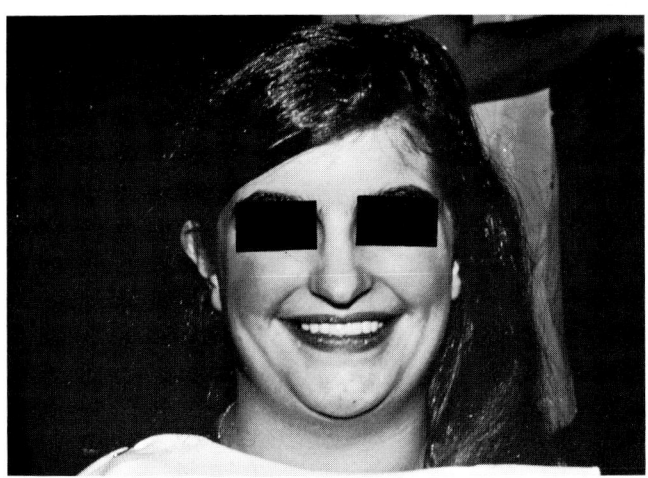

Figure 15-22 Improved appearance of patient with congenital heart defect. Following extensive dental treatment, the patient had an entirely new social outlook.

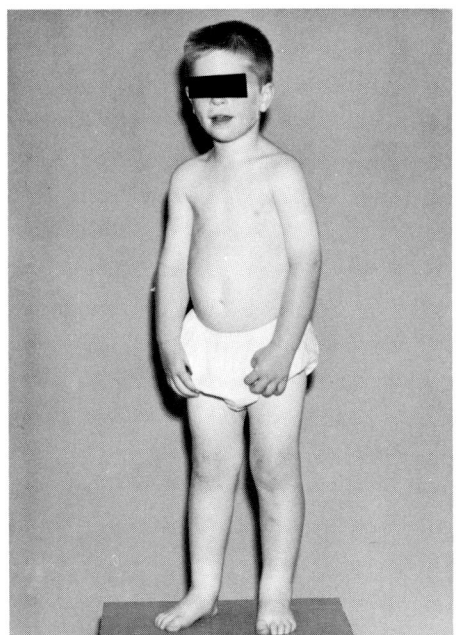

Figure 15-23 Typical stance of mongoloid child. Initial diagnosis should begin prior to the child's being seated in the dental chair. These children are usually most cooperative.

Figure 15-24 Palm of hands of mongoloid child shows deep simian crease. Extra care should be given in diagnosis of handicapped children to clearly identify their problems.

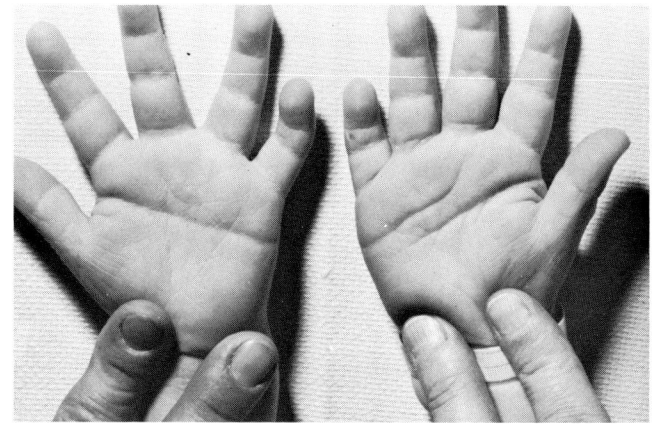

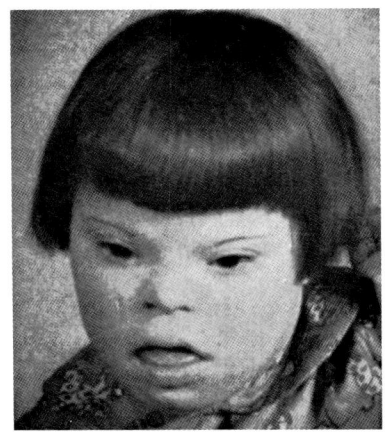

Figure 15-25 Seven-year-old mongoloid child. Facial appearance is typical. Parents must be particularly encouraged in home care for these children, since periodontal problems are usually severe. (From Nelson, W. E.: *Textbook of Pediatrics*. 8th ed., 1964, p. 1237.)

THE HANDICAPPED CHILD

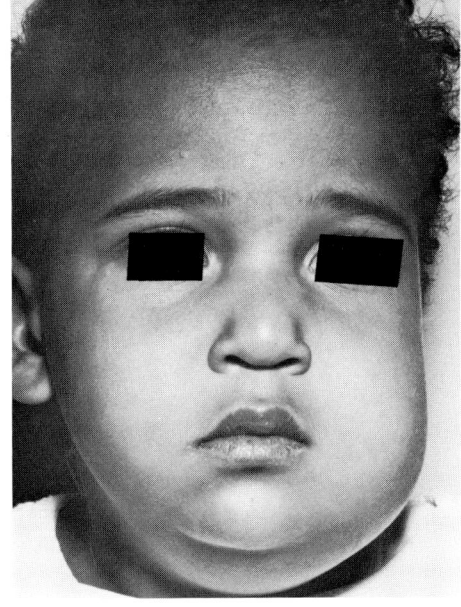

Figure 15-26 Abscess of a primary molar, a relatively common condition, presents a major threat to the child with a blood dyscrasia such as sickle cell anemia or hemophilia. A careful case history should be taken prior to surgery on any such patient. Proper treatment involves close cooperation with a hematologist.

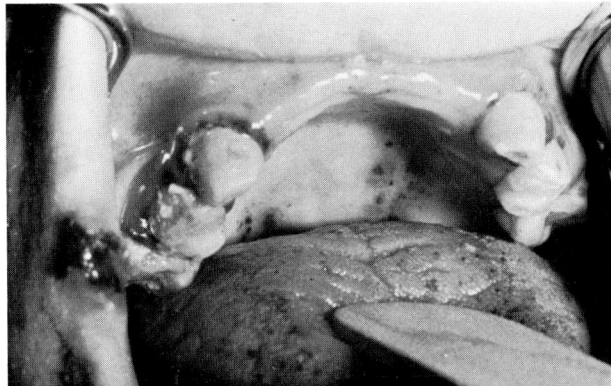

Figure 15-27 The first sign of leukemia may appear in the mouth in the form of petechiae. All such findings should be thoroughly investigated. Again, early care with emphasis on preventive measures is important. In acute leukemia, the dentist can render a very comforting service by giving palliative treatment to the irritated tissues.

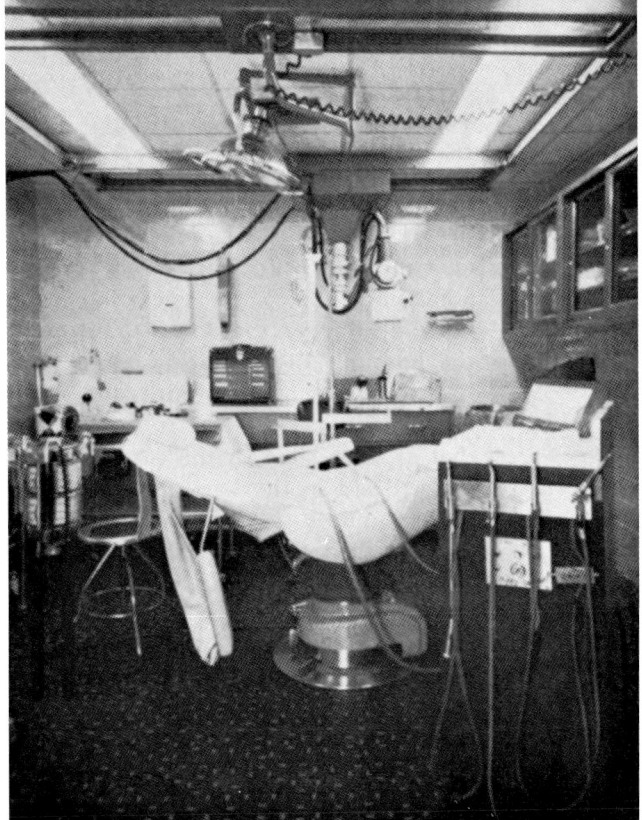

Figure 15-28 A hospital operatory designed exclusively for the treatment of dental cases. The hospital operatory is the preferred location for treatment of physically and mentally handicapped patients who are unable to cooperate as necessary for satisfactory treatment in the dental office. (From Boller, R. J., and Posnick, I. H.: Fifteen years of hospital dentistry. J. Dent. Child. 34:56-64, January, 1967.)

MANAGEMENT OF THE CHILD PATIENT

Chapter 16

> *"We approach all problems of children with affection.*
> *Theirs is the province of joy and good humor.*
> *They are the most wholesome part of the race for they are the freshest from the hands of God."**

The Preschool Child

The successful management of the preschool patient is not only essential to accomplishment of treatment procedures, but it is even more important in laying a foundation for future acceptance of dentistry as a health service. The child who is comfortable in the dental environment during his early years will also usually be a good patient in the school-age and teen period. While some persons have intuitive skill in understanding and directing the behavior of small children, any dentist who has a sincere desire to treat them can be very successful by following known guidelines and principles of behavior modification.

To obtain rapport with the preschool child and carry out dental operations it is necessary to have some idea of his language and motor and social development. Utilizing this knowledge, step by step procedural acquaintance, accompanied by constant reinforcement of good behavior will result in positive conditioning.

Fear and anxiety are probably the most important emotional blocks with which the dentist contends. Small children may acquire fear of the dentist from conversations overheard at home and also from discussion with

---
*From Herbert Hoover's White House Conference on Children, 1930.

playmates. In some cases they may have been actually exposed to a traumatic situation in the hospital or physician's office. First visits to the dentist, therefore, should be structured so that the child will have a pleasant and interesting experience. Definitive treatment should not be attempted on the first appointment. Time must be spent in getting acquainted with the child and in carrying out routine diagnostic procedures: examination, prophylaxis, radiographic survey. Small children need to know and have confidence in their dentist. For this reason the first appointment should not be delegated to auxiliary personnel.

Making the preschooler feel comfortable and confident in the dental office requires that all personnel with whom he comes in contact reflect an aura of friendliness and personal interest. The dentist should be pleased to see the child patient and should express this feeling in voice and demeanor. Positive statements such as, "It's nice to see you today," or "What a lovely dress," are preferable to thoughtless questions or remarks directed primarily to parent figures. Voice inflection, too, can be a factor in gaining rapport and cooperation. Certainly there is much to be gained by courteous remarks such as "Thank you for opening your mouth so widely," and use of the word "Please." At all times lavish praise is effective with preschool children and helps to build their confidence in the dentist. At this age level it is advisable to use some verbal distraction by conversation about topics appropriate to the child's interests. This could include his clothes, pets, favorite foods, or reference to his birthday or similar event. Avoid discussion of school, athletics or other subjects beyond his experience.

The dentist who sees small children needs to establish friendly physical contact also since his eventual treatment will certainly involve intimate physical contact. This can be achieved by such devices as taking the child's hand when entering the operatory, helping him into the chair, and giving him a gentle hug when the appointment is over. It should be pointed out, however, that at the time of the initial contact with the preschool child the dentist should maintain a distance and avoid too precipitous physical advances.

Whether the parent should be in or out of the dental operatory has been a controversial subject among pedodontists. Certainly with a very young child, two or three years of age, it is advisable to have the parent present for the first two or three appointments. The decision to allow the parent of an older child in the operatory is up to the dentist himself. Most successful pedodontists, however, do prefer to exclude the parent if the child is uncooperative. Management of the uncooperative child involves firmness on the part of the dentist and positive communication of the behavior limits acceptable while treatment is being carried out. In this regard, the use of drugs to modify child behavior is largely a matter of individual preference. The experienced operator, who structures his appointments carefully, and who gains the confidence and trust of his patients, will encounter few behavior problems serious enough to interfere with the accomplishment of dental treatment. The very young child who has a complex dental problem, or the preschooler who is seriously disturbed and does not respond to the usual approach, constitutes a group that should be considered for treatment under a general anesthetic in the hospital operatory.

Giving the preschooler a small gift or token of his visit after each dental appointment is a sound procedure from a psychological standpoint as long as there is no implication of its being a bribe or reward for good behavior. The young child cannot be expected to appreciate the long-term benefits of oral health and, therefore, the prospect of dental appointments is not especially rewarding. The anticipation of receiving a small gift changes this attitude, however, and in many instances results in the child eagerly looking forward to seeing his dentist.

Much has been written concerning the physical arrangement of offices in which children are treated. Although this is largely a matter of personal taste, there should be some attention given to creating an attractive environment in which the child will feel welcome and comfortable. The dentist must be careful not to allow his decorating theme to be exclusively devoted to the interest level of the preschooler, however, or older children will feel out of place. The reception room should be cheerfully furnished with the possible inclusion of a corner with a child size chair and table. Books appropriate for various age levels should be available and in good condition. The operating areas should be uncluttered and free of visible instruments which may create unnecessary anxiety. Highly antiseptic odors are undesirable as well as medicinal soaps and hand creams. A pleasant flavored mouthwash can be beneficial to both patient and dentist alike.

In conclusion it should be emphasized that while the physical aspects of the reception room and operatory should be carefully structured to create a favorable atmosphere, no amount of unusual decor will take the place of a sympathetic and friendly operator who has secured the trust and confidence of his small patient.

The School-Age Child

Children in the mixed dentition period, between the ages of 6 and 12, are usually more amenable to reason than their younger counterparts; and consequently, less problems are encountered in their behavior management. As in dealing with the preschool child, however, it is equally important to establish rapport and to follow the principles of procedural acquaintance, although necessarily on a more sophisticated level.

Reinforcement of acceptable behavior is still a desirable approach, especially if complicated procedures are anticipated. Verbalization can be effected on a more adult basis with children at this age, and school is a favorite topic of discussion. Comments on dress are quite appropriate for girls, while boys enjoy talking about sports or hobbies. A noncooperative school-age child may be more difficult to manage than a preschooler because his emotional problem has had more years to develop. It is extremely important in these cases to allow more time for getting acquainted and gaining the confidence and respect of the patient. It is possible to explain long-term objectives of treatment at this age and to point out the consequences of negligence.

Tranquilizers are frequently of benefit if these children are unduly apprehensive. In some instances, where fear of injection is the chief hurdle to be surmounted, alternative procedures can be suggested. With some children an agreement can be reached to proceed with treatment without local anesthesia. In others, nitrous oxide-oxygen analgesia may be an acceptable alternative. The use of the new pressure anesthetic device is another approach that may be helpful. Rarely is it necessary to resort to general anesthesia and the hospital operating room in order to complete the required dentistry for this age group of patients. Exceptions to this would include the very disturbed child with urgent dental needs, and the mentally retarded or otherwise handicapped child.

The Adolescent Patient

Management problems with the adolescent dental patient are likely to be in the nature of non-cooperation in home care recommendations and failure to keep appointments, rather than in outright refusal of treatment or overt expressions of anxiety such as temper tantrums. Since children in this age group, however, often manifest severe dental problems associated with a high caries rate, they represent an extremely important area of concern for the dentist.

Some guidelines for the practitioner who treats this age group are necessary, and yet there is a dearth of pertinent information in the literature. Tjossem[1] warns against the dentist persisting in patterns of interaction developed during the earlier child care years of the patient. There is a clear need to realize that during the adolescent period the dentist must change certain aspects of his approach.

The adolescent is characterized by a desire for personal independence and an aversion to adult authority. Recognizing these facts, the dentist can structure his management of these patients to avoid unnecessary problems. Tjossem suggests that the role of the parent be de-emphasized, and that as much as possible the adolescent himself be involved in the dental office procedures. For example, appointments, whenever possible, should be made directly with the adolescent thus making him feel important and providing him with the opportunity to work out his own schedule. There should be no criticism or unsympathetic remarks concerning dress, hair styles or teenage fads. Instructions on oral hygiene should be carried out on an adult level without assuming an authoritarian position. If the adolescent equates the dentist with parent or teacher in a concept of a reprimanding or critical adult figure, he will not accept treatment readily and may fail to cooperate at all. A supportive understanding approach will be far more successful at these age levels, and every effort should be made by all members of the dental office team to work towards this end.

It is axiomatic, however, that the fundamental principles of behavior modification successful with young children should be utilized with the adolescent as well. Reinforcement of good behavior, step by step procedural acquaintance and courtesy, all help in creating a favorable dentist-patient relationship.

---

[1]Tjossem, T. O., Psychologic considerations in the care of the adolescent dental patient. *Dental Clinics of North America*, July, 1966, p. 149, W. B. Saunders Co., Philadelphia.

Sedative Drugs in the Management of the Child Patient

The experienced dentist does not find the use of drugs necessary in the majority of the children he treats. However, there are occasions when it is helpful to employ adjuncts to reduce the anxiety level of the child patient prior to operative procedures. A variety of drugs have been suggested to aid in relieving tension and emotional stress, but it is not within the scope of this ATLAS to review in detail all of these preparations. One safe and effective sedating agent for children is a combination of hydroxyzine hydrochloride and chloral hydrate. For office use, it is suggested that the appropriate dosage be given orally about 45 minutes before the time of the dental appointment.

Basic Dosage for Sedative Effect
For 40 Pound Child

(Hydroxyzine hydrochloride and Chloral hydrate)

  20 mg. Atarax* .... (2 teaspoons)
500 mg. Noctec** .... (1 teaspoon)

Give orally 45 minutes before appointment. The dosage may be proportionately increased or decreased according to the weight of the child. Each teaspoon of Atarax syrup equals 10 mg. and each teaspoon of Noctec syrup equals 500 mg. A teaspoon is specified as the equivalent of 5 cc.

---

*Atarax, (hydroxyzine hydrochloride), J. B. Roerig Division, Chas. Pfizer & Co., Inc.
**Noctec, (chloral hydrate), E. R. Squibb & Sons, Inc.

INDEX

Note: Page numbers in *italics* represent illustrations. The letter *t* after page numbers refers to a table.

Abscess, of mandibular primary incisor, following traumatic injury, *276*
  of maxillary second primary molar, in patient with blood dyscrasia, *317*
  periapical, of mandibular right primary second molar, *39*
    of maxillary right primary second molar, face swelling due to, *29*
Adams clasp, in interceptive orthodontics, *243*
Alveolar anesthesia injections, *148, 149*
Amalgam condensers, alterations of, *165*
Amalgam restoration(s), approximating, *170*
  gingival, *179, 180*
  in mandibular arch, *170*
  in primary dentition, 164
  occlusal, on second primary molars, *166*
  of distal surface of mandibular cuspid, *178*
  of mandibular first permanent molar, *166*
  of mandibular second primary molar, *169, 171*
  proximo-occlusal, *170*
    marginal ditching in, *173*
  well-contoured, *175*
Amelogenesis imperfecta, 78t, 80-90
  delayed eruption and, *99*
Anesthesia, 143-152
  general, 144
    neotracheal intubation of, *152*
    orotracheal intubation of, *152*
  local, 143-144
    equipment for, *145*
    lip biting following, *151*
    resuscitation equipment for, *148*
    techniques for, 143

Anesthesia (*Continued*)
  needles in, 143
  nerve location and, 145t
  storage of, *146*
Anesthesia injection(s), alveolar, *148, 149*
  long buccal, *148*
  nasopalatine, *150*
  of maxillary area, *147*
  palatal, *149*
Angle's classification of malocclusion, 23
Ankyloglossia, 33
Ankylosis, of maxillary first permanent molar, *110*
  of mesial root of second primary molar, *109*
  of primary molars, *108*
  of replanted maxillary permanent central incisor, *297*
Anodontia, hereditary anhidrotic ectodermal dysplasia and, 53
Anomalies, of color of teeth, 72-76
  of dentition, 51-111
  of dentin, 79t, 91-97
  of enamel, 78t, 80-90
  of eruption and exfoliation of teeth, 98-102
  of number of teeth, 51-64
  of position of teeth, 98, 103-110
  of shape of teeth, 65-72
  of structure and texture of teeth, 77-97
Antibiotics, in exodontia of primary dentition, 209
Aphthous ulcers, recurrent, of oral mucosa of upper lip, *32*
Arch. See specific name of arch.
Atarax, in management of child patient, 323

"Baby bottle syndrome," 134
Ball clasps, in interceptive orthodontics, 243
Band remover, proper use of, 225
Band restoration, 177
Bicuspid(s), eruption of, space maintainer for, 225
  mandibular, right, missing, 59
  mandibular second, blocked, due to loss of arch length, 223
    dentigerous cyst of, 48
    idiopathic internal resorption of, pulpotomy and, 46
    in abnormal position, 105
    indirect pulp capping of, 190
    missing, 58
    rotated, 105
  maxillary second, lingual eruption of, 223
Bite, open, anterior, finger-sucking and, 40, 41
Bite, open, caries due to, 136
Bitewing(s), 115
  carious areas in, 42
  posterior, radiographic technique in, 124
Blind patient, dental technique in treatment of, 312
Blood dyscrasia, dental care and, 317
Brass wire, in interceptive orthodontics, 241
Bridging, dentin, 202, 203
Brushing, of child's teeth, technique for, 137, 138, 139
Bruxism, effects of, 42
  occlusal wear and, in primary dentition, 10

Calcification, dental, in eight-month fetus, 3
  in newborn, 3
Calcium hydroxide, in pulp therapy, 188, 192, 202
Calculus deposits, gingivitis and, 36
Canker sore, of oral mucosa of upper lip, 32
Capillary hemangioma, on inferior surface of tongue, 34
Capping, pulp, 188
Carbon markings, reduction and, 172
Cardiac disease, dental care and, 315
Caries, arrested, of primary molars, 45
  due to open bite, 136
  fluorides in prevention of, 131
  gingival, 44
    amalgam restorations in, 179
    of maxillary permanent incisors, 46
    of primary molars, 134
  in bitewings, 42
  interproximal, 176
    in lower permanent incisors, 135
    in maxillary primary molars, 134
Caries, loss of arch length due to, 43
  occlusal, of mandibular permanent first molars, 45
    mandibular primary second molar, 44
  oral hygiene in prevention of, 131
  of primary anterior teeth, 134, 177
  prevention of, 131-142
  prosthodontic treatment for, 263
  proximal, on mandibular incisors, 179
  rampant, of primary dentition, 43, 44, 45, 133
  sucrose and, 131
Cavernous hemangioma, of tongue, 34

Cavity preparation, in primary dentition, 163
  lingual dovetail, and restoration, in primary cuspid, 178
  of mandibular first primary molar, 167
  proximal and restoration, 168
Cephalometric exposure, lateral, radiographic technique for, 129
Cerebral palsy, dental care and, 313
Child patient, handicapped, 307-317
  management of, 319-322
Cingula, exaggerated, of maxillary central incisor, 70
Clamps, and rubber dam, 156, 157
Clasps, in interceptive orthodontics, 243
Cleft, of lip, bilateral, 310
  unilateral, 309
  of lip, alveoli, and palatal bone, unilateral, dental approach in, 311
  of maxillary arch, bilateral, dental approach in, 311
  of palate, hard and soft, 311
  soft, 310
Cleidocranial dysostosis, delayed eruption of permanent teeth and, 99
  supernumerary teeth and, 57
Concrescence, of teeth, 66, 69
Condensers, amalgam, alterations of, 165
Crossbite, acrylic guide plane in correction of, 236, 237
  anterior, 41, 103
    correction of, 234, 235
  posterior, 41, 103
    correction of, 238
Crown, fracture of, of maxillary primary central incisor, 274
Crown restoration, gold three-quarter, of permanent young incisor, 298
  jacket, of permanent incisor, 293
  stainless steel, in dentin and pulpal fractures, 291
    of molars, procedure for, 182-185
    of primary dentition, 181
Cuspid(s), mandibular, amalgam restoration in, 178
  radiographic technique for, 122
  maxillary, radiographic technique for, 119
  permanent, in horizontal position, 106
  permanent mandibular, ectopic eruption of, 104
  primary, clamp for, 156
    lingual dovetail cavity preparation and restoration in, 178
  primary mandibular, crown restoration of, 181
    extraction of, 216, 217
    fusion of, with lateral incisor, 68
    geminated, 67
  primary maxillary, extraction of, 212, 213
Cyanosis, dental care and, 315
Cyst, dentigerous, of mandibular bicuspid, 47, 48
  epithelial, in newborn, 7
  eruption, in newborn, 6
Cystic fibrosis, dental care and, 314
  teeth color and, 76

Deaf patient, dental treatment of, 312
Dens-in-dente, of maxillary left permanent central incisor, 70

INDEX

Dental calcification, in eight-month fetus, 3
  in newborn, 3
Dental floss, in polishing interproximal contact areas, 140
Dental surgery, rubber dam in, 155
Dentigerous cyst, of mandibular bicuspid, 48
Dentin, hereditary anomalies of, 79t
Dentin bridging, 202, 203
Dentin fractures, of maxillary permanent central incisor, 287
    treatment for, 286
  of maxillary primary incisor, treatment and prognosis of, 272
Dentinal dysplasia, 97
Dentinogenesis imperfecta, 79t, 91-97
  effects of, on bite closure, 93
  prosthodontic treatment for, 250-258
  teeth color and, 93
Dentistry, operative, 163-186
Dentition, anomalies of, 51-111. See also *Anomalies of teeth.*
  development of, 4, 5
  growth and development of, 1-24
  mixed, crowding of, in mandibular arch, 12
  normal, 12
  permanent. See *Permanent dentition.*
  primary. See *Primary dentition.*
Dentures, complete, 249, 251, 258, 262, 263
  partial, 249, 259, 262, 263
    acrylic temporary, 303
    chrome cobalt, 250, 262, 304
    for mandibular incisors, 259
    for maxillary primary incisor, 264-267, 278
Diagnosis, oral, 25-29
Diastema, between maxillary central incisors, correction of, 240
Diet, following exodontia in primary dentition, 211
  in caries prevention, 136
Dilaceration, of permanent central incisors, 69
Dilantin hyperplasia, 38
Disclosing solution, for prophylaxis, 140
Down's syndrome, missing teeth and, 53
Drugs, in exodontia in primary dentition, 210
  in management of child patient, 323
  in pulp therapy, 188
Dyscrasia, blood, dental care and, 317
Dysplasia, anhidrotic ectodermal, 62, 63, 64
  anodontia and, 53
  dentinal, 97
  ectodermal, prosthodontic treatment for, 259, 260, 261, 262

Ectodermal dysplasia, 53
  prosthodontic treatment in, 259, 260, 261, 262
Enamel, effects of fluoride on, 90
Enamel fracture(s), of maxillary permanent central incisors, treatment for, 285
  of maxillary primary incisor, treatment and prognosis of, 272
Enamel hypocalcification, hereditary, 78t, 86, 87
  snow-capped teeth in, 88
Enamel hypoplasia, due to fall, 88
  due to febrile disease, 89
  hereditary, 80

Enamel hypoplasia (*Continued*)
  hereditary, atypical, 85
    delay of eruption of permanent teeth due to, 81
    hard, pitted type, 83
    with horizontal wrinkling and grooving, 84
    with vertical grooving, 84
  in primary dentition, 90
  local, due to virus infection, 89
Epithelial cyst, in newborn, 7
Eruption, delayed, conditions associated with, 98
  in amelogenesis imperfecta, 99
  in hypothyroidism, 101
  of maxillary permanent central incisor, 13
  of permanent teeth, cleidocranial dysostosis and, 99
    hereditary, enamel hypoplasia and, 81
    posterior, 100
  ectopic, of mandibular first permanent molar, 106
    of mandibular permanent cuspids, 104
    of maxillary first permanent molar, 107
  exfoliation and, anomalies of, 98-102
  labial, of permanent maxillary left central incisor, 13
  lingual, of mandibular permanent central incisors, 11, 12
  of maxillary second bicuspids, 223
Eruption cyst, in newborn, 6
Eruption hematoma, in infant, 8
Erythroblastosis fetalis, discoloration of teeth due to, 75
Exfoliation, eruption and, anomalies of, 98-102
  precocious, of primary dentition, in hypophosphatasia, 102
  delayed, of maxillary left primary second molar, 102
Exodontia, in primary dentition, 209-220. See also *Extraction.*
  antibiotics in, 209
  diet following, 211
  postoperative procedures in, 210
  radiographs in, 209
Expansion screw, palatal, 238
Extraction(s), in primary dentition, 209-220. See also *Exodontia.*
  forceps for, 212, 214, 216, 218
  tray set up for, 211
  of anterior maxillary primary teeth, 212, 213
  of mandibular primary cuspids, 216, 217
  of mandibular primary molars, 218, 219
  of mandibular primary incisors, 216, 217
  of maxillary primary molars, 214, 215
  of natal teeth, 6, 7

Fibromatosis, gingival, idiopathic, 37, 38
Finger-sucking habit, anterior open bite and, 40, 41
Fluoride(s), effects of, on enamel, 90
  in caries prevention, 131
  topical, application of, 141
    adaptable trays in, 142
Fluoride supplements, administration of, 142t

Fluorosis, 90
  teeth color and, 75
Forceps, for extractions, 212, 214, 216, 218
Formocresol, in pulpotomy, 188
Fracture(s), bilateral, of roots of maxillary primary incisors, 275
  dentin, of maxillary permanent central incisors, treatment for, 286
    of maxillary primary incisor, treatment and prognosis of, 272
  dentin and pulpal, stainless steel crown restorations in, 291
  diagonal, of maxillary right permanent central incisor, restorations of, 299
  enamel, of maxillary permanent central incisors, treatment for, 285
    of maxillary primary incisor, treatment and prognosis in, 272
  of amalgam, of mandibular first primary molar, 172
  of crown, of maxillary primary central incisor, 274
  of enamel and dentin, of protruding maxillary permanent central incisors, 284
  pulpal, of maxillary permanent central incisor, 290
    treatment for, 288
    of maxillary primary incisor, treatment and prognosis in, 273
  stainless steel crowns, in treatment of, 291
Fusion, of teeth, 66, 68, 69

Gemination, of teeth, 66, 67, 68
Geographic tongue, 33
Germicidal solution, for anesthesia storage, 146
Gingival amalgam restorations, 179, 180
Gingival caries, 44
  of maxillary permanent incisors, 46
  of primary molars, 134
Gingival fibromatosis, idiopathic, 37, 38
Gingival hyperplasia, due to Sodium Dilantin, 314
Gingival margin, stripping of, around mandibular permanent central incisors, 40
Gingival recession, localized, 39
Gingivitis, calculus deposits and, 36
  due to poor oral hygiene, 35
  marginal, 35
  pubertal, 37
  ulcerative, necrotizing, 36
Gingivoplasty, dilantin hyperplasia following, 38
Gingivostomatitis, primary herpetic, on lower face, 31
  of lower lip and oral mucosa, 32
Gold foil restorations, 179, 180
Guide plane, acrylic, in correction of crossbite, 236, 237

Habits, finger-sucking, 40, 41
  lip-sucking, 29-31
Handicapped child, 307-317
Hawley space maintainer, for protruding incisors, 239

Hemangioma, capillary, on inferior surface of tongue, 34
  cavernous, of tongue, 34
Hematoma, eruption, in infant, 8
Hemophilia, dental care in, 317
Herpetic gingivostomatitis, primary, on lower face, 31
  on lower lip and oral mucosa, 32
Hospital operatory, for dental treatment of handicapped child, 317
Hutchinson's incisors, 71
Hyperplasia, Dilantin, 38
  gingival, due to Sodium Dilantin, 314
Hypocalcification, enamel, hereditary, 86, 87, 88
Hypodontia, incidence of, 52. See also Teeth, missing.
Hypophosphatasia, precocious exfoliation of primary dentition in, 102
Hypoplasia, enamel. See Enamel hypoplasia.
  of maxillary right permanent central incisor, 279
  of permanent incisors, due to injury, 280
  Turner's, of mandibular permanent central incisor, 279
Hypothyroidism, delayed eruption and, 101

Incisor(s), Hutchinson's, 71
  mandibular, brushing methods for, 138
    central, gold foil restorations of, 179
    lateral, odontoma obstructing eruption of, 48
    partial acrylic dentures for, 259
    proximal caries on, 179
    radiographic technique for, 121
  maxillary, abnormal position of, 104
    brushing methods for, 139
    enamel hypoplasia, hereditary and, 83
    fractured, dentin bridge, following calcium hydroxide pulpotomy, 203
    hypoplasia of, due to facial injury, 88
    radiographic techniques for, 118
  maxillary central, correction of anterior crossbite of, 234
    correction of diastema between, 240
    left, nonvital, treatment of, 204, 205
    with exaggerated cingula, 70
  permanent, hypoplastic defects, due to injury, 280
    immature, 298
    restoration of, with jacket crown, 293
    young, gold three-quarter crown for, 298
    pulpotomy procedure for, 289
  permanent mandibular central, lingual eruption of, 11, 12
    right, dilaceration of, 69
    stripping of gingival margin around, 40
    Turner's hypoplasia of, 279
  permanent mandibular interproximal caries in, 135
  permanent maxillary, gingival caries of, 46
    gold foil restoration of lingual pit on, 180
    lateral, lingual position of, 104
      missing, 60, 61
      right, peg-shaped, 70
  permanent maxillary central, abnormal position of, 103
    avulsed, treatment for, 296, 297

Incisor(s) (*Continued*)
  permanent maxillary central, delayed eruption of, *13*
    dentin fractures of, *287*
      treatment for, *286*
    diastema between, *15*
    enamel fractures of, treatment for, *285*
    intruded, treatment for, *295*
    labial eruption of, *13*, *103*
    left dens-in-dente of, *70*
      dilaceration of, *69*
      gemination of, *67*, *68*
    porcelain fused-to-gold restoration of, *300*, *301*, *302*
    protruding, dental injuries and, *284*
    pulpal fractures of, treatment for, *288*, *291*, *292*
    replanted, ankylosis of, *297*
    right, diagonal fracture of, restoration of, *299*
      hypoplasia of, *279*
      pulpal fracture of, *290*
    root canal therapy in, *208*, *292*
    root fracture of, treatment for, *294*, *295*
    stainless steel crowns for, in pulpal fractures of, *291*
  primary, abrasion of, due to bruxism, *42*
    band restoration in, *177*
    discoloration of, due to hereditary porphyria, *73*
  primary mandibular, abscess of, following traumatic injury, *276*
    extraction of, *216*, *217*
    supernumerary, *54*
  primary maxillary, bilateral fracture of roots of, *275*
    dentin fracture of, treatment, *272*
    enamel fracture of, treatment, *272*
    extraction of, *212*, *213*
    internal resorption following traumatic injury to, *275*
    intrusion of, treatment for, *274*
    lateral, endodontic therapy for, *206*
      gemination of, *67*
    pulpal exposure of, treatment, *273*
  primary maxillary central, discoloration of, due to trauma, *276*
    fracture of crown of, *274*
    partial denture for, *278*
    protruding, retraction of, with Hawley appliance, *239*
Infant, eruption hematoma in, *8*. See also *Newborn*.
Inlays, silver, *173*
Injections, anesthesia. See *Anesthesia injections*.

Jacket, crown restoration, of permanent incisor, *293*
Jaundice, teeth color and, *76*
Jaw, lateral exposure of, radiographic technique for, *115*, *125*
Klinefelter's syndrome, taurodontism and, *71*

Leukemia, dental care and, *317*
Lingual eruption, of mandibular permanent central incisors, *11*, *12*

Lip, cleft of, bilateral, *310*
  unilateral, *309*
  mucocele of, *34*
  primary herpetic gingiovastomatitis of, *32*
Lip-biting, anesthesia and, *151*
  prevention of, following extraction, 211
Lip-sucking habit, effects of, *29*, *30*, *31*

Malocclusion, Angle's classification of, *23*
Mandibular arch, crowding in, *12*
  idiopathic gingival fibromatosis of, *38*
  loss of length of, *6*
  with amalgam restorations, *170*
Mandibular area, posterior, radiographic technique in, *123*
Mandibular growth sites, *2*
Mandibular occlusal exposure, radiographic technique in, *127*
Marginal ditching, *173*
Marginal gingivitis, 35
Matrix, faulty, results of, *174*
  T-band, *174*
Matrix holder, Tofflemire, *174*
Maxillary arch, idiopathic gingival fibromatosis of, *37*
Maxillary area, posterior, anesthesia injection in, *147*
  radiographic technique in, *120*
Maxillary growth sites, *2*
Maxillary occlusal exposure, radiographic technique for, *126*
Maxillary permanent teeth, normal developmental patterns of, *14*
Mesial root, of second primary molar, ankylosis of, *109*
Mesiodens, *54*, *55*, *56*. See also *Supernumerary teeth*.
Mizzy Syrijet, *150*
Molar(s), brushing method for, *138*, *139*
  clamps for, *156*
  maxillary, natal, *7*
  Mulberry, *71*
  permanent first, gold foil restoration in buccal pit, *180*
  permanent mandibular first, ectopic eruption of, *106*
    occlusal amalgam restoration of, *166*
    occlusal caries of, *45*
    space maintainer and, *227*
  permanent maxillary first, ankylosis of, *110*
    ectopic eruption of, *107*, *241*
  primary, amalgam restoration of, *171*
    ankylosis of, *108*
    caries of, arrested, *45*
      gingival, *134*
    failure of restorations in, *176*
    pulp exposure in, *195*
    pulps of, *207*
    with roots enclosing crown of bicuspid, *220*
  primary first, formocresol pulpotomy and, *201*
  primary mandibular, anatomy of, *166*
    ankylosis of, *108*
    calcium hydroxide capping of, *192*
    extraction of, *218*, *219*
    root canals of, *207*
    stainless steel restoration of crowns of, *181*

Molar(s) (*Continued*)
  primary mandibular first, cavity preparation of, *167*
    formocresol pulpotomy of, failure in, *199*
    formocresol pulpotomy of, *47*
    fracture of amalgam of, *172*
    indirect pulp capping of, *189, 190*
    reduction of distolingual cusp in, *171*
    left, taurodontism of, *71*
  primary mandibular, second, amalgam restoration of, *171*
    caries of occlusal pit of, *44*
    mesio-occlusal cavity preparation and restoration in, *169*
    occlusal amalgam restorations, *166*
    proximo-occlusal cavity preparation in, *169*
    right, crown restoration procedure for, *182-185*
      periapical abscess of, *39*
      pulpotomy and, *199*
      reduction of mesiobuccal cusp of, *171*
  primary maxillary, extraction of, *214, 215*
    interproximal carious lesions in, *134*
    root canals of, *207*
  primary maxillary first, following endodontic treatment, *208*
  primary maxillary second, abscess of, in patient with blood dyscrasia, *317*
    left, delayed exfoliation of, *102*
    mesial migration of, *43*
    occlusal amalgam restorations of, *166*
    without grooves and fissures, *168*
  primary second, ankylosis of, *108, 109*
    flat plane relationship of distal surfaces of, *10*
    pulpotomy in, calcium hydroxide, *203*
      formocresol, *193, 194, 200, 201*
    step relationship of distal surfaces of, *10*
Molt mouth prop, *147*
Mongolism, dental care and, *316*
  missing teeth and, *53*
Moniliasis, *314*
Mouth prop, Molt, *147*
Mouth protectors, in athletics, *305*
Mucocele, of lip, *34*
Mulberry molars, *71*

Nasopalatine anesthesia injection, *150*
Natal teeth, *6*
  extraction of, *6, 7*
Needles, in anesthesia, *143*
Neonatal teeth, *6*
Neotracheal intubation, of general anesthesia, *152*
Nerves, anesthesia and, *145t*
Newborn, dental calcification in, *3*
  epithelial cyst in, *7*
  eruption cyst in, *6*
  with maxillary molar, *7*
Noctec, in management of child patient, *323*

Occlusal radiograph, *115*
Occlusal wear, bruxism and, in primary dentition, *10*
Odontoma, *48*

Oligodontia, hereditary anhidrotic ectodermal dysplasia and, *53*
Open bite, caries due to, *136*
Operative dentistry, 163-186
Operatory, hospital, for dental treatment of handicapped patient, *317*
Oral diagnosis, 25-49
  procedure in, 25
Oral hygiene, in caries prevention, 131
  poor, effects of, *135*
Orotracheal intubation, of general anesthesia, *152*
Orthodontics, interceptive, space maintenance and, 221-247
Overbite, in primary dentition, *11*

Palatal anesthesia injection, *149*
Palatal expansion screw, *238*
Palate, hard and soft, cleft of, *311*
  soft, cleft of, *310*
Partial denture, as space maintainer, *233*. See also *Denture, partial.*
Patient, handicapped, 307-317
Permanent dentition, supernumerary teeth in, 52
  trauma to, 281-306
    causes of, 282t
    incidence of, 281
    treatment of, 282
Pituitary dwarfism, delayed eruption of teeth in, *101*
Pliers, crown crimping, *184, 185*
  in space maintenance and interceptive orthodontics, *245*
Pneumonia, enamel hypoplasia due to, *89*
Polishing, of teeth, *140*
Porphyria, hereditary, *73, 74*
Pressure anesthesia, in exodontia in primary dentition, *210*
Primary dentition, amalgam restoration in, *164*
  bruxism and occlusal wear in, *10*
  caries in, *43, 44, 45, 133*
  caries-free, *132*
  cavity preparation in, 163
  crowding of, 9
  crown restoration in, stainless steel, *181*
  enamel hypoplasia in, *90*
  exodontia in, 209-220
  normal, *9, 10*
  overbite in, *11*
  supernumerary teeth in, 52
  trauma to, 269-280
    dental procedure in, 269
    incidence of, 269
  tetracycline staining of, *41*
Prophylaxis, disclosing solution for, *140*
Prosthodontics, 249-267
  for caries, 263
  in ectodermal dysplasia, *259, 260, 261, 262*
  in hereditary dentinogenesis imperfecta, 250-258
Protrusions, maxillary, dental injuries and, *282, 284*
Pubertal gingivitis, *37*
Pulp, of primary molars, *207*
Pulp capping, 188
  indirect, 188, *189, 190, 191*
Pulp exposure, primary molars with, *195*

Pulp therapy, 187-207
Pulpal exposure(s), in maxillary central permanent incisors, *290*
   in maxillary primary incisor, treatment and prognosis in, *273*
   stainless steel crowns in, in treatment of, *291*
Pulpectomy, 188
Pulpotomy, 188
   calcium hydroxide, of mandibular second bicuspid, *46*
     of primary second molar, internal resorption in distal canal following, *203*
     successful, *202*
     procedure for, on young permanent incisor, *289*
   contraindications for, *195*
   formocresol, burn due to, *199*
     contraindications for, *193*
     in primary molars, *47, 193, 194, 199, 200, 201*
       failure of, *199*
     procedure for, *196, 197, 198*
     success rate of, *199*

Questionnaire, health, in oral diagnosis, 25

Radiograph(s), bitewing, *115, 124*
   in exodontia, in primary dentition, 209
   occlusal, *115*
   panoramic, *116*
   periapical, *115*
Radiography, 113-129
   as diagnostic tool, 26, 113
   considerations in, 114
   in children, 114, *117*
   technique in, for bitewing exposure, posterior, *124*
     for lateral cephalometric exposure, *129*
     for lateral jaw exposure, *115, 125*
     for mandibular central and lateral incisors, *121*
     for mandibular cuspid area, *122*
     for mandibular occlusal exposure, *127*
     for mandibular posterior area, *123*
     for maxillary area, posterior, *120*
     for maxillary central and lateral incisors, *118*
     for maxillary cuspid, *119*
     for maxillary occlusal exposure, *126*
Ranula, 35
Replantation, 283, *296, 297*
Restoration(s), amalgam, in primary teeth, 164. See also *Amalgam restorations.*
   band, *177*
   crown. See *Crown restoration.*
   lingual dovetail cavity preparation and, in primary cuspid, *178*
   porcelain fused-to-gold, of maxillary permanent central incisor, *300, 301, 302*
   proximal cavity preparation and, *168*
Resuscitation equipment, for local anesthesia, *148*
Rickets, vitamin D-resistant, dental radiographs of child with, *49*
Root(s), mesial, of second primary molar, ankylosis of, *109*
   of maxillary primary incisors, bilateral fracture of, *275*

Root canal therapy, in maxillary permanent central incisors, *208, 292*
Root canals, of mandibular primary molar, *207*
   of maxillary primary molars, *207*
Root fracture, of maxillary central permanent incisor, treatment of, *294*
"Rootless teeth," 97
Rubber dam, 153-161
   advantages of, 153
   clamps and, *156, 157, 158, 159, 160*
   technique for use of, 153, *157, 158*
   tray setup for placement of, *156*
Rubber elastic therapy, in correction of diastema, *240*

Sedation, 323
Shell teeth, 97
Silver inlays, *173*
Snow-capped teeth, hereditary, *75*
   in enamel hypocalcification, *88*
Sodium Dilantin, gingival hyperplasia due to, *314*
Space maintainer, band and loop, 225
   bilateral, acrylic, *230*
   distal shoe, 227
     bilateral, *228*
     failure of, *226*
     unilateral, *226, 228*
   equipment for, *246, 247*
   Hawley, for protruding incisors, *239*
   mandibular, acrylic, removable, *232*
   mandibular lingual arch, *229*
   maxillary lingual arch, *229*
   partial denture as, *233*
   removable, acrylic, *231, 232, 235*
   unilateral, cast gold crown and bar, *224*
     distal shoe, *226, 228*
     fixed, *225*
     stainless steel, *224, 225*
Space maintenance, and interceptive orthodontics, 221-247
   stainless steel wire in, *244*
Space regainer, acrylic, with recurved helical finger spring, *242*
   split acrylic, *242*
Staining, tetracycline, of primary dentition, *41*
Sucrose, caries and, 131
Supernumerary teeth, 51, *53, 54, 55, 56*
   cleidocranial dysostosis and, *57*
   in permanent dentition, 52
   in primary dentition, 52
Surgery, dental, rubber dam in, *155*

Taurodontism, Klinefelter's syndrome and, *71*
   of mandibular left first primary molar, *71*
T-band matrix, *174*
Teeth, anomalies of, 51-111. See also *Anomalies.*
   concrescence of, *66, 69*
   fusion of, *66, 68, 69*
   gemination of, *66, 67, 68*
   maxillary permanent, normal development of, *14*
   missing, *58, 59, 60, 61*
     clinical management of, 53

Teeth (*Continued*)
  missing, incidence of, 52
    syndromes with, 53
  natal, 6
    extraction of, 6, 7
  neonatal, 6
  permanent, delayed eruption of, due to cleidocranial dysostosis, 99
  polishing of, *140*
  posterior, fracture of, due to injury, *280*
  primary, anterior, caries in, *134, 177*
    exodontia in, 209-220
  shell, *97*
  snow-capped, hereditary, 75
    in enamel hypocalcification, 88
  supernumerary, 51. See also *Supernumerary teeth.*
Tetracycline staining, *41, 76*
Tofflemire matrix holder, *174*
Tongue, ankyloglossia and, 33
  capillary hemangioma on inferior surface of, *34*
  cavernous hemangioma of, *34*
  geographic, *33*
Trauma, to permanent dentition, 281-306
  to primary dentition, 269-280

Treacher-Collins syndrome, dental care and, *312*
Turner's hypoplasia, of mandibular permanent central incisors, *279*

Ulcer(s), aphthous, recurrent, of oral mucosa of upper lip, *32*
Ulcerative gingivitis, necrotizing, *36*

Vitamin D-resistant rickets, dental radiographs of 3-year-old with, *49*

Wire, brass, in interceptive orthodontics, *241*
  stainless steel, in space maintenance and interceptive orthodontics, *244*

X-ray unit, panoramic, *128*